W9-BWQ-634

Date: 6/4/14

616.8582 WAL
Walsh, Barent W.
Treating self-injury : a
practical guide /

TREATING SELF-INJURY

TREATING
SELF-INJURY
A Practical Guide

SECOND EDITION

BARENT W. WALSH

THE GUILFORD PRESS
New York   London

© 2012 The Guilford Press
A Division of Guilford Publications, Inc.
72 Spring Street, New York, NY 10012
www.guilford.com

Printed in the United States of America

This book is printed on acid-free paper.

Last digit is print number: 9 8 7 6 5 4 3 2 1

The authors have checked with sources believed to be reliable in their efforts to provide
information that is complete and generally in accord with the standards of practice that
are accepted at the time of publication. However, in view of the possibility of human error
or changes in behavioral, mental health, or medical sciences, neither the authors, nor
the editor and publisher, nor any other party who has been involved in the preparation
or publication of this work warrants that the information contained herein is in every
respect accurate or complete, and they are not responsible for any errors or omissions or
the results obtained from the use of such information. Readers are encouraged to confirm
the information contained in this book with other sources.

Library of Congress Cataloging-in-Publication Data

Walsh, Barent W.
  Treating self-injury: a practical guide / by Barent W. Walsh. — 2nd ed.
    p. cm.
  Includes bibliographical references and index.
  ISBN 978-1-4625-0539-5 (hardback : acid-free paper)
  1. Self-mutilation—Treatment.   I. Title.
  RC552.S4W36 2012
  616.85′82—dc23

                                                                2012006503

For Benjamin Edward Frank Walsh
and Anna Kim Hwa Yung Walsh
with love

About the Author

Barent W. Walsh, PhD, is Executive Director of The Bridge of Central Massachusetts in Worcester and Teaching Associate in Psychiatry at Harvard Medical School. The Bridge specializes in implementing evidence-based practice models according to protocol in public-sector settings. It comprises over 40 programs serving persons with mental health or developmental disability challenges, including special education; residential treatment; wraparound services; supported housing services; a drop-in center for gay, lesbian, bisexual, and transgender teens; and a program for homeless people.

A recipient of the Lifetime Achievement Award from the Massachusetts chapter of the National Association of Social Workers in 2011, Dr. Walsh has worked with self-injuring persons for over 40 years and has conducted research, written extensively, and presented internationally on self-injury. He has consulted on this topic at numerous schools, outpatient clinics, group homes, psychiatric hospitals, and correctional facilities, and has also served on the clinical and research faculties of the Simmons and Boston College Schools of Social Work.

Contributing Authors

Kenneth L. Appelbaum, MD, Professor of Clinical Psychiatry and Director, Correctional Mental Health Policy and Research, Center for Health Policy and Research, Commonwealth Medicine, University of Massachusetts Medical School, Shrewsbury, Massachusetts

Amy M. Brausch, PhD, Assistant Professor of Psychology, Western Kentucky University, Bowling Green, Kentucky

Leonard A. Doerfler, PhD, Professor and Director, Counseling Psychology Program, Assumption College, and Adjunct Associate Professor of Psychiatry, University of Massachusetts Medical School, Worcester, Massachusetts

Gordon P. Harper, MD, Associate Professor of Psychiatry, Harvard Medical School, and Medical Director, Child/Adolescent Services, Massachusetts Department of Mental Health, Chestnut Hill, Massachusetts

Michael Hollander, PhD, Day Hospital Director and Director of Training, 3East DBT Program, McLean Hospital, Belmont, Massachusetts

Jennifer J. Muehlenkamp, PhD, Assistant Professor of Psychology, University of Wisconsin–Eau Claire, Eau Claire, Wisconsin

Ariana Perry, BA, Outcomes Manager, The Bridge of Central Massachusetts, Worcester, Massachusetts

Acknowledgments

Writing a book involves sacrifice for the author and those around him. My profound thanks to my wife, Valerie, and my children, Ben and Anna, who did without my presence for many hours as I sat sequestered, tapping out words on the computer.

Special thanks to Jennifer J. Muehlenkamp, Michael Hollander, Amy M. Brausch, and Kenneth L. Appelbaum for contributing four of the eight new chapters in this book. I also am grateful that Gordon P. Harper was willing to update his chapter on psychopharmacology. Two other individuals helped me cowrite chapters: Leonard A. Doerfler and Ariana Perry. Len Doerfler deserves special recognition, as he not only supports research efforts at my agency, The Bridge of Central Massachusetts, but also serves as a member of the Board of Trustees.

My thanks also to all my long-time colleagues at The Bridge; they have supported and contributed to this effort, helping me in overseeing more than 40 programs for persons with mental health or developmental challenges. Specifically, I wish to thank my committed management team of Fred Battersby, Nancy Bishop, Carol Tripp-Tebo, Erica Robert, Milt Bornstein, Steve Murphy, Donna Bradley, Tina Wingate, and Doug Watts; my talented service or division directors, including Jen Eaton, Kerrin Westerlind, Margaret Crowley, Pam Hanam, Jennifer Megas, Jill Macarelli, Kelli Durocher, and Marcia Almeida; and the Board of Trustees, including Board President Charley O'Neill.

I also wish to thank the major funders of The Bridge, who are supportive in so many ways. These include Susan Wing, Susan Sprung, Ted Kirousis, Babs Fenby, Sue Sciaraffa, Jack Rowe, and Richard Breault from the Massachusetts Department of Mental Health; Terry O'Hare and Margaret Grey from the Massachusetts Department of Developmental Services;

Jan Yost from the Health Foundation of Central Massachusetts; and Marty Cohen from the Metrowest Community Health Care Foundation.

Beyond those directly involved in my day-to-day professional work, many others have had an impact on this project. I wish to thank long-time colleagues in the field of self-injury for their scholarship and wisdom. These include Paul Rosen, Wendy Lader, Karen Conterio, Tracy Alderman, Jane Hyman, Caroline Kettlewell, Daphne Simeon, Armando Favazza, Kate Comtois, Milton Brown, Sarah Shaw, Efrosini Kokaliari, and Jan Sutton. I also want to acknowledge the major contributions of more recent scholars, including Matthew Nock, David Klonsky, Janis Whitlock, Karen Rodham, Nancy Heath, Mary Kay Nixon, Jason Washburn, Mitch Prinstein, Peg Andover, Kim Gratz, Alex Chapman, and Paul Plener. I am especially grateful for collaborations with two Japanese scholars, Yoshitomo Takahashi and Toshihiko Matsumoto.

I also wish to thank those who have assisted me in learning mindfulness, including Marsha Linehan, Charlie Swenson, Zindel Segal, and the late Cindy Sanderson. I am particularly indebted to my meditation teachers: Issho Fujita, a Soto Zen priest, and the Venerable Lobsang Phuntsok, a Tibetan monk.

My greatest inspiration in writing on the topic of self-destructive behavior has been an intellectual giant, suicidologist Edwin Shneidman. As the saying goes, he has forgotten more than I will ever know about the topic of self-harm. In the same vein, I wish to acknowledge the profound influence of Thomas Joiner, who is arguably the most influential suicidologist alive today. I also want to thank Lanny Berman, Executive Director of the American Association of Suicidology, for enabling me to present on self-injury for many years at the Association's annual conference.

It is also very important to recognize two close friends who have listened to me talk on and on about self-injury, showing far greater interest and patience than anyone could reasonably expect. Thank you to Michael Addis and Effie Malley.

Finally, I want to acknowledge those who have taught me the most about self-injury: people struggling with self-injury. The secret to understanding and treating self-injury is first and foremost developing an ability to really listen. Adopting a nonjudgmental, respectful, and compassionate approach with people who self-injure puts one in a position to learn from them. Based on that learning, a therapist can facilitate growth, problem solving, and healing. The role of the therapist with these individuals is primarily one of intermediary. They are some of the most inspiring people I have known. Many of them have worked so hard to overcome so much in order to move to a better, stronger place. I appreciate the learning they have sent my way, and I hereby pass it on.

Preface

This second edition of *Treating Self-Injury: A Practical Guide* is substantially different from the first. It includes the work of four new authors and eight new chapters on subjects not considered in the first edition. The new chapters are:

> "The Relationship between Self-Injury and Suicide" (Chapter 2)
> "Formal Assessment of Self-Injury" by Jennifer J. Muehlenkamp (Chapter 8)
> "Family Therapy" by Michael Hollander (Chapter 13)
> "Treating Persons with Multiple Self-Harm Behaviors" (Chapter 17)
> "Residential Treatment Targeting Self-Injury and Suicidal Behavior in Adolescents" with Leonard A. Doerfler and Ariana Perry (Chapter 18)
> "Asphyxial Risk-Taking (the 'Choking Game')" by Amy M. Brausch (Chapter 22)
> "Understanding, Managing, and Treating Foreign-Body Ingestion" with Ariana Perry (Chapter 23)
> "Self-Injury in Correctional Settings" by Kenneth L. Appelbaum (Chapter 24)

This new edition also employs a "stepped-care model" to assist in matching client needs to a specific roster of interventions. A stepped-care approach is appropriate for this volume because a broad array of interventions are now available for the treatment of self-injury. A stepped-care approach helps clinicians and clients decide which treatments are best for the needs of each individual.

Key points within a stepped-care model are that (1) each client's needs should be matched with the level of intensity of the intervention; and (2) client outcomes should be carefully monitored, allowing treatments to be "stepped up" if required. In a stepped-care approach, clients usually move through less-intensive interventions before receiving more-intensive interventions (if the latter become necessary). Moving up the steps is generally associated with increasing behavioral risk, intensity of interventions, and expense in delivering the service.

In this new edition, all chapters that are carried over from the first edition have been fully updated with references to the most recent research and intervention methodologies. This edition builds on the knowledge base of the first, but makes full use of the great expansion of knowledge about self-injury since the first edition was published.

Finally, this book includes many reproducible forms that can be used by clinicians and program staff members with their clients. Purchasers may download larger versions from the book's page on The Guilford Press website.

I am pleased to be able to offer this much more comprehensive version of *Treating Self-Injury: A Practical Guide* to professionals, persons who self-injure, and their families.

BARENT W. WALSH

Contents

PART I

Definition and Contexts for Self-Injury

INTRODUCTION

Part I of this volume has six chapters. The first defines self-injury and spends time carefully differentiating self-injury from suicidal behavior. The second chapter shows how complicated the relationship between self-injury and suicide has become. Although the two behaviors are distinct in many ways, recent research has revealed that self-injury appears to be an important predictor of suicide attempts. The clinical implications for these findings are discussed here.

Chapter 3 reviews the full range of direct and indirect self-harm behaviors. This chapter emphasizes the need for conducting a thorough assessment of all self-harm behaviors in clients who self-injure. Chapter 4 discusses the surprising emergence of self-injury in nonclinical populations. Various forms of self-injury (e.g., cutting, burning, picking, and self-hitting) are now commonplace in community groups, particularly students in middle schools, high schools, and universities. A review of recent research on self-injury in these groups is provided, along with some speculations as to why self-injury is so common among our youth today.

Chapter 5 discusses the always interesting topic of body modifications, such as tattoos, piercings, brandings, and scarifications. The conclusion is that these behaviors are generally not self-injurious in nature, but are related to cultural influences and self-expression. However, notable exceptions are also discussed, such as piercing or tattooing in the service of self-injury.

Part I of this book concludes with the discussion in Chapter 6 of understanding self-injury by using a simple, experience-near, biopsychosocial theory. This book is intended above all to be a practical guide. All the topics in Part I are linked to the pragmatics of understanding and treating self-injury.

CHAPTER 1

Definition and Differentiation from Suicide

The most important point should be stated at the outset: Self-injury is a conundrum. In many ways it is separate and distinct from suicide, and should be managed as such. Yet self-injury is also an important risk factor for suicide attempts. In this chapter, I define self-injury and differentiate it from suicidal behavior. In the next chapter, I discuss self-injury as a risk factor for suicide attempts, with specific suggestions for how to prevent the most extreme of all self-destructive acts.

TERMINOLOGY

Since the mid-1990s, the language used to refer to such behaviors as self-inflicted cutting, scratching, burning, hitting, and excoriation of wounds has changed. These were previously referred to as "self-mutilation," but the more common and popular term has become "self-injury" or "nonsuicidal self-injury." Both self-injuring people and those who treat them have protested that "self-mutilation" is too extreme and pejorative a term (e.g., Hyman, 1999; Connors, 2000; Simeon & Favazza, 2001). These advocates have argued that most people who self-injure employ the behavior as a coping mechanism to deal with psychological distress; therefore, the behavior has adaptive features. Moreover, they have correctly stated that the large majority of self-inflicted wounds involve only modest physical damage that leaves little if any long-term scarring. The wounds do not result in a "mutilation" of the body. The *Merriam-Webster Dictionary* (1995) defines "mutilate" as "to cut up or alter radically so as to make imperfect" and "to maim,

3

cripple" (p. 342). I accept the contention that the term "self-mutilation" is derogatory, stigmatizing, or even sensationalistic in referring to the behavior (Simeon & Favazza, 2001), and therefore I use the term "self-injury" in this text.

FORMAL DEFINITION

In this book, self-injury is defined in the following way:

> *"Self-injury" is intentional, self-effected, low-lethality bodily harm of a socially unacceptable nature, performed to reduce and/or communicate psychological distress.*

The components of this definition require some explication. As explained above, the term "self-injury" is descriptive and nonpejorative. It is also nonexaggerative. The word "intentional" specifies that self-injury is deliberate; it is not accidental or ambiguous as to intent. Self-injury is also "self-effected." This term is chosen rather than "self-inflicted," because many individuals self-injure with the assistance of others. Not uncommonly (especially among adolescents), two or more people may take turns hurting or simultaneously hurt each other. For quite a few people, self-injury is an interpersonal experience.

The next term in the definition is "low-lethality." Self-injury, by definition, involves those forms of self-harm that do modest physical damage to the body and pose little or no risk to life. The distinction of self-injury from suicide is explicit and fundamental, as discussed in detail later in this chapter.

Self-injury is primarily about "bodily harm." The behavior alarms others because of the tissue damage. A person may present with talk or planning about self-injury, but until he or she crosses the line into actively damaging the body, there is no self-injury.

The phrase "of a socially unacceptable nature" is included in the definition to emphasize social context. Favazza (1996) has written extensively about the multifarious body modifications that occur around the world. In most cultures, body modification is symbolically meaningful and culturally endorsed. It may have profound religious significance and be part of a complex rite of passage. This is not the case for common self-injury, which, although it may have many meanings for its perpetrators, is not endorsed by the prevailing culture. Granted, self-injury can often seem to be part of an adolescent expression of angst and alienation; among teens, there may be considerable social reinforcement for the behavior. However, there are no organized, culturally endorsed rituals that surround it. Self-injury is not connected to any socially sanctioned rite of passage.

The final phrase in the definition is "performed to reduce and/or communicate psychological distress." Self-injury is enacted primarily because of its ability to modify and reduce psychological discomfort. It is usually immediately and substantially effective, and therefore it is often repeated. The behavior is not suicidal, but it is psychologically motivated. Self-injury is a behavior that cannot be explained via biological mechanisms alone. Rather, it is a self-conscious, self-intentioned form of distress reduction behavior.

To a lesser degree, self-injury also often has interpersonal features. Self-injury frequently serves such interpersonal functions as communicating pain, influencing others to change their behavior, or demonstrating courage or toughness. As discussed later in this volume, social contagion can also play a role in the occurrence of self-injury.

DIFFERENTIATING SELF-INJURY FROM SUICIDE

This portion of the chapter discusses 11 points of distinction between self-injury and suicide. These points are provided to justify the contention that self-injury and suicide should be understood, managed, and treated differentially. All too often, self-injury is inappropriately labeled "suicidal," resulting in unnecessary psychiatric hospitalizations and other poorly designed interventions. The 11 points of distinction presented here provide a practical roadmap for determining whether a self-destructive behavior is suicidal or self-injurious. This distinction has major implications for all the assessment and treatment that follow. A concise summary of 10 of these 11 points is provided in Table 1.1. (Prevalence, the first point discussed below, is omitted from the table, since its importance is demographic rather than clinical.)

Prevalence

The prevalence for suicide versus self-injury is very different. The prevalence for completed suicides in the U.S. population is well established via ongoing epidemiological studies: Suicide occurs at a rate of 11.5 per 100,000 (American Association of Suicidology [AAS], 2008). In contrast, the prevalence rate for self-injury is unknown, in that large-sample epidemiological studies have yet to be conducted. Estimates have ranged from 400 (Pattison & Kahan, 1983) to 1,000 per 100,000 (Favazza, 1998). Even if the low estimate is correct (and this is very unlikely, given the rising prevalence in

TABLE 1.1. Differentiating Suicide Attempts from Self-Injurious Behavior

Assessment focus	Suicide attempt	Self-injury
What was the expressed and unexpressed intent of the act?	To escape pain; terminate consciousness	Relief from unpleasant affect (tension, anger, emptiness, deadness)
What was the level of physical damage and potential lethality?	Serious physical damage; lethal means of self-harm	Little physical damage; nonlethal means used
Is there a chronic, repetitive pattern of self-injurious acts?	Rarely a chronic repetition; some overdose repeatedly	Frequently a chronic, high-rate pattern
Have multiple methods of self-injury been used over time?	Usually one method	Usually more than one method over time
What is the level of psychological pain?	Unendurable, persistent	Uncomfortable, intermittent
Is there constriction of cognition?	Extreme constriction; suicide as the only way out; tunnel vision; seeking a final solution	Little or no constriction; choices available; seeking a temporary solution
Are there feelings of hopelessness and helplessness?	Hopelessness and helplessness are central	Periods of optimism and some sense of control
Was there a decrease in discomfort following the act?	No immediate improvement; treatment required for improvement	Rapid improvement; rapid return to usual cognition and affect; successful "alteration of consciousness"
Restriction of means	Important, often life-saving	Impractical, often inadvertently provocative
What is the core problem?	Depression, rage about inescapable, unendurable pain	Body alienation; exceptionally poor body image in clinical populations

community samples), the rate of self-injury is almost 40 times higher than that for completed suicide.

Intent

A fundamental place to start differentiating suicide from self-injury clinically is the topic of intent. A clinician needs to know what a person is intending to accomplish via the behavior. What are his or her goals in acting self-destructively? Some people are quite insightful and articulate in explaining the intent of their self-harming behavior. They provide clinicians with explanations of their behavior that are clear and concise. For example, some self-injuring people say, "I cut myself to feel better. I don't want to die. I just want to get the anger out." In a similar vein, suicidal individuals make their motives quite evident. They may say, "If I don't have this relationship in my life, it's not worth living. My life is over. That's why I took the overdose." In both examples, intent could not be more clear.

However, more frequently than not, clinicians find it difficult to elicit a clear articulation of intent. Self-destructive persons are emotionally overwhelmed and often very confused about their own behavior. When asked why they acted self-destructively, many individuals provide ambiguous responses, such as "I'm not sure why I took the overdose; it just seemed like the thing to do." Others speak with considerable vagueness, such as "I wouldn't cut myself now, but I had to do it then," and refuse (or are unable) to say more.

Some individuals seem to be disconnected from conscious thought processes when they hurt themselves, such as the individual who said, "At one point, I looked down at my arms, saw a lot of blood, and had no idea how it happened." Another variation is the all-too-common encounter with adolescents who, when asked why they performed some self-destructive act, reply with that classic roadblock to psychological progress: "I don't know."

Intent can be successfully elicited from both suicidal and self-injuring persons, but the process often requires a combination of profound compassion and investigative persistence.

Suicidal Intent

In his classic work *Definition of Suicide,* Shneidman (1985) identified a number of salient points that differentiate suicide from self-injury. The first of these is intent. Shneidman stated that the intent of the suicidal person is generally not so much to kill the body; rather, the intent is to "terminate consciousness." The suicidal person wants to stop the psychological pain—to escape the "psychache," as Shneidman (1993) calls it. The suicidal person will do whatever it takes to make the pain go away *permanently*.

Self-Injurious Intent

In contrast, the intent of the self-injuring person is not to *terminate* consciousness, but to *modify* it. The overwhelming majority of self-injuring individuals report that they harm themselves in order to relieve painful feelings. The type of emotional distress they want to relieve falls into two basic categories. The majority of those who self-injure report hurting themselves in order to relieve *too much* emotion (Favazza, 1987; Walsh & Rosen, 1988; Brown, 1998, 2002; Brown, Comtois, & Linehan, 2002; Klonsky, 2007, 2009; Nock, 2010). The minority report harming themselves in order to relieve either *too little* emotion or states of dissociation (e.g., Conterio & Lader, 1998; Shapiro & Dominiak, 1992; Simeon & Hollander, 2001). Those who report feeling too much emotional distress identify such feelings as these:

- Anger
- Shame or guilt
- Anxiety, tension, or panic
- Sadness
- Frustration
- Contempt

Studies differ regarding the order of these uncomfortable emotions. See Brown (2002) and Klonsky (2007) for thorough reviews of studies on emotions that precede self-injury.

A smaller proportion of self-injurers report feeling too little emotion. They state that they feel "empty," "zombie-like," "dead," or "like a robot." These individuals self-injure to alleviate this absence of feeling. As a young adult female once told me, "When I cut myself and see the blood, it's very reassuring, because I can see for myself that I'm still alive." Many of these individuals may be experiencing states of dissociation immediately prior to self-injuring.

The key point regarding intent is that a suicidal person wants to eliminate consciousness permanently; a self-injuring person wants to modify consciousness, to reduce distress, in order to live another day.

Method and Related Level of Physical Damage and Potential Lethality

Given the difficulty of eliciting clearly articulated intent from clients, clinicians often have to focus on the acts of self-harm in order to perform an accurate assessment. Fortunately, the chosen method of self-harm often tells us a great deal about the intent of a self-destructive person. Certain behaviors convey suicidal intent; others suggest self-injurious motivation.

Suicide Methods

Research has shown repeatedly that people who die by suicide use a rather short list of high-lethality methods. For example, statistics from the Centers for Disease Control and Prevention (CDC, 2010) identify death by suicide as occurring via six basic methods: use of a firearm (50.7%); hanging (23.1%); pill or poison ingestion (18.8%); jumping from a height (1.6%); use of a sharp instrument (1.7%); and death involving motor vehicles, such as cars, trains, or buses (1.1%). Note that the most common form of self-injury (cutting or use of a sharp instrument) is reported to result in death for only 1.7% of those who die by suicide. That is to say, *98.3% of individuals who die by suicide in the United States use methods other than cutting.* Furthermore, it should be emphasized that those who die by cutting use very specific and uncommon methods: (1) severing the carotid artery or jugular vein in the neck, (2) piercing the heart, or (3) performing a massive incision to the abdomen (CDC, 2010). The most common form of self-injury, cutting the arms or legs, is not listed as a method that results in death; nor are other forms of common self-injury listed below.

Moreover, if the statistics for cause of death by suicide are reviewed for the age group of 15–24 years, the percentage of those dying by cutting becomes even lower. This is the age group in which self-injury is most common. The proportion of 15- to 24-year-olds who die by cutting/piercing is 0.6% (CDC, 2010). *Thus 99.4% of youth who die by suicide use methods other than cutting.* The methods of suicide are highly distinct from those of self-injury.

Self-Injury Methods

There are no comparable data from large samples regarding the methods of self-injury. Favazza and Conterio's (1988) study employed a convenience sample that responded to an episode of *The Phil Donahue Show* devoted to self-injury. Responding to a request to complete a mail-in questionnaire, 250 people (96% of whom were female) did so. The results indicated that respondents used the following self-injury methods: cutting (72%), burning (35%), self-hitting (30%), interference with wound healing (22%), hair pulling (trichotillomania; 10%), and bone breaking (8%).

Some additional data regarding types of self-injury are available from a small-sample study I conducted in the late 1990s (Walsh & Frost, 2005).

The study sample consisted of 70 adolescents who were receiving intensive treatment in either special education or residential programs. Of these, 34 had a history of suicide attempts and recurrent self-injury, as well as multiple forms of indirect self-harm (including risk-taking, substance abuse, and eating disorders). These youth reported that their self-injury took the following forms: cutting (82.4%), body carving (64.7%), head banging (64.7%), picking at scabs (61.8%), scratching (50%), burning (58.8%), self-hitting (58.8%), and self-piercing (apart from properly sterilized ornamental piercings) (52.9%). Other less common forms of self-injury for these youth were self-inflicted tattoos (47.1%), self-biting (44.1%), and hair pulling (38.2%). Although many of these behaviors were alarming, it is important to emphasize that none was life-threatening. Note also that when the categories of cutting, scratching, and carving were combined, body incising (91.2%) was by far the most popular method of self-injury for this sample.

Whitlock, Eckenrode, and Silverman (2006) reported somewhat different findings in their study of college students. The self-injury in their sample of over 2,800 students, 17% of whom self-injured, consisted of the following:

Severely scratched or pinched with fingernails or objects causing skin to bleed	51.6%
Punched objects to the point of bruising or bleeding	37.6%
Cut	33.7%
Punched oneself to the point of bruising or bleeding	24.5%
Ripped or tore skin	15.9%
Carved words or symbols into skin	14.9%
Interfered with the healing of wounds	13.5%
Burned skin	12.9%
Rubbed glass or sharp objects into the skin	12.0%
Engaged in trichotillomania	11.0%

Note that when cutting and carving are combined for the Whitlock et al. study, this new category is second only to scratching and pinching in frequency. What is clear is that across the literature on self-injury (e.g., Favazza, 1987; Walsh & Rosen, 1988; Alderman, 1997; Conterio & Lader, 1998; Brown, 1998; Briere & Gil, 1998; Simeon & Hollander, 2001; Klonsky, 2007; Nixon & Heath, 2009; Nock, 2010), the most common methods of self-injury are as follows:

- Cutting, scratching, and carving
- Excoriation of wounds
- Self-hitting
- Self-burning
- Head banging
- Self-inflicted tattoos
- Other (e.g., self-biting, abrading, foreign-body ingestion, inserting objects, self-inflicted piercings, hair pulling)

These are presented in the general order of frequency, although the exact order varies from study to study. Cutting is by far the most common form reported.

It is important to emphasize that none of these behaviors is likely to result in death, except in the most extreme circumstances (e.g., self-burning that takes the form of self-immolation, an exceedingly rare behavior). If cutting behaviors are unlikely to result in death—particularly the most common forms of cutting arms, wrists, and legs—it is quite reasonable to conclude that the behavior is generally about something *other than suicide*. If self-injury is generally not about trying to end one's life, then what is it about? This is the question I attempt to address in the rest of this book.

Chapter 3 discusses the broad category of direct self-harm, which can be divided into two groups: suicide and self-injury. When clients discuss plans to use (or actually employ) such methods as shooting, hanging, self-poisoning, jumping from a height, cutting the neck, stabbing through the heart, or performing massive abdominal puncture, it is appropriate to conclude that their intent is suicidal. These are high-lethality behaviors that frequently result in death. In contrast, if clients discuss performing, or actually perform, acts of cutting, excoriation, self-hitting, self-burning, or self-biting on themselves, it is appropriate generally to view the behaviors as self-injurious rather than suicidal.

Frequency of the Behavior

Another point of distinction between suicide and self-injury is the frequency with which the behaviors occur. In general, self-injury occurs at much higher rates than suicide attempts. The large majority of people who attempt suicide do not do so recurrently or frequently. The most common pattern is that people attempt suicide once or twice when they are in a particularly stressful period in their lives (Nock & Kessler, 2006). For most persons, this type of crisis period passes, and they move on with their lives. Most individuals are resilient and/or obtain professional help and are unlikely to attempt suicide again.

However, there are others—those in the minority—who attempt suicide recurrently over extended periods of time (years or even decades). These are usually persons who have a serious and persistent mental illness (e.g., major depression, bipolar disorder, borderline personality disorder [BPD]). Most frequently, it appears that those who recurrently attempt suicide employ pill overdose as their methods. These individuals appear to know how much prescribed or over-the-counter medication they can ingest and still survive. Or they may take serious, even lethal dosages, but quickly disclose their actions to others, resulting in protective intervention. However, even for these individuals, the rates of their attempts pale in comparison to rates of self-injury in many persons.

Many, probably the majority, of self-injuring persons perform the behavior frequently. A commonly reported frequency by self-injuring clients is 20–100 times over a multiple-year period (Walsh & Rosen, 1988). Even adolescents who are in their early teens describe a several-year course of self-injury, with as many as 20–30 episodes per year. For example, in my own clinical experience, I have encountered two 14-year-olds who cut themselves over 150 times in a single week! It is very common for self-injury to be a high-rate behavior.

Sometimes the frequency of self-injury can be hard even to count for some clients. Consider this example:

Eloise's favorite form of self-injury was to cut many finely executed parallel lines on her left forearm. She would begin near her wrist and cut progressively up her forearm until she reached the inside of her elbow. On one occasion, as part of a behavioral assessment, we attempted to count the exact number of separate and distinct cuts executed during a single episode. The count was about 78. Also, several days after inflicting such self-injury, Eloise would tend to reopen the wounds by scraping a razor blade "across the grain" repeatedly. This type of self-harm defied any attempts at counting.

Many persons self-injure many (even hundreds of) times. Almost no one attempts suicide at such rates.

Multiple Methods

Another point of distinction between suicide and self-injury is whether the perpetrators use multiple methods. Research has shown that individuals who repeatedly attempt suicide tend to use the same method (Berman, Jobes, & Silverman, 2006). Although there are no precise statistics on these individuals, clinical experience suggests that most of them employ one method over time, that being overdose. In contrast, most self-injuring persons use more than one method. Note that in my small-sample study of adolescents mentioned above, over 70% employed more than one method. In the Favazza and Conterio (1988) study cited above, 78% of 250 responders had used multiple methods. And Whitlock, Muehlenkamp, and Eckenrode (2008) also reported a rate of 78% using multiple methods in their young adult community sample.

The use of more than one method may be related to at least two factors: preference and circumstances. Many self-injuring persons state that they use different methods of self-injury because they prefer to do so. For example, some self-injuring people say that they cut when they are anxious and burn when they are enraged. Others say that they cut when dissociating but hit themselves when angry. The range of links between types of affective distress and forms of self-injury is almost infinite. An important detail in the assessment and treatment of self-injury is determining whether an individual uses more than one method and, if so, how he or she decides on a specific method at any point in time.

Sometimes the decision on method of self-harm is more related to circumstance than personal preference. For example, adolescents placed in a group home or an inpatient unit may have difficulty obtaining a razor to cut because of close staff supervision. Although cutting may be their preferred method, they may have to resort to scratching, hitting, or biting due to the unavailability of the preferred tool.

Level of Psychological Pain

Shneidman (1985) emphasized that "unendurable, persistent pain" drives the suicidal crisis. The misery of the suicidal person is so profound, deep, and excruciating that it is intolerable—unlivable. Moreover, the pain is persistent, wearing down the person and producing profound psychic fatigue. Given the phenomenological experience of this pain, it is no wonder that the suicidal person contemplates a permanent escape. For the large majority of suicidal persons, this experience of intense pain is fraught with significant cognitive and emotional distortions. Nonetheless, within the mindset of suicidal persons is a certain logic that compels them in the direction of suicide in order to escape.

In contrast, a different type of psychic distress characterizes self-injury. The pain of the self-injuring person is intense and uncomfortable, but it does not reach the level of a suicidal crisis. The psychological anguish is interruptible and intermittent, rather than permanent and unalterable. One reason for the difference is that the self-injury itself offers a method to interrupt and reduce the pain, rendering it temporary and partial.

Muehlenkamp and Gutierrez (2007) conducted a study of adolescents that compared those who self-injured with those who had attempted suicide.

They found that those who self-injured, but had not attempted suicide, had lower ratings on hopelessness, more developed reasons for living, a stronger future orientation, and more fear of suicide than those who had attempted to kill themselves. These important findings support the clinical impression that the levels of psychological pain are different for the two forms of self-harm.

Constriction of Cognition

Another key feature of a suicidal crisis is cognitive constriction. Shneidman (1985) has used several terms to explain this mindset, including "constriction," "tunnel vision," and "dichotomous thinking." They all mean essentially the same thing: In a suicidal person, life is channeled down to an all-or-nothing option. The person thinks in a radically narrow or constricted way. A particularly common example is the belief "I must have this relationship with this person, or I must die," but there are many other scenarios. Here are some other examples encountered in clinical practice:

> "If I lose my fortune, I will kill myself."
> "If this disease is incurable, I will end it all."
> "I can't tolerate getting a bad grade. If I get a mere B, I'll overdose."
> "If I can't get this job back, I'll kill my boss and myself."
> "If I can't have custody of my children, no one will."

(Note that the last two are murder–suicide scenarios.) However diverse the content, all these examples have constricted thinking in common. The basic formula is "X must happen, or I must die."

Self-injury is not characterized by dichotomous thinking. More frequently than not, the thought process of self-injuring individuals is disorganized rather than constricted. They do not reduce their lives to an all-or-nothing predicament. Rather, they still perceive themselves to have choices in their lives and options from which to select. One of these options—and not the best one—is to self-injure. For self-injuring persons, the option to cut or burn is oddly reassuring.

Helplessness and Hopelessness

Suicide research has long identified both hopelessness and helplessness as important components of depression and suicidal behavior (Beck, Rush, Shaw, & Emery, 1979; Seligman, 1992; Milnes, Owens, & Blenkiron, 2002). "Helplessness" refers to a loss of controllability (Seligman, 1992). People who feel helpless believe that they have no real influence or control over their situations. They are convinced there is nothing they can do to affect or improve their lives. Such cognitive pessimism is very conducive to the "giving up" that suicide entails.

"Hopelessness" is the counterpart to helplessness. When people feel hopeless, they believe that their pain is endless, permanent; they have no future. Persons in a suicidal crisis feel unendurable pain that seems infinite and over which they believe they have no control. Within such a bleakly pessimistic mindset, it is no wonder that people consider suicide as the remaining option.

Another way to describe the helpless and hopeless world view of the suicidal person is in terms of the "cognitive negative triad of depression" (Beck et al., 1979). Within this perspective, suicidal people think, "I'm no good [self], everything around me is terrible [world], and nothing will ever change [future]."

In contrast, helplessness and hopelessness do not characterize the self-injury scenario. Self-injuring persons generally do not feel that they have no control over their psychological pain. In fact, the option of self-injury provides a key sense of control. Most self-injuring people find it reassuring that cutting, burning, or some other form of self-harm is available whenever they may need it to reduce distress. The control that self-injury offers is antithetical to hopelessness. The future is not one of endless inescapable pain, because self-injury often works as a tension-reducing mechanism. Granted, self-injuring persons may be episodically pessimistic and despair that their lives include so much discomfort. But their distress lacks the sense of inescapability and permanency that is fundamental to the suicidal crisis.

Psychological Aftermath of the Self-Harm Incident

The aftermath of suicidal behaviors also differs from that of self-injury. Most people who survive a suicide attempt report feeling no better following the attempt. Instead, they often report feeling even worse. They may make bitterly self-critical comments, such as "I even screwed this up—I'm such a loser," or "I didn't even kill myself right." Other statements include "I didn't have the guts to do it, but next time I will," or "Now I feel even worse than I did before I took the pills." These are people who, despite the attempt at suicide, have in no way diminished their psychological pain and their intent to kill themselves. One case vignette conveys the tone and content of the suicidal aftermath quite well:

Erin was a 17-year-old with a history of depression and recurrent suicide attempts by overdose. Recently released from a psychiatric unit where she was deemed to be safe, Erin became enraged and despondent when her mother was critical of her. Erin walked to a nearby bridge and jumped from a 30-foot height into frigid winter water. She survived only because an off-duty policeman saw the incident and pulled her out. Once medically cleared, Erin was immediately placed on a locked psychiatric unit.

Interviewed the next day on the ward, Erin was asked if she was feeling any better. In a bitter, sarcastic tone, she spat out her reply: "My only regret is that I didn't jump off something higher onto something harder!"

This vignette points to the common features of a suicide attempt's aftermath. The person often shows persistent, intense psychological pain and high-lethality intent even after the attempt.

The aftermath of self-injury behavior is often the *direct opposite* of the reaction following a suicide attempt. The "draw" of the self-injury episode is its effectiveness in reducing emotional distress. Moreover, the relief obtained is *immediate*. Self-injuring persons emphasize the importance of the relief obtained and the accessibility of the effect. They make such comments as these:

> "As soon as I cut, it was like all the anger was let out, and I felt so much better."
> "After cutting my arms or legs, all the tension leaves my body, and I can go to sleep."
> "Once I burn myself, I can see my rage on the outside, so I don't have to feel it inside any more."

Clinicians should be especially alert when clients report that their self-injury is no longer producing the desired outcome. When self-injury fails to provide its usual "therapeutic" effect, persons who rely on it for relief can begin to feel hopeless and helpless and may start to panic, feeling that the pain is inescapable. This loss of escape can catapult such persons into a suicidal crisis. The pain is no longer manageable and within their control. As the pain escalates and they are unable to reduce it, the conditions for a suicidal crisis may emerge, and protective intervention may be necessary. In such cases, the individuals will switch methods from those associated with self-injury to those associated with acts of suicide.

Restriction of Means

Another key distinction between suicide and self-injury has to do with restriction of means. It has long been established that restriction of means is an important, often life-saving intervention with suicidal behavior (Jacobs, Brewer, & Klein-Benheim, 1999; Berman et al., 2006). Examples include confiscating firearms and pills, erecting protective barriers on bridges, and moving from coal gas to natural gas as a heating fuel in the United Kingdom (Kreitman, 1976). Every graduate student is taught that a basic aspect of performing a suicide assessment is to ask the client (and significant others) about access to lethal means. And if the answer is affirmative, a first course of action is to restrict those means.

In contrast, it is not at all clear that restricting means is an effective strategy in responding to self-injury. In fact, in my experience, restriction often appears to be counterproductive. There are two main problems with attempting to restrict means with those who self-injure. First, it is impractical. It is virtually impossible to remove all means of self-injury. I have often encountered staff members from inpatient units or residential programs who are intensely, even fiercely, committed to preventing self-injury. Although their intentions are good, the results are often less than effective. In consulting to workers in these settings, I often make the point: "If you are so committed to preventing self-injury, don't forget to remove your clients' fingernails, fists, and teeth. And in the environment, don't forget to remove every staple, CD case, hard floor, or wall." In other words, it is impossible to provide such safety and prevention.

A second and related problem with using coercive and intrusive methods of supervision is that they often inadvertently provoke those who self-injure. It can be immensely triggering to have one's body, room, and/or belongings searched for "sharps" or "weapons." The mere process of "preventing" self-injury can paradoxically produce it. A far more promising strategy is to emphasize the collaborative teaching of skills with clients to replace self-injury. This approach is discussed in detail in Chapter 11.

The Core Problem

The core problem for the suicidal person is usually some combination of depression, sadness, and rage about his or her primary source of unendurable pain. Maltsberger (1986) has emphasized that the despair that drives a suicidal crisis is not only about sadness, loneliness, and isolation, but also includes elements of "murderous hate." This hatred provides much of the energy for the suicidal behavior and is often directed both at the self and at others.

The challenge in assisting suicidal individuals is therefore to identify the primary source of unendurable pain and to reduce it. Shneidman (1985) stresses that if a professional can add a third term to the dichotomous thinking of a suicidal person, then suicide risk will be reduced. For example, if the constricted thinking of such an individual is "I must have this relationship, or I will die," adding a third term might mean introducing the option of counseling with a focus on the relationship. The dichotomous scenario of "This must happen, or I will die" is expanded (and lethality simultaneously diffused) by adding a third term: "This must happen, or I will die, *or* I will address the relationship in counseling."

Finding the *specific* source of the unendurable, inescapable pain is the primary focus in working with suicidal persons. The more precisely defined the source, the more effective the work is likely to be. Moving from the global (e.g., "All of my life is terrible") to the idiosyncratic (e.g., "I'm tired of being humiliated by my boss at work") is at the heart of the therapeutic work.

In contrast, the core problem for many self-injuring persons often involves their body image. Not surprisingly, many people who repeatedly hurt their bodies often have especially negative attitudes toward their bodies (Walsh & Rosen, 1988; Alderman, 1997; Hyman, 1999). For many, a profound sense of body alienation or body hatred drives them to self-injure. Key questions that become central foci in the treatment of self-injury are "Why do you repeatedly inflict harm on your body?" and "What are the origins of this relationship with your body?" The relationship between body alienation and self-injury is discussed at length in Chapter 15.

However, one emerging group of self-injuring persons does not appear to have significant body image problems. This group appears to consist of healthier individuals from community samples (as opposed to clinical samples), who have surfaced only since the late 1990s as a self-injury phenomenon. The core problem for these individuals appears to be a combination of intense stress, inadequate self-soothing skills, self-denigrating thoughts, and peer influences that endorse self-injury. The challenges that drive these individuals to self-injure are reviewed in Chapter 4.

CONCLUSION

This chapter has set the stage for the rest of the book. A formal definition of self-injury has been provided and explained. In addition, suicide has been differentiated from self-injury in terms of 11 key characteristics:

- Prevalence
- Intent
- Level of physical damage and potential lethality
- Frequency
- Use of multiple methods
- Level of psychological pain

- Constriction of cognition
- Helplessness and hopelessness
- Psychological aftermath
- The utility of restriction of means
- The overall core problem

The next chapter deals with self-injury as a risk factor for suicide attempts.

CHAPTER 2

The Relationship between Self-Injury and Suicide

For many years, self-injury specialists such as myself, Favazza (1996, 1998), Conterio and Lader (1998), and Alderman (1997) have argued that self-injury should be considered separate and distinct from suicide. All too often, we and other professionals have seen clients inappropriately hospitalized for forms of self-injury that are deemed to be suicide attempts. One of the great myths of American popular culture is that wrist cutting is suicidal behavior. As Chapter 1 has emphasized, common forms of self-injury are generally about emotion regulation and social influence rather than a desire to die.

The repercussions of hospitalizing those who present with common, low-lethality self-injury are significant. First of all, psychiatric inpatient stays are among the most expensive of all behavioral health interventions. Second, being admitted to a "mental hospital" can be both frightening and stigmatizing for clients and families. Third, being immersed in an inpatient unit exposes individuals to a wide range of dysfunctional behaviors they might not otherwise encounter; this exposure can result in substantial iatrogenic effects. Fourth, inpatient stays can have dire consequences in terms of school, employment, or other meaningful activities. Clearly, it is important not to misdiagnose self-injury as suicidal behavior.

RECENT RESEARCH LINKING SELF-INJURY WITH SUICIDE ATTEMPTS

However, recent research has indicated that the relationship between self-injury and suicide may be much more complicated than we thought. This research has shown that self-injury may be distinct from suicide, but it is also an *important risk factor for suicide attempts* (but not necessarily completed suicides). For example, in a study of 89 inpatient adolescents, Nock, Joiner, Gordon, Lloyd-Richardson, and Prinstein (2006) found that 70% of the subjects who had recently self-injured had also made a suicide attempt during their lifetimes. In addition, 55% reported having made multiple suicide attempts.

In a similar vein, Klonsky and May (2010) reported on the relationship among self-injury, suicidal ideation, and suicide attempts in three different samples. The first consisted of a random sample of 442 U.S. adults contacted by phone. For this sample, 6% reported having self-injured, 17% reported experiencing suicidal ideation, and 3% reported having made a suicide attempt. Additional statistical analyses revealed that both suicide ideation and self-injury contributed uniquely to the prediction of attempted suicide.

Klonsky and May's second study focused on a community sample of 428 high school students. Of these youth, 21% reported having self-injured, 16% reported experiencing suicidal ideation, and 5% disclosed a suicide attempt. An especially striking finding was that the strongest association with attempted suicide was suicidal ideation (.51), followed by self-injury (.39). Self-injury had a stronger relationship with suicide attempts than a diagnosis of BPD (.29), emotion dysregulation problems (.22), loneliness (.20), and impulsivity (.11).

Klonsky and May's third study employed a sample of 171 adolescent inpatients. Of these, 58% reported having self-injured, 60% reported suicidal ideation, and 40% reported having attempted suicide. As with the study of high school students, suicidal ideation had the strongest association with suicide attempts (.55), followed by self-injury (.50). The associations for BPD, emotion dysregulation, impulsivity, and loneliness were substantially weaker.

Thus, in all three studies conducted by Klonsky and May (2010), which included both community and inpatient samples, self-injury was one of the top two predictors of suicide attempts. Clearly, such findings and the work of others (e.g., Muehlenkamp & Gutierrez, 2007; Jacobson & Gould, 2007) argue for giving serious consideration to the relationship between self-injury and suicide.

JOINER'S INTERPERSONAL THEORY OF SUICIDE AND SELF-INJURY

Another way to explicate the relationship between self-injury and suicide is through the "interpersonal theory of suicide" posited by Thomas Joiner. His seminal work *Why People Die by Suicide* (Joiner, 2005) is arguably the most important contribution to suicidology since *Definition of Suicide* (Shneidman, 1985). Joiner is eminently qualified to present his theory, as he is a rigorous empirical researcher, a practicing clinical psychologist, and a suicide survivor (his father died by suicide).

Joiner contends that there are three necessary and sufficient conditions for a suicide to occur:

1. Habituation to pain
2. Perceived burdensomeness and incompetence
3. Thwarted belongingness

I briefly explain each of these points and link them to self-injury as a risk factor for suicide. I also suggest interventions that match the dimensions of Joiner's theory.

Habituation to Pain

Joiner defines suicide as a monumental act. He contends that there are no impulsive suicides; rather, for suicides to occur, a great deal of *habituation* is required. He suggests that people must acquire the ability to commit suicide over time. This process occurs via a myriad of preparatory, disinhibiting activities. Deliberate acts of self-harm or other extreme experiences such as recurrent violence, intravenous drug use, eating disorders, and risk-taking behaviors allow a person to acquire the "courage" or "fearlessness" to commit suicide (Joiner, 2005, p. 52). Such practice is necessary in order to "beat down" or override the instinct for self-preservation.

Joiner notes that habituation to pain can be facilitated by any activity that allows a person to become inured to physical discomfort and mental anguish. Self-injury is one such example. Thus Joiner's theory offers an explanation as to why self-injury may be so strongly related to suicide attempts. Recurrent self-injury, particularly that which is extensive and prolonged, provides just the habituation to pain that Joiner is describing. Self-injury is an especially good way to beat down self-protection and preservation, because (1) it involves deliberate tissue damage; and (2) it tends to occur frequently, thereby providing lots of "practice." This conclusion points to the importance of intervening early with self-injury before it becomes an established pattern. Successful treatment can fend off the habituation necessary for a suicide to happen.

Habituation can occur cognitively as well as behaviorally. Nock and Kessler (2006) reported in an analysis of National Comorbidity Study data that individuals who cited suicide as their "reason" for self-injuring (as opposed to emotion regulation or interpersonal functions) were ultimately more likely to die by suicide. Thus clinicians should be especially alert to those who self-injure and refer to suicidal intent as their motivation. These individuals are at greater risk of moving from self-injury to suicide. One way to understand this shift is that cognitive habituation to and rehearsal for suicide are occurring.

Joiner explains another aspect of habituation that can be linked to self-injury. He discusses "opponent process theory," in which "with repetition, the effects of a provocative stimulus diminish and the opposite effect, or opponent process, becomes amplified and strengthened" (Joiner, 2005, p. 59). One example of opponent process theory is a trajectory often found with self-injury. Most individuals, when they first contemplate self-injuring, are quite ambivalent and afraid. Not infrequently they ask themselves, "Will it hurt?", "Will it work?", or "Will others condemn me?" However, over time, that which is initially feared can be transformed into something eagerly anticipated (i.e., an opponent process has occurred). These are the individuals who "can't wait to get home to self-injure," or find the anticipation of self-injuring exhilarating. Although this major shift can occur *within* the self-injury sequence, it can also manifest itself in *moving from self-injury to suicide*. That is to say, with sufficient repetition, endorsement, and anticipation, self-injury can help transform suicide into something attractive and alluring. Joiner refers to an extreme example of an opponent process when he says, "People who are near death by suicide view death in a very peculiar way—namely that death is somehow life-giving" (Joiner, 2005, p. 86).

Perceived Burdensomeness and Incompetence

According to Joiner, the second necessary and sufficient condition for suicide is *perceived burdensomeness*. He emphasizes the word "perceived," in that suicidal people often have cognitive distortions not supported by evidence. He proposes that people contemplating suicide believe themselves to be a burden on others and society. Quite often this belief takes the form of such statements as "My loved ones will be better off if I am dead." Coupled with this feeling of being an albatross is a bitter, self-denigrating sense of complete and utter *incompetence*. For example, a client of mine with major suicidal depression once described himself as "a burden on society. I make no contribution whatsoever, and the world would be better off without me."

Of particular interest is that there is some evidence that depressed people actually can be "burdensome." Joiner reviews several studies of depressed individuals who have been found to "speak more slowly, and with less volume and voice modulation; . . . and to take longer to respond when someone else addresses them" (Joiner, 2005, p. 104). Thus individuals who are depressed may receive subtle feedback that they are challenging to engage, thereby supporting their self-perceived burdensomeness.

This component of Joiner's theory is congruent with recent research on self-injury by Nock (2010) and Klonsky and Glenn (2009b), who have pointed to the important role of self-criticism or self-derogation in those who self-injure. This dimension resonates with Joiner's concepts of burdensomeness and incompetence. If we are to inoculate people who self-injure from progressing to suicidality, it may be crucial to target their self-denigrating cognitions. This aspect of treatment is discussed in Chapter 12.

Thwarted Belongingness

Joiner contends that the third necessary and sufficient condition for suicide is *thwarted belongingness.* He explains that the desire for death stems from feeling disconnected and alienated from others. He notes, "Thwarted belongingness is more than just loneliness; rather, it is the sense that sustaining connections are *obliterated*" (Joiner, 2005, p. 120; my emphasis). He adds that even when habituation and burdensomeness are in evidence, a sense of belongingness can mitigate risk. By the same token, when the basic human need for connection is thwarted, risk increases markedly.

Joiner also points out that once an individual is habituated to pain or extreme circumstances, there is no reversing it. People remain habituated for the lifespan; they are wired to remember and retrieve these experiences should major distress reemerge. The opportunity for prevention and intervention lies especially in the realm of belongingness—which is a major protective factor vis-à-vis suicide. This notion points to importance of supporting the social connections in those who self-injure; this can take the form of encouraging informally occurring relationships in the real world. Or, from a psychological treatment perspective, interventions such as social skills training and family therapy can enhance the social connectedness of clients and reduce their isolation. These aspects of treatment are discussed in Chapter 11 on replacement skills training and Chapter 13 on family treatment.

WHAT TO DO ABOUT THE RELATIONSHIP BETWEEN SELF-INJURY AND SUICIDE

The studies reviewed here, as well as Joiner's theory, suggest that it is important to develop strategies for managing self-injury in relation to suicide. Good clinical practice suggests the following guidelines:

- In beginning treatment with anyone who self-injures, it is important simultaneously to assess for suicidal thoughts, plans, and past behavior.
- In treating self-injury over time, it remains important to assess consistently for suicidality, even when suicidal content has been absent for extended periods of time. Once habituation has occurred, it persists.
- As noted in Chapter 1, self-injury tends to be a high-rate behavior, whereas suicide attempts are low-rate. It is important not to be lulled into forgetting about suicide risk because the behavior is rare.
- Evidence suggests that those with a repetitive history of self-injury are at greater risk of suicide attempts (Nock et al., 2006). We should strive to alleviate self-injury early in its trajectory, because treatment success may not only solve one problem, but also prevent another.
- Evidence also suggests that hypervigilance is warranted for those who self-injure and state that their motivations are suicidal. This explanation is much rarer than intent involving emotion regulation and social influence. Nock and Kessler (2006) have provided evidence that these self-injuring individuals are significantly more likely to die by suicide.
- We need to be alert for individuals who report that their self-injury has "stopped working." These individuals may be prone to switch to more lethal methods (e.g., firearm, overdose, hanging, jumping, vehicle) if they perceive their pain to be "unendurable and inescapable" (Shneidman, 1985).
- We also need to be alert for individuals who switch methods of self-injury in a way that is atypical for them. This may be another signal that the effectiveness of the self-injury is diminishing.
- Finally, we need to be vigilant for the main warning signs of suicide as outlined by the American Association of Suicidology (AAS). AAS employs the acronym IS PATH WARM, which represents:
  o <u>I</u>deation
  o <u>S</u>ubstance abuse
  o <u>P</u>urposelessness

- o <u>A</u>nxiety
- o <u>T</u>rapped
- o <u>H</u>opelessness
- o <u>W</u>ithdrawal
- o <u>A</u>nger
- o <u>R</u>ecklessness
- o <u>M</u>ood changes

The AAS website (*www.suicidology.org*) provides a full explanation of this terminology.

CONCLUSION

The overall messages regarding the relationship between self-injury and suicide are as follows:

- Self-injury is substantially different from suicide.
- Yet self-injury is a major risk factor for suicide attempts.
- Good clinical practice suggests that we should:
  - o Understand, manage, and treat the behaviors differentially.
  - o Carefully cross-monitor and assess interdependently.

CHAPTER 3

An Overview of Direct and Indirect Self-Harm

In this chapter, I move from discussing self-injury and suicide to reviewing all the forms of self-harm. A clinician assessing for self-injury should (1) seek to differentiate it from suicide (as discussed in Chapter 1); (2) assess for suicide risk (as reviewed in Chapter 2); and (3) evaluate for other self-destructive behaviors, such as substance abuse, an eating disorder, risk-taking, and medication discontinuance. A competent clinical assessment should look at *all* the forms of self-harm, in order to provide a full understanding of the clinical challenges ahead.

A CLASSIFICATION SCHEME FOR DIRECT AND INDIRECT SELF-HARM

Farberow (1980) provided a classic formulation of self-destructive behaviors that is still relevant today. In his discussion of the entire spectrum of self-destructive acts, he made the distinction between *direct* and *indirect* self-harm. Pattison and Kahan (1983) elaborated on this distinction and proposed a classification scheme that remains the best of its kind. In this framework, the concept of direct versus indirect self-harm is combined with the dimensions of lethality and number of episodes. I have employed a modified version of the Pattison and Kahan classification scheme, because it provides an excellent framework for organizing information regarding the entire spectrum of self-destructive behavior (see Figure 3.1). The schema shown in Figure 3.1 can be easily used in conducting an assessment of self-destructive behavior, regardless of client or setting. A checklist based on this conceptual model is provided in Figure 3.2 on page 29.

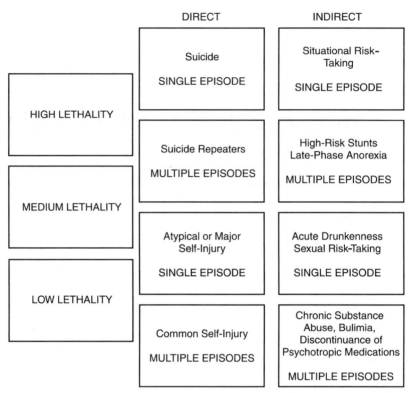

FIGURE 3.1. Differential classification of self-damaging behavior. After Pattison and Kahan (1983).

Direct Self-Harm

The first dimension in the schema is the distinction between *direct* and *indirect* self-harm. "Direct self-harm" is behavior that involves immediate tissue damage and for which intent is generally unambiguous. The category of direct self-harm applies to people who deliberately and concretely hurt themselves, and the damage inflicted is immediate. As shown in Figure 3.1, the main types of direct self-harm are suicidal behavior, major or atypical self-injury, and common self-injury. These range from high-lethality behaviors (suicide) to medium-lethality behaviors (recurrent suicide attempts and atypical or major self-injury) to low-lethality behaviors (common forms of self-injury). As shown in Figure 3.1, the behaviors can involve either single or multiple episodes.

Check those that the client reports having done at any time.

Direct Self-Harm

____ Suicide attempts (e.g., overdose, hanging, jumping from a height, use of a gun)

____ Major self-injury (e.g., self-enucleation, autocastration)

____ Atypical self-injury (mutilation of the face, eyes, genitals, breasts, or damage involving multiple sutures)

____ Common forms of self-injury (e.g., wrist, arm, and leg cutting, self-burning, self-hitting, excoriation)

Indirect Self-Harm

Substance abuse
____ alcohol abuse
____ marijuana use
____ cocaine use
____ inhalant use (e.g., glue, gasoline)
____ hallucinogens, ecstasy, etc.
____ IV drug use
____ other; specify:

Eating-disordered behavior
____ anorexia nervosa
____ bulimia nervosa
____ obesity
____ use of laxatives
____ other; specify:

____ Physical risk-taking (e.g., walking on a high-pitched roof or in high-speed traffic)

____ Situational risk-taking (e.g., getting into a car with strangers, walking alone in a dangerous area)

____ Sexual risk-taking (e.g., having sex with strangers, unprotected anal intercourse)

____ Unauthorized discontinuance of psychotropic medications

____ Misuse/abuse of prescribed psychotropic medications

____ Other forms of indirect self-harm; specify:

FIGURE 3.2. Checklist for direct and indirect self-harm behaviors.

Indirect Self-Harm

Substance Abuse and Eating Disorders

"Indirect self-harm" is behavior in which the damage is generally accumulative (and/or deferred) rather than immediate. In addition, with indirect self-harm, intent is often very ambiguous. Common examples of indirect self-harm are patterns of substance abuse and eating disorder that damage physical health. For both types of behavior, the physical harm is usually accumulative rather than immediate in nature (acute alcohol or drug overdoses are exceptions). In addition, individuals who abuse substances or have eating disorders tend to deny self-destructive intent. Those with substance abuse may justify their behavior by saying that they "just like to get high" or "live to party." Those with eating disorders may explain their behavior by stating that they are "too fat" or "out of shape."

The following vignette is an excellent example of indirect self-harm. The person described had an eating disorder that had reached life-threatening proportions, and yet she adamantly denied any self-destructive intent:

Alyssa had struggled throughout her teen years with anorexia nervosa. She was hospitalized multiple times on specialized eating disorder units, due to dangerously low body weights, unstable vital signs, and other related health problems. Appearing to have made progress by the time she reached age 18, Alyssa left home to attend college in a nearby state. At the time she left for school, she had a marginally acceptable body weight of 90 pounds (at a height of 5 feet 2 inches).

Three weeks later, Alyssa returned for a therapy meeting utterly transformed. When she walked into the therapist's office, her appearance resembled that of a concentration camp victim. The skin on her face was stretched tightly across her skull, giving her a skeletal appearance. The skin on her hands and limbs was tautly stretched across the bones. Shocked by Alyssa's appearance, the therapist insisted that she go to an emergency room immediately. The hospital found her vital signs to be extremely unstable and her weight to be 72 pounds. She was admitted directly to an intensive care unit.

Several days later, the therapist interviewed Alyssa at the hospital. When the therapist asked her quite directly why she was trying to kill herself, Alyssa replied indignantly, "I'm not trying to kill myself! I'm too fat!"

Alyssa's dilemma is a classic example of indirect self-harm. It took years for her anorexia to become life-threatening. When Alyssa went to college, she was unsupervised by family or professionals for the first time. Without oversight from others, Alyssa's anorexia quickly careened out of control. Yet when she was asked about the potential lethality of her eating disorder, she vehemently denied self-destructive intent. Her eating disorder met both conditions of indirect self-harm: The damage was accumulative rather than immediate in nature, and the intent was very ambiguous.

Substance abuse also can result in serious health risks. Use of street drugs may result in death via overdose or the contraction of HIV. The deleterious effects of chronic alcoholism are well known, ranging from damage to the liver, heart, and other organs to Korsakoff's syndrome (with its related memory loss and dementia). Yet it is a rare individual who acknowledges that his or her substance abuse has self-destructive motivations.

Risk-Taking

Risk-taking behavior is another major type of indirect self-harm. There are three main types of risk-taking behavior: "situational," "physical," and "sexual." Situational risk-taking includes behaviors that are not risky in and of themselves; The behaviors become potentially harmful only in relation to a particular context. For example, taking a walk is not a dangerous activity per se; however, choosing to walk alone at night in a high-crime area of a city is potentially quite dangerous. Some people tend to put themselves in harm's way because of poor judgment and/or minimal investment in life (Orbach et al., 1991; Orbach, Lotem-Peleg, & Kedem, 1995). Consider the following as a representative example of situational risk-taking:

Tiku was a seriously self-destructive individual who not only frequently cut herself, but also had the habit of going off with strangers. On one occasion she was walking alone in a city late at night when a car occupied by four young men pulled up. They showed her a supply of beer they had in the car and asked if she'd like to "party with them." She thought, "This sounds like fun!" so she jumped into the car. Later that evening, after some heavy drinking, she was gang-raped by the four men. After the sexual assaults were over, the four men drove off with her clothes, leaving her to fend for herself naked.

Tiku's poor judgment and failure to take reasonable precautions in dealing with strangers constitute an example of situational risk-taking. It is important to emphasize that labeling a behavior as risk-taking is not tantamount to blaming a victim. In Tiku's case, the rapists were reprehensible and responsible for their assaults. Nonetheless, the young woman's failure to protect herself played a role in the outcome. Moreover, her tendency to take such risks repeatedly represented a self-destructive pattern.

Physical risk-taking is a second type of such behaviors. Many self-injuring youth and adults take notorious physical risks (Lightfoot, 1997; Ponton, 1997). They may walk in high-speed traffic, sit on the edge of a roof of a multistory building, or straddle an open stairway at a high elevation. Here the risk is not situational but concrete. A slight miscalculation could result in serious injury or even death. Many youth report feeling exhilarated when they take physical risks. As one adolescent once told me, "I feel most alive when I flirt with death. It's so cool!"

Sexual risk-taking behavior comes in many forms. Some involve having multiple partners within a short period of time or unprotected sex with strangers. Others entail having sex with individuals who are known to use drugs intravenously or to have sexually transmitted diseases. Still others include having sex while intoxicated and being unaware of one's activities. Unprotected oral, vaginal, or anal sex can represent serious risks, particularly when the partner's sexual history is not well known. A person's sexual behaviors can be so impulsive and erratic that they assume self-destructive proportions. Granted, the actual extent of physical risk is often ambiguous at the time of the act. It is generally impossible to know whether a particular sexual encounter will lead to genital herpes, gonorrhea, syphilis, chlamydia, or HIV/AIDS. However, some individuals have so many random or impulsive sexual encounters that they markedly increase their risk of disease and even death.

Few individuals deliberately attempt to get HIV/AIDS or other sexually transmitted diseases. Nonetheless, when individuals repeatedly fail to protect themselves, such behavior should be viewed as sexual risk-taking that is potentially self-destructive in nature. The self-destructive intent of the individual may be more of omission than commission, but the results are the same. The following anecdote is an example of sexual behavior that has self-destructive motivations:

Early in treatment, Jim described himself as "wild and crazy." One of his favorite weekend activities was to drink heavily at a gay bar and have sex with several partners. Jim's pattern was to give oral sex and receive anal sex, usually in a restroom stall. He took precautions only when a partner demanded it. Jim complained, "Using condoms takes the spontaneity out of it. Besides, I lose them most of the time."

Over time in treatment, Jim admitted to being depressed about being thrown out of his parents' house for being gay. He also said that he didn't really care if he lived or died, so "the sexual precaution stuff is irrelevant." This minimal investment in life reflected Jim's depression and hopelessness.

After Jim had been in treatment for several months, he began to acknowledge that his drinking and unprotected sexual behaviors were both self-demeaning and self-destructive in nature. He identified that his real goal was to have an ongoing stable relationship. He also discussed his pain related to his family's rejection; eventually, he came to accept that reconciliation was unrealistic for the time being, due to his family's homophobia.

ASSESSING FOR RISK-TAKING BEHAVIORS

A thorough assessment of self-destructiveness explores all three types of risk-taking behaviors. This can be accomplished by asking a few very basic questions, as outlined below:

Situational Risk-Taking

"Do you ever walk in a dangerous area of a city alone at night?"

"Have you ever gotten into a car with strangers?"

"Do you ever hitchhike alone?"

"Do you place yourself in risky situations?"

Physical Risk-Taking

"Do you ever take physical risks, such as walking in high-speed traffic or standing on the edge of a roof?"

"Have you done risky things, such as walk on train tracks in a tunnel?"

"Do you find physically risky activities thrilling?"

Sexual Risk-Taking

"Have you ever had sex with people you barely know?"

"Have you ever had sex while you were very intoxicated and had little or no memory of the experience afterward?"

"Have you ever had unprotected anal sex?"

"How many sexual partners have you had in the last year?"

"Do you think that any of your sexual behavior is risky?"

Some individuals respond quite enthusiastically to questions about risk-taking, indicating that they relish such activities. Motivations are complex in those who report high rates of risk-taking (Lightfoot, 1997; Ponton, 1997). For many, the payoff appears to involve enjoying the adrenaline rush associated with the risk-taking, while simultaneously indulging a desire to demean or destroy the self. A recurrent pattern of situational, physical, and/or sexual risk-taking should be viewed as potentially life-threatening—indeed, as much so as high-lethality suicidal behavior.

Asking a series of questions about risk-taking behaviors should be done with great care and compassion. A therapeutic alliance usually has to be well established before reliable information can be obtained, especially about sexual behaviors. Inquiring about these behaviors should be done in a supportive, nonjudgmental manner. Clients should not feel that they are being subjected to an evaluation of their morality; the goal is to assess their self-destructiveness in all its manifestations. The presence of these major forms of indirect self-harm points to significant distress and a lack of important coping skills. Both should be targeted in treatment.

Medication Discontinuance or Abuse

Yet another form of indirect self-harm is the unauthorized discontinuance or abuse of prescribed medications. It is well known that many people do not comply with medication regimens completely. For example, significant percentages of people who are prescribed an antibiotic for a bacterial infection fail to complete the entire course. This is *not* the type of medication discontinuance deemed to be self-destructive here.

Many self-injuring people are on psychotropic medications, be they antidepressants, antianxiety agents, antipsychotics, or mood stabilizers. Unfortunately, many clients episodically discontinue or abuse these medications. The noncompliance with prescribed regimens is part of a recurrent self-destructive pattern for some individuals. Consider this example:

In the course of treatment, Erika identified a number of key steps that preceded her self-injuring behavior. She found that some sort of relationship disappointment generally triggered the downward spiral. Once this had occurred, she began drinking or smoking pot heavily. Before long, Erika would abruptly stop taking her antipsychotic medication without telling her doctor. This decision quickly led to paranoid thinking and increased anxiety. As her cognitive and affective distress increased, she became more and more focused on "the solution." This was to cut herself on her forearms and legs, after which she felt calm for several days.

In the course of treatment, Erika recognized that it was important for her to stay on her medication. Her impulse to discontinue was part of a self-destructive pattern that culminated in cutting behavior. She decided that if she were to give up cutting, she needed to remain on her medication and to avoid heavy drinking and pot smoking. She also had to work on her relationship skills in order to reduce the frequency of her disappointments.

Erika was involved in multiple forms of indirect self-harm, including alcohol and marijuana use and discontinuance of prescribed medications. All three behaviors were part of a web of self-harm that led to cutting. Untangling this web enabled her to reduce her cutting behavior while she also worked on acquiring new skills.

COMORBIDITY OF INDIRECT SELF-HARM WITH SELF-INJURY

Thoroughness is one reason to assess for all forms of direct and indirect self-harm. Another is that the various forms of direct and indirect self-harm have frequently been found to co-occur. The relationships have been reported both within and across the categories of direct and indirect self-harm. More specifically, as discussed at length in Chapter 2, self-injury has frequently been found to be associated with suicidal behavior. Persons who frequently self-injure may turn to suicide when their self-injury stops working as an effective affect management technique.

Self-injury has also frequently been found to be associated with the major forms of indirect self-harm. In an early study of 52 self-injuring adolescents (Walsh, 1987), the number one predictor of self-injury was the presence of an eating disorder. Favazza, DeRosear, and Conterio (1989) described a sample of 65 self-injuring clients in which 50% reported having a past or present eating disorder. Within the Favazza et al. (1989) sample, 15% identified their eating disorder as anorexia nervosa, 22% as bulimia nervosa, and 13% as both. Paul, Schroeter, Dahme, and Nutzinger (2002) reported that in a sample of 376 inpatient women being treated for eating disorders, 34.4% had self-injured at some point in their lifetimes.

In an unpublished study I conducted in the 1990s (Walsh & Frost, 2005), over 60% of a sample of 34 poly-self-destructive adolescents reported having vomited in order to lose weight. Favaro and Santonastaso (1998), Muehlenkamp, Engel, et al. (2009), and Whitlock et al. (2006) have also reported an association between eating disorder and self-injury.

Another important relationship has been reported between self-injury and substance abuse. In the unpublished study cited above (Walsh & Frost, 2005), many of the 34 poly-self-destructive adolescents reported having major problems with substance abuse: 77% reported sniffing glue; 53% stated that they drank alcohol frequently; 85% reported having used marijuana; 32%, cocaine; and 42%, LSD.

Other publications have pointed to the comorbidity of self-injury and substance abuse. Simeon and Hollander (2001) reviewed studies of skin picking, hair pulling (trichotillomania), and nail biting, and reported associations with substance abuse. Greilsheimer and Groves (1979) reviewed reports of male genital self-mutilation and cited acute intoxication as a precipitant in a number of cases. Linehan (1993a), Alderman (1997), Hyman (1999), and Connors (2000) have also linked substance abuse with self-injurious behaviors.

For many individuals, the affect-modulating effects of substances may complement the tension reduction capabilities of self-injury. Emotionally dysregulated people tend to seek relief from their distress in multiple directions. Sometimes they may self-injure to deal with anxiety, anger, sadness, or shame; at other times they may drink or use drugs to deal with the same or different feelings. Relatively few individuals report self-injuring while they are under the influence of a substance. For example, Linehan (1993a) reported that 13.4% of a sample of 119 self-injuring persons had used alcohol shortly before the act. An example of this atypical scenario is described below:

Sarah had been self-injuring a few times a year for about a 3-year period. She stated that she only cut herself when she was high on marijuana or alcohol. She explained that she "really didn't like doing it." She added that it hurt when she cut, and because of that, she was scared to do it. However, sometimes "the pressure just got to be too much" and she "just *had to*." Being high helped her "to build up the courage."

Yet another relationship exists between self-injury and risk-taking behaviors. In the Walsh and Frost (2005) study, 94% of the sample of 34 poly-self-destructive adolescents reported physical risk-taking and 85% situational risk-taking. In addition, 41% reported having had sex with strangers; 15%, anal sex without a condom; 18%, sex with no memory afterward due to intoxication; and 32%, who averaged 15.81 years of age, had had eight or more sexual partners.

CONCLUSION

This chapter has reviewed the spectrum of self-destructive behaviors in relation to the categories of direct and indirect self-harm. The interrelationships between various self-destructive behaviors have also been discussed. The checklist in Figure 3.2 includes the major types of direct and indirect self-harm. This checklist is intended as a reference for clinicians; it is *not* suggested that it be distributed to clients to complete. Asking clients to complete it might be triggering and counterproductive. Clinicians who use the checklist will find that it can be quickly memorized and employed informally while interviewing clients. Inquiring about all of the items on the checklist should provide a reasonable degree of confidence that a thorough inventory of self-destructive behavior has been obtained.

Although the checklist is reasonably inclusive, I do not claim it to be exhaustive. Unfortunately, self-destructive people are creative and often come up with new forms of self-harm. One example of this creativity is the frequent emergence of new "designer drugs." Another is the development of new methods to disfigure or mar the body. Therefore, an "other" category is provided in several places within the checklist.

CHAPTER 4

Major Groups in Which Self-Injury Occurs

The prevalence of self-injury in the United States appears to be growing markedly. In the early 1980s, Pattison and Kahan (1983) estimated the rate of what they called "deliberate self-harm" in the U.S. population to be 400 per 100,000. By the late 1980s this estimate had grown to 750 per 100,000 (Favazza & Conterio, 1988), and by the late 1990s it had advanced to 1,400 per 100,000 (Conterio & Lader, 1998). If these estimates are correct, the rate of self-injury grew by 250% over a 15-year period. An alternative explanation is that self-injury is more in the public eye now, because it is better recognized as an important public health problem; as a result, the reporting may be more accurate. Or both may be true: The rate of self-injury may have increased, *and* the reporting may be more precise. Regardless of the explanation, it should be emphasized that these prevalence figures for self-injury are approximations only. One of the frustrations for those who desire to understand self-injury is that there have been no large nationwide epidemiological studies of the behavior to date.

It may be instructive to compare the rate of self-injury to rates of other forms of direct and indirect self-harm. The suicide rate in the United States is approximately 11.5 per 100,000 (AAS, 2008), and the rate of alcohol abuse is estimated to be about 5,600 per 100,000 (Grant et al., 1994). Thus, according to Conterio and Lader's (1998) estimate of 1,400 per 100,000 for self-injury, individuals are about 120 times more likely to self-injure than to commit suicide, and are about 4 times less likely to self-injure than to abuse alcohol.

SELF-INJURY IN CLINICAL GROUPS: EARLIER FINDINGS

What accounts for the increasing rate of self-injury nationally? One explanation is that the behaviors are now occurring in broader segments of the population. In the past, self-injury was reported primarily in the following groups of people:

- Outpatients with serious emotional disturbance or mental illness (Linehan, 1993a; Alderman, 1997; Deiter, Nicholls, & Pearlman, 2000)
- Persons presenting at psychiatric emergency rooms (Clendenin & Murphy, 1971; Weissman, 1975)
- Persons with serious and persistent mental illness who were in day treatment or partial hospitalization programs (Deiter et al., 2000)
- Adults with serious and persistent mental illness who were living in community-based residential or supported housing programs
- Patients in short- and long-term psychiatric and forensic units (Offer & Barglow, 1960; Phillips & Alkan, 1961; Pao, 1969; Podvoll, 1969; Kroll, 1978; Darche, 1990; Langbehn & Pfohl, 1993; Himber, 1994; Conterio & Lader, 1998; Gough & Hawkins, 2000; Paul et al., 2002)
- Youth in special education schools, residential treatment, or juvenile detention facilities (Ross & McKay, 1979; Walsh & Rosen, 1985; Rosen & Walsh, 1989; Chowanec, Josephson, Coleman, & Davis, 1991; Boiko & Lester, 2000; Heinsz, 2000; Walsh & Doerfler, 2009)
- Prison inmates (Virkkunen, 1976; Haines & Williams, 1997; Howard League for Penal Reform, 1999; Ireland, 2000; Motz, 2001)

These groups, of course, were not mutually exclusive. For example, individuals could be discharged from institutions (such as hospitals or prisons) and become clients in residential or outpatient settings, or vice versa.

Not surprisingly, people being treated in the above-described settings tended to have or to acquire major psychiatric diagnoses. These included, first and foremost, BPD (Gardner & Cowdry, 1985; Linehan, Armstrong, Suarez, Allmon, & Heard, 1991; Linehan, 1993a; Dulit, Fyer, Leon, Brodsky, & Frances, 1994; Zweig-Frank, Paris, & Guzder, 1994; Bohus, Haaf, et al., 2000), followed (in no particular order) by posttraumatic stress disorder (PTSD; van der Kolk, McFarlane, & Weisaeth, 1996; Briere & Gil, 1998; Simeon & Hollander, 2001), dissociative disorders (Briere & Gil, 1998), anorexia nervosa and/or bulimia nervosa (Walsh & Rosen, 1988; Favazza & Conterio, 1988; Warren, Dolan, & Norton, 1998; Favaro & Santonastaso, 2000; Rodriguez-Srednicki, 2001; Paul et al., 2002), depression (Ross & Heath, 2002), anxiety disorders in general (Ross & Heath, 2002), obsessive–

compulsive disorder (OCD; Gardner & Gardner, 1975; Favaro & Santonastaso, 2000; McKay, Kulchycky, & Danyko, 2000; Simeon & Hollander, 2001), antisocial personality disorder (McKerracher, Loughnane, & Watson, 1968; Virkkunen, 1976), and a variety of psychoses (Menninger, 1938/1966; Green, 1968; Rosen & Hoffman, 1972; Greilsheimer & Groves, 1979; Favazza, 1987; Walsh & Rosen, 1988).

During the period from the 1960s through the 1980s, the assumption (correct or not) was that a person who self-injured was probably suffering from serious mental disturbance and considerable functional impairment, including compromised social functioning and a diminished ability to deal with the demands of school and/or work. This level of impairment was often linked to aversive childhood experiences. Self-injuring persons were described as having experienced various forms of major family dysfunction. These included sexual abuse (Walsh & Rosen, 1988; Darche, 1990; Shapiro & Dominiak, 1992; Miller, 1994; van der Kolk et al., 1996; Alderman, 1997; Favazza, 1998; Briere & Gil, 1998; Turell & Armsworth, 2000; Rodriguez-Srednicki, 2001; Paul et al., 2002); physical abuse (van der Kolk, Perry, & Herman, 1991; van der Kolk et al., 1996; Briere & Gil, 1998; Low, Jones, MacLeod, Power, & Duggan, 2000); parental loss and divorce; and exposure to family violence, family alcoholism, or family mental illness and suicidality (Walsh & Rosen, 1988; Turell & Armsworth, 2000).

In short, until recently, self-injuring persons were deemed to be seriously disturbed, to be functionally impaired, and to have come from seriously dysfunctional family backgrounds. Moreover, consistent with these profiles, these persons were seen as requiring intensive and expensive long-term treatment.

SELF-INJURY IN THE GENERAL POPULATION: MORE RECENT FINDINGS

Surprisingly, this pattern changed in the late 1990s, when self-injury began to appear in ever-greater numbers in people who did not fit the profiles described above. This is not to say that self-injury declined in the usual populations thought to be associated with the behavior. Persons with major psychiatric diagnoses continued to have high rates of self-injury. But, at the same time, a new generation of self-injuring persons was emerging from the general population rather than from clinical settings.

Self-Injury in Middle and High Schools

The first decade of the new century saw a substantial increase in research on self-injury in young community samples, including students in middle schools and high schools. An important early contribution to this literature was an empirical study of 440 self-injuring students from urban and suburban high schools in Canada (Ross & Heath, 2002). It is important to note that these youth were students in *regular education* classes, not special education. Ross and Heath (2002) found that 61 (or 13.9%) of the students reported having self-injured. Of these, 39 (or 64%) were girls, and 22 (or 36%) were boys. At the time this was a very startling finding! Initially, these results appeared to be anomalous. But a large number of studies have since confirmed that self-injury is now commonplace in public schools.

One such example comes from Massachusetts Youth Risk Behavior Survey data collected from a large random sample (Massachusetts Department of Elementary and Secondary Education, 2008). Data indicated that 17% of high school students and 16% of middle school students reported having self-injured *during the past year*. Thus, in Massachusetts (as in many other U.S. states), the behavior has become a significant public health problem.

There are numerous other studies documenting that self-injury occurs at high rates in middle and high schools (e.g., Rodham, Hawton, & Evans, 2004; Muehlenkamp & Gutierrez, 2007; Klonsky & May 2010). For thorough reviews of these studies, see Heath, Schaub, Holly, and Nixon (2009) and Rodham and Hawton (2009).

The prevalence reported in diverse studies can be summarized as follows: The rates of self-injury found in community samples range from 13 to 45% of adolescents (Nock, 2010). On average, there is a prevalence rate of 15–20% for adolescents in community samples (Heath et al., 2009). To put these findings in perspective, consider that the estimated lifetime prevalence rates for self-injury appear to exceed the rates for many other important clinical problems, including anorexia nervosa and bulimia nervosa (<2%), panic disorder (<2%), OCD (<3%), and BPD (<2%) (Nock, 2010, p. 345).

Other important details regarding self-injury in community samples of youth include the following:

- The average age of onset is 12–14 years (Nock, 2010).
- Whereas in clinical samples more females report self-injury than males, in community samples there is usually no gender difference (Heath et al., 2009).
- Self-injury may be more common among European Americans and among gay, lesbian, bisexual, and transgender (GLBT) youth (Heath et al., 2009).
- Females may be more likely to cut or pick; males may prefer more aggressive methods, such as hitting themselves or punching walls (Laye-Gindhu & Schonert-Reichl, 2005).

Beyond the research findings reviewed above, two brief case examples may be representative of the new type of self-injuring youth encountered in middle and high school settings:

Amy is a 13-year-old seventh grader who attends a small private school for girls. She is a B+ student, a fine artist, and a talented musician who plays the cello in her school orchestra. Amy is articulate and personable. She is slightly underweight and engages episodically in bulimia, especially when her peers make an offhand remark about her size. Amy has close friends whom she sees every weekend. She poses no disciplinary problems for her mother, who is a single parent. Recently, friends at school disclosed that Amy has been cutting herself once or twice a week for about 6 months. She tends to cut when exam pressures mount or she has an upcoming cello performance. She reports that the cutting relaxes her and is "no big deal." Amy usually inflicts the cuts on her left forearm with a razor blade. The cuts draw blood, but do not require sutures and do not appear to be leaving permanent scars.

Sean is a 17-year-old junior in a large urban public high school. He is a C student and a member of the football team. Most of Sean's friends are also team members. Sean lifts weights daily as part of his training for football. He is an attractive young man who is meticulous about his appearance. He is not talkative in therapy, but he is cooperative and responsive when asked direct questions.

Sean lives with his parents and a younger brother. His self-injury started about a year ago. He has carved designs into his upper arms with a razor and has burned his forearms and legs with cigarettes (although he does not smoke). Sean's self-injury appears to be linked to intense anger. He resents parental curfews and is frequently infuriated by the dictatorial style of his football coach. Sean reports that cutting or burning himself helps him "not to hit people." He states that if he were to get into a physical altercation with his parents or coach, he "would have too much to lose," so he handles it in his own way. Sean says he can't wait to get to college, where he will run his own life.

Many of this new generation of youth who self-injure have a substantial circle of friends. In some cases, their friends may self-injure as well. An example of this type of peer interaction and influence is described in the following vignette.

The principal of a middle school in a middle-class suburb was alarmed to discover that her students were experiencing an epidemic of self-injury. All the more surprising were the specific students involved in the self-harm. None of these students had been in trouble at school, and most were doing well academically. The students primarily involved in this behavior were eight females in the seventh grade. All eight knew each other, but only about half were close friends. The principal learned that the two most influential leaders in the group had been cutting themselves for about 9 months—sometimes alone, sometimes together. The others had begun to cut more recently, within the last 6 weeks. Asked about the family lives of these girls, the principal replied that the large majority of the students had concerned and involved parents. The principal said that when the parents learned of the cutting, they were horrified and sprang into action, looking for professional services. The response from the parents was everything the principal could have hoped for.

It should be emphasized that although this new group of self-injuring adolescents often has major strengths, the students are nonetheless experiencing serious distress. Self-injury in middle and high school students should not be minimized or dismissed as "attention seeking" or "just a fad." When people take the radical step of harming their bodies, they should be taken seriously, and the sources of their stress should be addressed.

Usually a friend has introduced these youth to self-injury (although most adolescents will deny imitating others). Once they have tried self-injuring, they may quickly come to rely on it as a preferred way of managing and reducing emotional pain. Almost always these youth lack the healthy coping skills necessary to acknowledge and reduce emotional distress.

Another interesting feature regarding this new generation of self-injuring youth is what is *not* wrong with them. In the past, I have argued that body alienation is central to understanding self-injury (Walsh, 1987, 2001; Walsh & Rosen, 1988; see also Chapter 15). Time and again, when encouraged to tell their stories, self-harming persons from the 1970s and 1980s disclosed histories of trauma, especially sexual and/or physical abuse. Very consistently, those who had been abused reported a profound sense of bodily hatred or alienation derived from the trauma. These persons had suffered greatly at the hands and organs of others and had come to view their bodies as contaminated, dirty, and broken. Moreover, they often blamed themselves (irrationally) in some way for the abuse, and they seemed to condemn their bodies as the culprits or co-conspirators in their trauma histories.

Many of the new group of self-injuring persons do not report high rates of sexual or physical abuse (Heath, Toste, Nedecheva, & Charlebois, 2008). Moreover, when they are asked detailed questions about body image, they present with normative attitudes. Many exhibit no body alienation; that is, they do not loathe their bodies and do not report experiences of dissociation derived from trauma. One line of demarcation between the old and new groups of self-injuring individuals may be whether or not they present with negative attitudes regarding the body (see Chapter 15 for an extended discussion and some empirical data regarding this topic).

Not surprisingly, given that many of these youth are relatively psychologically healthy and have strengths in the areas of family, peers, and school, my impression is that they also tend to give up the self-injury behavior more quickly. Unlike individuals from clinical populations, who may self-injure for years, many of these youth cease doing so after 6 months to 2 years.

Treatment often has a key role in helping these individuals stop self-injuring. In therapy, these clients can be very responsive, cooperative, and motivated. They often are quite receptive to learning new self-soothing skills, which they may practice quite diligently.

Peer influences are often crucially important as well. If a small circle of friends stops self-injuring, an individual may give it up with or without treatment. Mutual support among peers can also be quite helpful in assisting self-injuring adolescents to stop. These considerable peer factors do not imply that these adolescents are not in real distress. They are in intense pain and need assistance until they mature and can handle their emotional distress more effectively through other means.

Another way to understand the world of this new group of self-injuring adolescents is to read Caroline Kettlewell's *Skin Game* (1999), the first book-length autobiographical memoir of a "cutter's journey." Kettlewell grew up living on the campus of a Virginia prep school where her father was an administrator. She lived in an intact family and was not subjected to abuse. She first cut herself in the seventh grade. She received little in the way of professional treatment until she was in her 20s, and that treatment pertained more to relationship issues than to the cutting. Throughout her youth, despite her emotional turmoil and persistent cutting, she was an exceptional student, as evidenced by her attending and graduating from Williams College (one of the more academically competitive colleges in the United States). After majoring in English at Williams, she obtained her master's degree in writing from George Mason University. Kettlewell is an exceptional writer, perhaps the most incisive and poignant voice ever to describe the act of self-injuring. An example of her ability to articulate the experience of self-injury is provided below:

> I intended to kill something in me, this awful feeling like worms tunneling along my nerves. So when I discovered the razor blade, cutting, if you'll believe me, was my gesture of hope. That first time, when I was twelve, was like some kind of miracle, a revelation. The blade slipped easily, painlessly through my skin, like a hot knife through butter. As swift and pure as a stroke of lightning, it wrought an absolute and pristine division between before and after. All the chaos, the sound and fury, the uncertainty and confusion and despair—all of it evaporated in an instant, and I was for that moment grounded, coherent, whole. *Here is the irreducible self.* I drew the line in the sand, marked my body as mine, its flesh and its blood under my command. (Kettlewell, 1999, p. 57; emphasis in original)

Kettlewell is a key spokesperson regarding self-injury, particularly for this new group of self-injuring youth who are often very capable and accomplished. She now lives in Virginia with her husband and son. Although she no longer self-injures, her ability to describe and share the anguish of the self-injuring experience is unique.

Self-Injury in Colleges and Universities

Youth from middle and high schools who self-injure eventually grow up and leave home. Some enter the general population as workers; others go to college. Youth who have harmed themselves during adolescence may continue or resume self-injuring in adulthood. Those who attend college may be more likely to come to the attention of professionals, because they often are referred to, or appear at, university health services. Of course, some youth do not begin to self-injure until college. In one study, Favazza and Rosenthal (1990) reported that 12% of a college-age sample claimed to have self-injured.

Shaw (2002), in a qualitative study, discussed a sample of six women in college who had extensive histories of self-injury. These women ranged in age from 18 to 21 years. They had self-injured for 1–5 years. The level of physical damage associated with their self-harm ranged from very modest self-injury to major self-injury. The number of episodes of self-injury for these women varied from about 10 to over 50. Their involvement in treatment also differed greatly. One had been hospitalized repeatedly, and three others had had extensive outpatient treatment; however, two of the six had received no treatment whatsoever.

The women in Shaw's study appear to be good examples of the new type of self-injuring college student. All six were functioning quite adequately in their college settings, and some were excelling academically. Most were engaged in serious relationships. Moreover, of particular interest is that all six had *ceased* self-injuring. These women were experiencing considerable distress in their lives and had repeatedly used self-injury in the past to manage emotional pain. Nonetheless, they had considerable strengths and were able to discontinue self-injury through the use of treatment and/or their own internal resources and naturally occurring external supports.

An especially influential empirical study of college undergraduates was conducted by Whitlock et al. (2006). They recruited a sample of almost 3,000 students from Cornell and Princeton universities, two very competitive Ivy League schools. Quite remarkably, they found that 17% indicated having self-injured, and 11% reported doing so repeatedly. Moreover, Whitlock and colleagues replicated this study in a research project involving eight colleges and more than 11,000 students (Whitlock, Eells, Cummings, & Purington, 2009). This time they found that 15.3% reported some nonsuicidal self-injury lifetime, and that 29.4% reported more than 10 episodes.

Adult Self-Injury in the General Population

For decades, self-injury was described as a type of behavior found in adolescents and young adults. Clinicians were aware of only a few relatively rare cases in which persons persisted in harming themselves into middle age. These tended to be people with serious and persistent mental illness who were part of an adult mental health system of care.

In an important study, Briere and Gil (1998) employed a national sampling service to generate "a stratified, random sample of the U.S., based on geographical location of registered owners of automobiles and individuals with listed telephones" (p. 611). The resulting sample consisted of 927 adults, with equal gender representation. The authors founds that 33 (or 4%) of the sample reported having self-injured at least occasionally, and that 3 (or 0.3%) reported *often* engaging in the behavior. The self-injuring participants had a mean age of 35 years, clearly indicating the adult nature of the sample. Also of note is that there was no significant gender difference for the 33 self-injuring participants, with 4% of the females and 3% of the males reporting self-harm. Briere and Gil concluded from their findings that self-injury is "relatively rare in the general population" (p. 612), given the rate of 4% obtained in their sample.

Although 4% of any group may not seem like a large proportion, we can reach a different conclusion if we consider national census data. The U.S. Census Bureau (2010) reported that there were approximately 104,492,000 persons between the ages of 20 and 44 in the country. (Note: I have selected this age range for adults as the one in which self-injury is more likely to occur. The age range may, in fact, be too narrow in discussing self-injury in the general population of adults, but I have used it here in order to be conservative.) If we use Briere and Gil's prevalence rate, 4% of the 20- to 44-year-old population in the United States equals 4,179,680 persons. Thus, based on the Briere and Gil (1998) study, we can estimate that there may be more than 4 million adults in the U.S. general population who have self-injured. If we consider only those who stated that they self-injured "often" in the Briere and Gil report, then the rate drops to 0.3% of the sample. This percentage (0.3%) yields an estimate of approximately 313,476 persons in the United States between the ages of 20 and 44 who have *often* self-injured. The results from the Briere and Gil study thus begin to suggest the true scope of the problem of self-injury in the general adult population.

Numerous other studies have focused on self-injury in adults (e.g., Favazza et al., 1989; Klonsky, Oltmanns, & Turkheimer, 2003; Nada-Raja, Skegg, Langley, Morrison, & Sowerby, 2004). In general, 2–4% of adults in community samples report self-injuring, while 19–25% in clinical samples do so (Nock, 2010).

One way to approach the problem of self-injury in adults is via epidemiological and clinical research; another is through qualitative methods. Hyman's (1999) book is an innovative and informative qualitative study of self-injury in adults. Her work focused on 15 women who had self-injured for years and were willing to tell their stories in detail. The women ranged in age from 26 to 51, with a mean of 36.9 years. Thus the ages of Hyman's group further dispel the notion that self-injury is solely an adolescent and young adult problem.

The women that Hyman came to know and wrote about had not had easy lives. All 15 had been sexually abused as children; all but one had been repeatedly sexually abused by a parent or stepparent. The trauma continued to be a focal point of their lives and a key antecedent in their long histories of self-injury. What are particularly instructive (and inspirational) about the lives of these women are their resilience and related levels of functioning. At the beginning of her book, Hyman (1999) identified each woman in terms of a pseudonym, age, and profession. This list bears repeating because it is inherently revealing:

Edith, 51, physical therapist
Karen, 49, human services worker
Elizabeth, 25, typist
Jane, 39, treasurer
Erica, 43, editor and writer
Peggy, 34, human services worker
Mary, 47, technology manager for communications company
Esther, 40, central security station operator and store sales associate
Jessica, 46, part-time social worker, in graduate school for social work
Rosa, 30, drafter for engineering and architectural firm
Meredith, 26, part-time social worker, in graduate school for social work
Caroline, 30, office staff worker and student in music school
Helena, 28, free-lance proofreader and copyeditor
Sarah, 27, part-time worker, in graduate school for pharmacy

Hyman's list dispels another myth about self-injury: that persons who self-harm well into adulthood must be seriously disturbed and suffering from considerable functional impairment. The 15 women described in Hyman's book displayed an impressive level of accomplishment in the workplace. In addition, most were engaged in ongoing relationships and had meaningful social networks. Although the stories of Hyman's informants were fraught with anguish and psychic pain, they nonetheless convey a crucially important message of hope and recovery. Toward the end of *Women Living with Self-Injury*, Hyman described her follow-up contact with 9 of the 15 women. Her conversations or correspondence with the women occurred 1½–5 years after the initial interviews.

> I often heard tales of improvement and recovery from voices that sounded full and cheerful, contrasting with the sometimes audible shame, anxiety, and distress of the original interviews. Two of my informants have decreased self-injury, five have stopped self-injury altogether, and four of these five have also stopped feeling the need to self-injure. (Hyman, 1999, p. 177)

EXPLANATIONS FOR THE INCREASED PREVALENCE OF SELF-INJURY

Transcultural, Feminist, and Modern Primitive Views

Why is there such a marked increase of self-injury in contemporary society? Why is the behavior surfacing in healthier segments of the populations of the United States, Canada, Europe, Japan, New Zealand, and Taiwan? To address questions such as these, we must inevitably go beyond the individualistic approach of psychology and talk about sociocultural factors. Favazza (1996) has written about self-injury from a transcultural perspective. He has reviewed the practice of self-induced body modification around the world and linked it to such themes as religious transformation, pubertal rites of passage, shamanistic magic, and the mythologies of garnering power over the natural and spiritual worlds. He writes:

> Because of their persistence and the "deep" meanings attributed to them by societies, self-mutilative rituals inform us about basic elements of social life. Examination of the rituals . . . reveals that they serve an elemental purpose, namely, the correction or prevention of a destabilizing condition that threatens the community. A few examples of destabilizing conditions are diseases; angry gods, spirits or ancestors; failure of boys and girls to accept adult responsibilities when they mature; conflicts of all sorts, for example, male–female, intergenerational, interclass, intertribal; loosening of clear social role distinctions; loss of group identity and distinctiveness; immoral or sinful behaviors; ecological disaster.
>
> Self-mutilative rituals (and some practices) serve to prevent the onset of these conditions and to correct or "cure" them should they occur. The rituals work by promoting healing, spirituality, and social order. (Favazza, 1996, p. 226)

It is not difficult to cull from Favazza's discussion of worldwide phenomena many aspects that fit our own situation. These include the challenging problems of worldwide economic recession, disease (e.g., HIV/AIDS and the impact on youthful sexuality); conflict between the sexes, generations, and classes; loss of cohesiveness in the social order; confusion regarding the moral order; and widespread ecological disaster. Moreover, if we use Favazza's (1996) three dimensions, we can say that the contemporary version of self-injury entails aspects of *healing* (ironically, via hurting the body), *spirituality* (or at least an alteration of consciousness), and the *promotion of the social order* (by provoking a response in the social network). Thus the self-injury of today may not be so far removed from the culturally endorsed body modifications of the past.

Feminist writers have advanced other explanations for self-injury. Shaw (2002) has provided an excellent summary of feminist formulations of self-injurious behavior. She emphasizes the link between self-injury and the cultural standards of "feminine beauty" that are imposed on, and used to exploit, women. Shaw writes:

> Women voluntarily undergo culturally sanctioned procedures which are painful and physically destructive for the sake of Western beauty ideals. Such behavior is not interpreted as pathological or deviant. Women pluck, cinch, inject toxic substances, and have cellulite vacuumed out of their thighs. As Dworkin asserts, "not one part of a woman's body is left untouched, unaltered. No feature or extremity is spared the art, or pain of improvement" (1974, p. 113). "Pain is an essential part of the grooming process . . . no price is too great, no process too repulsive, no operation too painful for the woman who would be beautiful" (Dworkin, 1974, p. 115). (Shaw, 2002, p. 32)

Through the feminist lens, self-injury can even be viewed as an act of empowerment and body reclamation. Shaw states:

> Self-injury is uniquely distressing because it reflects back to the culture what has been done to girls and women. Whether or not it is a conscious process, by refusing to remain silent, by literally carving, cutting, and burning their experiences of violation and silencing in their arms and legs, girls and women claim ownership of their bodies and their subjectivity. They refuse to relinquish what they experience as true. This is a radical and threatening act because part of what holds patriarchy in place is girls' and women's silence. (2002, p. 35)

One problem with feminist formulations such as Shaw's, however, is that they provide little in the way of explanation regarding *male* self-injury. Given that self-injury is increasing for both genders (and in community samples is equally distributed), a feminist articulation explicates only about half the problem. Interestingly, the perspective of Fakir Musafar closely matches the feminist view, despite the gender difference. Musafar is an originator (perhaps *the* originator) of the "modern primitive movement" of body modification. He has pierced, tattooed, corseted, suspended, cinched, and winched virtually every part of his body. He is featured in the publication *Modern Primitives* (Vale & Juno, 1989), which influenced the popularity of piercing and tattoos that emerged in the late 1980s and continues to this day. Musafar reports that these various forms of body modification and stimulation produce not pain and torture, but "a state of grace" in him and others (Musafar, cited in Favazza, 1996, p. 325). Musafar writes about his and his colleagues' commitment to body modification:

> We had rejected the Western cultural biases about ownership and use of the body. We believed our body belonged to us. We had rejected the strong Judeo-Christian body programming and emotional conditioning to which we had all been subjected. Our bodies did not belong to . . . a father, mother, or spouse; or to the state or its monarch, ruler, or dictator; or to social institutions of the military, educational, correctional, or medical establishment. And the kind of language used to describe our behavior ("self-mutilation"), was in itself a negative and prejudicial form of control. (Cited in Favazza, 1996, p. 326)

Although I find the feminist and "Musafarian" formulations regarding self-injury to be intriguing and insightful, my own view comes from a more "experience-near" psychotherapeutic perspective.

Speculations on Reasons for the Increased Prevalence of Self-Injury

As a clinician, I am not so much concerned with broad cultural influences (over which I have little influence) as with the day-to-day forces directly affecting my clients' lives. I believe that many factors play a role in their decisions to self-injure. These elements fall into four broad categories: (1) environmental influences, (2) direct media influences, (3) peer group dimensions, and (4) internal psychological elements. This list is particularly pertinent to adolescents and young adults, for whom self-injury appears to be growing most rapidly. *I would like to emphasize that this list is no more than a set of speculations or hypotheses.*

Environmental Influences
- School and work environments are fraught with high stress.
- Multitasking lifestyles are conducive to persistent low-level stress and anxiety.

- Heavy emphasis on competition in schools and the workplace is conducive to isolation and distrust.
- The mass media heavily market a reliance on over-the-counter and prescription medications to alter mood, achieve desired feeling states, induce sleep, and so forth. The media infrequently pay attention to emotion regulation and self-soothing skills and activities.
- Modification of consciousness is viewed as something that can be achieved quickly and affordably via use of alcohol or street drugs.
- Many adolescents and adults believe that celebration requires intoxication.
- Families, schools, and peers rarely teach healthy self-soothing skills.
- The culture emphasizes acquisition of material goods over quality of life.
- With both parents working, children are left alone for substantial portions of each day. When parents are home, they are often exhausted and psychologically unavailable. Children are left with little soothing time with either parent.
- The divorce rate of 50% stresses not only children, but single parents, day care personnel, teachers, and many others.
- There is an overall diminished sense of community and social supports to assist those in distress.
- The prevailing culture overemphasizes physical appearance and sets impossible standards of beauty for its youth (in terms of weight, breast size, muscular configuration, etc.). That which is unattainable can easily become a negative self-attribution.

Direct Media Influences
- Many popular television shows and movies portray and sensationalize self-injury (e.g., *Girl Interrupted; Thirteen; Intervention*).
- Music videos frequently portray and glorify self-injurious acts.
- People prominent in the media have publicly discussed self-injuring (e.g., Angelina Jolie, the late Princess Diana, Johnny Depp, Shirley Manson, Christina Ricci) (Whitlock, Purington, & Gershkovich, 2009).
- Most television talk shows have featured self-injury as a topic.
- Many Internet chat rooms are dedicated to the topic of self-injury.
- Many websites focus on self-injury; all too many of these provide examples of poetry, artwork, and even photographs describing or depicting self-injury acts, wounds, or scars.
- A search for the term "self-injury" on YouTube instantly provides videos of individuals actually self-injuring (see Lewis, Heath, St. Denis, & Noble, 2011, for a detailed discussion).

Adolescent Peer Group Dimensions

- Adolescents routinely experience powerful emotions and lack the coping skills to manage them.
- Adolescent peer groups view extensive substance use as a normative rite of passage.
- Substance use often begins at early ages, in middle and even grammar school.
- Substance use forestalls normative problem solving and the development of healthy self-soothing skills.
- Adolescents place high value on being viewed as "outrageous outsiders" by peers and adults.
- Peer group cohesion is enhanced by behaviors that adults condemn or fear.
- Youth are action-oriented; self-injury is dramatic, is often highly visible, and produces immediate results.
- Adolescents are desensitized to self-injury because of the peer group's endorsement of body piercings, tattoos, brandings, and scarifications.
- Self-injury is viewed as "not much different" from these popular forms of body art or modification.

Internal Psychological Elements

- Self-injury works; it (temporarily) reduces tension and restores a sense of psychological equilibrium.
- Self-injury has powerful communication aspects.
- Self-injury provides a sense of control and empowerment.

There are, of course, many more internal psychological factors than those listed above. These additional factors are discussed at length in Parts II and III of this book. Let us now turn to the topic of when body modification should be considered self-injurious.

CONCLUSION

The major points covered in this chapter are as follows:

- Self-injury has been reported in clinical populations for decades, in such settings as inpatient units, residential schools, group homes, and correctional facilities.
- Since the 1990s, self-injury has been reported at high rates in the

general population in the United States and many other developed countries. Numerous studies have found high rates of self-injury (e.g., 6–25%) in samples of middle school, high school, and college students.

- Speculations as to why self-injury is markedly increasing in youth in the general population include such factors as environments of high stress and competion, underdeveloped emotion regulation skills, parental unavailability, and peer social contagion influences.

- The spread of self-injury may also be related to provocative content on the Internet regarding self-injury (on websites, message boards, chat rooms, YouTube, etc.).

CHAPTER 5

Body Piercings, Tattoos, Brandings, Scarifications, and Other Forms of Body Modification

Since the late 1980s, a remarkable cultural phenomenon has emerged internationally: the increased popularity of body piercings, professional tattoos, scarifications, brandings, and other forms of body modification. Clinicians often ask whether these forms of "body art," as they are sometimes called, should be considered self-injurious. There is no simple answer to this question.

One way to address the issue is to refer to the definition of self-injury provided in Chapter 1. Body piercings, professional tattoos, scarifications, and brandings may, at first glance, seem to meet some of the elements of this definition. Tattoos and piercings, for example, are acquired intentionally and are self-effected, in that they are deliberately obtained by going to a professional. These forms of body modification are also very low in lethality if typical sterile procedures are employed.

Whether tattoos, body piercings, and other body modifications meet the definition of self-injury becomes a more complex determination for the remainder of the definition. Should tattoos and piercings be considered a form of "bodily harm" (and therefore self-injury)? This judgment is in the eye of the beholder. Most people who select and acquire professional tattoos consider them to be attractive and to improve their appearance greatly. Certainly, many professional tattoo artists are very skilled and produce exceptional body art. As for body piercings, it seems unlikely that these should be considered disfiguring, in that the large majority of the perforations created for body jewelry fully heal and fill in if left unadorned over time. Brandings and patterned scarifications are another matter, in that the designs are permanent. However, those who obtain them often do so because they wish to proclaim affiliation to some group (e.g., football players to a team or fraternity, or gang members to a gang). In these latter cases, the body modification is symbolically meaningful and endorsed by an influential social group.

SOCIAL CONTEXT AND BODY MODIFICATION

In the international culture of the early 21st century, tattoos and piercings (and, to a lesser extent, brandings and scarifications) have widespread acceptance in diverse social contexts. In the late 1980s, when I showed slides of elaborate tattoos and body piercings to professional audiences and asked whether they considered them to be examples of self-injury, 80–90% said yes. In the decade 2000–2010, when I showed similar audiences the very same slides, the yes response dropped to 5–10%. Clearly, there has been a major shift toward the acceptance of body modification as normative, or even socially desirable, behavior; therefore, it seems inappropriate to consider such body modification to be self-injurious, because of the social endorsement. Body art is distinguishable from self-harming behavior in many instances because the tissue damage is viewed as either symbolically meaningful or beauty-enhancing, or both.

INTENT AND BODY MODIFICATION

Very few individuals would state that they acquire tattoos or piercings to reduce psychological distress. Some talk of an "addiction to ink" or piercings, but they seem to be speaking figuratively rather than literally. Therefore, if the behaviors are not pursued to manage psychological distress or crisis, then it would appear that body modification can clearly be distinguished from self-injury. And that would appear to be the end of the story.

Of course, it turns out to be not quite that simple. There is also the matter of *self-inflicted* tattoos, piercings, scars, and brands. These almost always lack the aesthetic accomplishment of the professional versions. Moreover, in some cases, the self-infliction is linked to distress management. Two examples from clinical practice make the point.

Naomi was a 16-year-old living in a group home. She was referred due to recurrent suicide attempts via overdose and multiple episodes of self-injury (wrist, arm, and leg cutting). In addition, on one occasion, Naomi had mutilated her genitals. In the group home Naomi was working hard to learn dialectical behavior therapy (DBT) skills to deal with her depression and rage (see Chapters 17 and 18). She was especially motivated to earn weekend passes to visit her friends and her mother. One of the conditions for these passes was that she be free of self-harm incidents during the previous week.

During one time period, Naomi seemed especially agitated and restless. The staff learned from Naomi's roommate that she might have pierced her body. Subsequently, a staff nurse discovered that Naomi had used a sewing needle to pierce one of her nipples. On examination, the wound appeared to be in the early stages of infection. Naomi argued that there should be no consequences for the self-inflicted piercing, because "everyone is doing it these days." The staff denied Naomi's request for a weekend pass, saying that professional piercings acquired under sterile conditions are different from self-inflicted piercings under nonsterile conditions. Staff members continued to work with Naomi regarding alternative ways to deal with agitation and restlessness.

In Naomi's case, the staff correctly viewed the behavior to be self-injury rather than body modification. Naomi's piercing was clearly related to psychological distress and was also unsafe medically. Naomi was astute enough to try to exploit the current climate of acceptance regarding body modification, but the staff did not accept her line of reasoning because of the details of her piercing behavior.

Ian, an 18-year-old living with his parents, stated that his goal in life was to become the most famous tattoo artist of all time. He said he intended to top the great names of Don Ed Hardy, Lyle Tuttle, and Hanky Panky. No one in Ian's family had a problem with his goal, but they had serious reservations about his plan to achieve it. Ian said he was "an innately gifted artist" and was quite capable of being "self-taught" as a tattooist. He was adamant that he needed no training in the technical art of tattooing, claiming that he could learn everything he needed on the Internet or in books. Trouble was, Ian started out on his own body, using third-hand equipment, and the results weren't promising. Ian discovered that what looked great on paper turned out differently on skin. He became enraged and depressed at the unsightly mess he had made of his arms.

Despairing that he had failed at his life's goal, Ian agreed grudgingly to see a family therapist with his parents. In treatment, no one challenged Ian's overall plan—even though it involved dropping out of junior college. Through a process of negotiation, the family worked with Ian to find a way to move him closer to his goal. Eventually, Ian agreed to become an apprentice at a well-known tattoo shop. Once he started work, Ian was relieved to learn that the owner could cover the mistakes on his arms with attractive professional tattoos.

In Ian's case, the problem wasn't so much psychological distress as poor planning and impulsivity. Some family ingenuity turned behavior that resembled self-injury into a vocational plan with some promise.

BODY MODIFICATION AND MENTAL HEALTH STATUS

Favazza (1998) has suggested that heavily pierced and tattooed individuals may have more psychopathology than members of the general public may. Not many data are available to support or disconfirm this hypothesis, but one study suggests that tattoos may have both advantages *and* disadvantages. Drews, Allison, and Probst (2000) studied differences between tattooed and nontattooed college students. In a sample of 235 they found that the tattooed students rated themselves as more adventurous, creative, and artistic than the nontattooed students rated themselves. The students with tattoos also viewed themselves as more likely to take risks.

Drews et al. (2000) also analyzed their results by gender. They found that the tattooed males viewed themselves as more attractive and reported having more sexual partners. These males also had higher rates of having been arrested and were more likely to have body piercings. The tattooed women in this sample were more likely to report using drugs other than alcohol, to have shoplifted, and to have piercings in body areas other than their ears.

What can we conclude from these results? Perhaps only that the students in this sample had a combination of strengths and weaknesses associated with tattooed status. The tattooed youth viewed themselves as being creative, free-spirited, attractive, and sexually engaged. These would appear to be strengths. However, they were also more likely to engage in illegal activity and risk-taking behaviors than their nontattooed peers. These would appear to be deficits.

DETERMINING WHEN BODY MODIFICATION IS SELF-DESTRUCTIVE

Although discussing people who are pierced and tattooed is an interesting diversion, there are also practical clinical issues that need to be addressed in a book on self-injury. One way to assess whether or not body modification is in the service of self-destructive motivations is to refer to the classification scheme regarding direct and indirect self-harm. A checklist for assessing direct and indirect self-harm is provided in Chapter 3 (see Figure 3.2). The clinician can employ this checklist (informally, at least) when speaking with a client who has extensive tattoos, piercings, or other forms of body modification. A useful rule of thumb is this: If an individual presents with multiple forms of direct and indirect self-harm, then the clinician should be alert for self-destructive motivations associated with the body modification. Otherwise, the client may just be participating in the cultural phenomenon of body art and enjoying it as a form of self-expression. In the latter instance, it would be a mistake to pathologize the behavior. Two examples from clinical encounters bring home the distinction between dysfunctional versus normative body modification.

Eugena was a 15-year-old teen brought into treatment by her parents because of her self-injury. For about 6 months, she had been cutting her forearms and legs with a razor blade. Eugena reported hurting herself when she fought with peers at school or when she broke up with a boyfriend. She conceded that her relationships tended to be stormy and short-lived. Asked about other forms of self-harm, Eugena acknowledged smoking pot almost daily and taking physical risks with some frequency. She denied suicide ideation or attempts.

The therapist noticed that Eugena had many pierced earrings in the outer cartilage of both ears. Asked about these, Eugena said that she had acquired some of these professionally but had done others herself. She admitted that sometimes she pierced an ear as a variation to cutting. The precipitants were strong, unpleasant feelings, and the results were emotional relief. The therapist concluded that Eugena occasionally used ear piercing as a self-injurious behavior. He decided to monitor both cutting and body piercing in his treatment with Eugena.

In the case of Eugena, the body modification was deemed to be a variant of the cutting behavior. In the case that follows, the conclusion was different.

For more conventional people, the first encounter with Buzz tended to produce shock. Buzz was a 30-year-old with tribal tattoos swirling about his face. He also sported a 3-inch bone-like protuberance through the cartilage at the base of his nostrils, as well as symmetrical piercings on his eyebrows, cheeks, and forehead. Although Buzz felt no need for psychological treatment, he would talk at length with anyone who was interested in his unusual appearance. Buzz was a professional tattoo artist and body piercer. He recognized that his extensive facial tattoos and piercings precluded him from interacting with a more conservative mainstream society. This was fine with Buzz. He spent the majority of his time working in his shop, having a beer in biker bars, or socializing with similarly body-modified peers. Buzz was quite comfortable within his niche in society. He had friends, a stable job, and little or no behavior that could be considered self-destructive.

THE EXTREME END OF THE CONTINUUM

What are we to make of individuals with *really* extensive tattoos and body piercings? As professionals, how should we view individuals who have scores of piercings on their faces, bodies, or genitals? What about those with multiple subcutaneous decorations, brandings, scarifications, and full-body tattoos? Some individuals suspend heavy objects from their nipples or genitals in order to induce intense body sensations. Others have multiple penile or labial piercings decorated with jewelry that they employ for extra stimulation during sexual contact.

My own opinion is that these individuals are quirky adventurers on the frontiers of body art and modification, and that there is much we can learn from them. Persons who push their bodies to their limits may have insights into the age-old mind–body dilemma that others cannot fathom. The mainstream is often informed and influenced by the extreme. Those who test the limits of body modification rarely end up in psychological treatment. They do not view the consultation room as a relevant resource, and therefore are neither a concern nor a challenge for psychotherapists.

CONCLUSION

Body modification, by and large, is different from self-injury. Key points discussed in this chapter include the following:

- Some body modifications, such as professionally obtained tattoos and piercings, are currently popular in the United States. They should not be unnecessarily pathologized or treated as forms of self-injury.
- Self-injury is usually performed by an individual, whereas body modifications such as tattoos and piercings are usually obtained from a trained professional.
- Self-injury is generally about emotion regulation and stress reduction; body modification is about self-expression and body enhancement.
- Some behavior may be ambiguous as to whether it is self-injury or body modification. Key questions in determining whether such behavior is self-injurious include these: Is the person emotionally dysregulated at the time? Does he or she have a history of self-harm, including self-injury? Did he or she use sterile procedures? Is he or she employing appropriate aftercare to wounds?
- Carefull attention to detail will clarify whether the behavior is culturally endorsed or self-destructive in nature.

CHAPTER 6

A Biopsychosocial Model for Self-Injury

Self-injury is conceptualized in this book as a biopsychosocial phenomenon. Based on this framework, the recommended approach to assessment and treatment is a bio-cognitive-behavioral one. The simple, streamlined model presented in this chapter is designed to be user-friendly and leads directly to the recommended assessment and treatment techniques discussed in subsequent chapters. A much more complex, comprehensive theoretical explanation of self-injury is Linehan's (1993a) biosocial model, which has been updated and applied exclusively to self-injury by Brown (2002). Nock (2009a, 2009b, 2010) has proposed a different complex formulation, which I also highly recommend.

Self-injury as a biopsychosocial phenomenon includes five interrelated dimensions:

1. Environmental
2. Biological
3. Cognitive
4. Affective
5. Behavioral

The etiology of the behavior can be understood by attending to the interrelationships among these five dimensions. For the large majority of individuals, all five dimensions play a role in the emergence and recurrence of self-injury. The mix of dimensions is unique for each individual. For some clients, environmental and biological dimensions may be most important; for others, cognitive, affective, and behavioral dimensions may predominate. The task of assessment is to identify which are most important and to prioritize these in the course of treatment—although all relevant dimensions need to be addressed eventually.

The five dimensions in the biopsychosocial model of self-injury are discussed in the sections that follow.

ENVIRONMENTAL DIMENSION

The environmental dimension contributing to the occurrence of self-injury includes three basic categories: family historical elements, client historical elements, and current environmental elements. These elements, as contextual or environmental, are in some sense "outside" the individual, but nonetheless have a salient impact on the individual and his or her pattern of self-injury.

Family Historical Elements

The term "family historical elements" refers to key aspects of the history of the nuclear, extended, or surrogate family that have been observed but not directly experienced. (Although relationships beyond the family can have a major influence on children, they tend to be less important than daily living environments.) For example, observing violence or substance abuse in the family is different from being assaulted or ingesting substances oneself. The former may have a powerful *indirect* impact; the latter, a profound *direct* impact. Many aspects of family history have been linked in empirical research to the emergence of self-injury later in life. These include such variables as mental illness, substance abuse, violence, suicide, and self-injury in the family (e.g., Walsh & Rosen, 1988; Shapiro & Dominiak, 1992; Favazza, 1996, 1998). Nock (2009b) has also identified family hostility as a distal risk factor for self-injury.

On a daily basis, family environments teach children behaviors via modeling, reinforcement, punishment, and extinction. For example, when family members tend to express emotions explosively, a child may learn to be explosive (or markedly inhibited). When family members deal with distress by using substances heavily, the child may acquire a pattern for this behavior and implement it at a later time. Clinicians are all too familiar with the latency-age child who swears he or she will never use alcohol or drugs, due to observing the effects of a parent's addiction. Then years later, as if on automatic pilot, the now-adolescent child begins abusing substances, unmindful of his or her previous convictions.

A particularly ominous pattern in family environments is self-destructive behavior. When parents or other family members model self-destructive behavior, such as suicide attempts or self-injury, these acts tend to have significant repercussions for children. Observing this behavior can have many connotations for a child. Witnessing self-destructive behavior in family members can convey such messages as these:

> "Life is overwhelmingly painful."
> "Life is not worth living."
> "Distress can be relieved by behaving self-destructively."
> "Others cannot help my pain."
> "My pain negates responsibilities I have to others."

These are only a few of the possible interpretations that children may attach to seeing family members behave self-destructively. Although such behavior in the family must be understood and responded to with compassion, the long-term effects on children cannot be ignored. Children living with family members who behave self-destructively learn to consider self-harm as an option when life becomes challenging. Completed suicides are the most damaging of self-harm acts; their long-term profoundly negative effects on family and significant others are well documented (AAS, 2011). These effects include depression, despair, isolation, substance abuse, and the repetition of self-destructive behaviors across generations.

Client Historical Elements

"Client historical elements" include those elements in the individual's personal history that have been *directly* experienced, as opposed to observed. Those found to be associated empirically with self-injury include the death of a parent or other caregiver; parental loss through separation, divorce, or placement outside the home; and experiences of neglect and/or emotional, physical, and sexual abuse (Walsh & Rosen, 1988; Shapiro & Dominiak, 1992; Miller, 1994; van der Kolk et al., 1996; Alderman, 1997; Favazza, 1998; Briere & Gil, 1998; Turell & Armsworth, 2000; Rodriguez-Srednicki, 2001; Gratz, Conrad, & Roemer, 2002; Paul et al., 2002). Nock (2009b) has also identified recurrent parental criticism as a distal risk factor for self-injury.

Work by Gratz et al. (2002) has provided some new insights into family experiences associated with self-injury. In a racially diverse nonclinical sample of 133 college students, a remarkable 38% of the sample reported a history of direct self-harm (self-injury). Also striking was that the lifetime self-reported prevalence of self-injury was slightly greater for males than for females—a very rare finding, indeed: 36% of the women and 41% of the males reported having self-injured.

Gratz et al. (2002) hypothesized that self-injury would be associated with a number of aversive family experiences, including neglect, physical abuse, sexual abuse, separation, loss, and related attachment problems. They also predicted that these negative family experiences would be linked to dissociation experiences, which in turn would be predictive of self-injury. They found significant gender differences regarding family experiences. The predictors of self-injury for the *women* in the sample were, in order of importance, dissociation, insecure paternal attachment, childhood sexual abuse, maternal emotional neglect, and paternal emotional neglect (for which there was a significant inverse relationship). In contrast, for the *men* in the sample, the predictors of self-injury, in order of importance, were childhood separation (especially from father), dissociation, and physical abuse. Thus the findings suggested that a number of aversive experiences from childhood should be considered in the assessment of self-injury, including neglect, physical abuse, sexual abuse, separation, and loss. Also, the possibility of gender differences should be given serious consideration.

Invalidating Environments within the Family

Linehan (1993a) and Miller, Rathus, and Linehan (2007) have discussed somewhat subtler family antecedents to histories of self-injury (and other problems). They have described the "invalidating environment" in the family experiences of individuals diagnosed with BPD. They contend that in many of these families, the affective experiences of children are often ignored, denied, ridiculed, or condemned (i.e., "invalidated"). Such experiences often result in children's questioning the accuracy, and even the very existence, of their own internal feeling states. Moreover, such environments may differentially reinforce only the most extreme of affective responses. For example, if a child indicates in a subtle manner that he or she is distressed, the invalidating environment may ignore the communication. Only when the child presents with an extreme emotional behavior (e.g., a tantrum) does he or she receive a response. The entire pattern is conducive to reinforcing maladaptive behavior while extinguishing adaptive behavior. When such a pattern is repeated countless times for many years, the eventual result can be an emotionally dysregulated person. Such people may come to rely on self-invalidating behaviors such as self-injury to manage emotional distress (Linehan, 1993a; Miller et al., 2007).

Family and Environmental Strengths and Assets

Often missing in the discussion of the families of self-injurious individuals is an examination of their strengths. Even the most dysfunctional family has strengths that should be identified and reinforced. In many cases, the families of the "new generation" of self-injuring youth (see Chapter 4) have considerable assets. The fact that a person self-injures does not mean that he or she comes from a family with marked dysfunction. Unlike the families often described in the empirical research, families of self-injuring persons can often be validating, non-neglectful, and nonabusive. Stated more positively, the families of self-injurers are often loving, committed, compassionate, and skillful at problem solving. A clinician should not assume dysfunction; rather, the clinician should conduct a careful strength-based analysis of each family. The areas to be assessed should include strengths within the following:

- The home and extended family
- The neighborhood and related networks
- School and employment sectors
- Financial resources and management
- Cultural identity and resources
- Recreational activities and hobbies
- Religious and spiritual beliefs and institutional supports

The strengths within a family serve to mitigate the risk of self-injury. The more strengths that can be brought to bear within the family, the greater the positive impact on reducing self-destructive behavior. The family may often be a source of distress for a self-injuring member, but it can also provide the solutions to problems if all its members are respected and engaged as therapeutic allies.

Current Environmental Elements

"Current environmental elements" are circumstances in the present that tend to trigger self-injury. Many environmental conditions can precipitate self-injurious behavior. Common examples include experiencing loss or conflict in relationships, being abused by a present caregiver or partner, or being exposed to peers who self-injure. Performance problems in the functional areas of school, work, and athletics or other extracurricular activities can also be key elements. Persons who have experienced aversive conditions in the family and personal historical elements are especially sensitive to similar problems in the present. For example, an individual who has experienced loss of a parent during childhood may be especially reactive to losses in peer relationships during adolescence. In a similar vein, those who have been physically abused or sexually assaulted as children may be exquisitely sensitive to threats of abuse or assault in the present. They may also be reactive to even normative forms of sexual approach from others. Not surprisingly, poly-self-destructive individuals often come from histories of poly-abuse. The more complicated and aversive the individual's historical context, the more vulnerable he or she is likely to be in the present to negative experiences.

BIOLOGICAL DIMENSION

The understanding of self-injurious behavior from a biological perspective has changed with the increasing advances in brain imaging studies. For many years, clinicians accepted a distinction between so-called "organic" and "functional" disorders. It is clear today that such a distinction arose from the limits of assessment technology in a given era. For instance, in the days of Emil Kraepelin, some psychiatric disorders, such as general paresis (tertiary syphilis), were associated with changes in brain structure that were visible with the microscopy of the time. Those examining brain tissues from patients who died of schizophrenia or manic–depressive disease could find no differences from the appearance of the brains of healthy comparison subjects. So the "organic" versus "functional" distinction arose and lasted for most of the 20th century.

In the last 25 years, with the rapidly increasing pace of discovery in the brain sciences, these distinctions have become obsolete. Demonstration of altered brain structure or function in living subjects, as well as in postmortem brains through brain imaging or metabolic studies, suddenly removed some disorders previously judged "functional" (such as OCD or autism) from that category. OCD has, in fact, provided one of the most provocative findings: In preliminary studies, interventions were found to "move" brain imaging abnormalities in the direction of patterns seen in control subjects. Most strikingly, these changes with treatment were seen with both pharmacological and cognitive-behavioral interventions.

In retrospect, the old functional–organic distinction was faulty in principle, not just in the light of today's neuroimaging. All behavior arises in the brain. The old distinctions differentiated not disorders that were fundamentally different, but only those in which we could measure a difference in the brain from those in which we could not.

The complex relationships between biology and self-injury constitute an important and emerging focus of empirical research. A number of psychiatric diagnoses associated with self-injury have been shown to have biochemical components, including BPD, depression, bipolar illness, and schizophrenia. Many extreme forms of self-injury have often been found to be associated with schizophrenia and other psychoses (Simeon & Hollander, 2001; Grossman, 2001; Large, Babidge, Andrews, Storey, & Nielssen, 2008). Other physiological problems commonly associated with self-injury include physical illness (e.g., diabetes, asthma, orthopedic disease), sleep disorders, eating disorders, and a tendency to somaticize distress.

A thorough discussion of the biological dimensions of self-injury is beyond my expertise. However, two recent and comprehensive reviews are available (Osuch & Payne, 2009; Sher & Stanley, 2009). In addition, reviews of the psychopharmacology of self-injury are provided by Gordon Harper (Chapter 14, this volume), by Plener, Libal and Nixon (2009), and by Sandman (2009). In the sections that follow, I briefly describe three of the major hypotheses that have been proposed about the biology of self-injury.

Serotonin-Level Dysfunction

One area of research that appears promising in understanding the biology of self-injury concerns serotonin levels in the brain. A number of empirical studies have linked diminished serotonin levels with impulsive aggression and self-injury. See Osuch and Payne (2009) and Sher and Stanley (2009) for reviews of the research. Diverse reports have measured serotonin levels in self-destructive people and found these lower levels to be lower than average. Researchers have concluded that such levels may facilitate self-injury. The use of selective serotonin reuptake inhibitors (SSRIs; e.g., Prozac, Zoloft, Paxil, Celexa) is designed to assist the body in using existing serotonin levels (however diminished) most efficiently (*medinfo.co.uk/drugs/ssris.html*). Some indirect support regarding the possible role of serotonin in self-injury has been obtained via the reduction of depression, impulsivity, and self-injury in some individuals using SSRIs (Grossman & Siever, 2001).

Endogenous Opioid System Dysfunction

Another biological explanation for self-injury concerns the endogenous opioid system (EOS) (Osuch & Payne, 2009; Sher & Stanley, 2009). Many clients who self-injure report an absence of pain at the time of the act (Favazza, 1996, 1998; Alderman, 1997; Conterio & Lader, 1998). As noted by Grossman and Siever (2001), "Abundant evidence indicates EOS involvement in pain perception, particularly in stress-induced analgesia" (p. 125). A number of researchers have hypothesized that enhanced EOS activity may support self-injury. Stated in laypersons' terms, when an individual harms his or her body, the brain may release naturally occurring opiate-like chemicals (e.g., endorphins) that are experienced as pleasurable and/or as a relief from emotional distress.

As noted by Grossman and Siever (2001), there are two main hypotheses regarding the relationship between the EOS and self-injury: the "addiction hypothesis" and the "pain hypothesis."

The addiction hypothesis suggests that there exists essentially a normal EOS that has been chronically overstimulated by frequent SIB [self-injurious behavior] for the purpose of relieving dysphoria. The individual develops a tolerance for the outpouring of endogenous opioids, cyclically suffers a withdrawal reaction, and is driven to further EOS stimulation by means of impulsive SIB. (p. 125)

The pain hypothesis suggests a constitutional abnormality in the EOS that is unmasked by the environment such that pain sensitivity is diminished. This may involve a lack of negative feedback in the EOS and/or overproduction of endogenous opioids. This heightened opiatergic tone could eventually lead to dysphoric experiences of numbness and dissociation. SIB may present a stimulus that breaks through a self-alienating dissociative state, brought on by a environmental and/or intrapsychic stressors, and thereby allows the self-injurer to feel again. (p. 125)

Some support for the addiction hypothesis is provided indirectly by reported success in a few case reports in treating self-injury with naltrexone, a medication originally developed to block opiate "highs" in substance-abusing individuals (see Plener et al., 2009). The use of naltrexone for self-injuring clients is intended to block the positive sensations associated with endogenous opioid release. The hypothesis is that blocking the EOS response may eliminate the biochemical "payoff" of self-injury for the more "addicted" individuals. We might also speculate that when naltrexone fails to work, the pain hypothesis might be the more accurate explanation for those individuals.

Diminished Pain Sensitivity

There is also empirical evidence that some self-injuring individuals have diminished responsiveness to physical pain (Osuch & Payne, 2009; Sher & Stanley, 2009). Bohus, Limberger, et al. (2000) have reported that about 60% of those who self-injure report no pain at the time of the act. Russ and colleagues (Russ et al., 1992; Russ, Roth, Kakuma, Harrison, & Hull, 1994) have conducted experiments comparing physical pain tolerance in self-injuring persons who report an absence of pain during the act, self-injuring persons who report experiencing pain, and non-self-injuring controls. In experiments that deliberately induced closely measured physical pain, Russ and colleagues reported a significantly diminished experience of physical discomfort for the "no-pain" self-injuring participants.

Bohus, Limberger, et al. (2000) have also found diminished pain sensation in self-injuring persons with BPD. They compared a sample of 12 self-injuring females with BPD who reported analgesia during self-injury with

19 "healthy controls." They administered both the cold pressor test and the tourniquet pain test in order to measure perception of physical pain in the study participants. Participants were tested both when they were feeling calm and when they were markedly distressed. In order to control for possible effects of psychotropic medication on pain sensitivity, none of the participants were receiving pharmacotherapy. Bohus, Limberger, et al. (2000) reported:

> Even during self-reported calmness, patients with BPD showed a significantly reduced perception of pain compared to healthy control subjects in both tests. During distress, pain perception in BPD patients was further significantly reduced as compared with self-reported calmness. The present findings show that self-mutilating patients with BPD who experience analgesia during self-injury show an increased threshold for pain even in the absence of distress. (p. 251)

The Russ et al. and Bohus et al. studies are especially intriguing, in that they move beyond psychological hypothesizing about dissociation or pain tolerance to physiological experiments. Clearly, there is an emerging body of evidence regarding the biological underpinnings of self-injury. This conclusion points to pharmacotherapy as a promising tool in the treatment of self-injury. (This topic is addressed in Chapter 14.) However, as noted by Grossman and Siever (2001), pharmacotherapy is unlikely to be a sufficient treatment in and of itself. Complementary psychological interventions are usually required as well. They state:

> Histories of sexual abuse and other traumatic/chaotic experiences often populate these patients' formative years. The lack of appropriate interpersonal experiences and the attendant conflicts in the areas of trust, self-esteem, mood regulation, and self-soothing cannot be resolved with medication. Rather, appropriate pharmacologic treatment can lessen the intensity of certain experiences and create a more favorable setting for psychotherapy and long-term characterologic/behavioral changes. (p. 128)

These words are an appropriate segue to discussing the cognitive, affective, and behavioral dimensions of self-injury.

COGNITIVE DIMENSION

The cognitive dimension associated with self-injury falls into two basic categories: *cognitive interpretations of environmental events* and *self-generated cognitions*. Environmental events are problematic only if a self-injuring person interprets them to be aversive, painful, or disorganizing. Of course, some environmental circumstances are so overwhelming as to have very compelling cognitive implications. It is a very rare individual who can be on the receiving end of physical or sexual abuse and not end up with problematic, self-defeating thoughts. I did encounter one such individual, who had been sexually assaulted as a prisoner of war during the Desert Storm war in 1991. She dismissed the groping behavior she had received as insignificant, because "the death and destruction around me were so much worse." She stated that the assault had no untoward repercussions for her thereafter. However, most individuals who are sexually abused develop complicated thoughts and judgments regarding their experiences. Very common are irrational self-blaming thoughts, such as "I should have done something to stop the abuse," or "I must have wanted it to happen for it to go on so long." Assisting clients to give up such irrational self-blaming cognitions is often at the heart of treatment for self-injuring survivors of trauma.

Other dysfunctional thoughts may be derived from less powerful environmental conditions, and thus may be more within the immediate power of the individual to challenge and modify. Examples include such thoughts as "I must get an A on every paper and test," or "I have to get along with all my friends all the time, or I'll be totally alone." These are cognitions that can cause individuals untoward pain and discomfort because of their unattainable perfectionism.

Self-generated cognitions are triggered by internal cues, as opposed to external events and circumstances. On awakening, a client might start the day with this thought: "Another grim, empty day. How will I get through it?" These are cognitions for which there may have been no conceivable environmental triggers. The day has just begun; there has been no time for aversive environmental events. Some self-injuring individuals carry with them an extensive roster of thoughts and judgments that predict nothing but discomfort and pain. Assessment of these recurrent negative, pessimistic cognitions is fundamental to moving forward psychotherapeutically; they need to be identified and modified if the client is to experience more success and less anguish.

In addition, self-injuring persons generate a wide range of cognitions that trigger their acts of self-harm. Identifying these thoughts is another key step in assessment. Typical thoughts that precede self-injury include "I have to do something," or "I deserve this," or "I hate my body so much," or "This will show people that I'm really hurting," or "This is the *only* way to deal with this problem." Supplanting such thoughts with ideas regarding alternative courses of action is fundamental to moving away from lives of self-harm.

The cognitive dimension related to self-injury is discussed in much greater detail in Chapters 9 and 12.

AFFECTIVE DIMENSION

Closely linked to the cognitive dimension is the affective dimension. Emotions emerge from the irrational, self-blaming, distorted cognitions that precede them. Emotions are often centrally important in assessing and treating self-injury. Most individuals self-injure in order to reduce or eliminate affective distress. As noted in Chapter 1, self-injuring persons identify a wide range of emotions as preceding their acts of self-harm, including anger, anxiety, tension, sadness, depression, shame, worry, and contempt (Favazza, 1987; Walsh & Rosen, 1988; Alderman, 1997; Conterio & Lader, 1998; Brown, 1998; Simeon & Hollander, 2001; Klonsky, 2007, 2009; Nock, 2010). I have yet to encounter a self-injuring individual who identified a positive emotion as triggering self-harm. No one is likely to say, "I cut [or burned, etc.] myself because I was feeling too relaxed and happy." Self-injury is about negative emotion.

Assessment needs to identify, very specifically, the most important and recurrent affective triggers for each individual. In turn, treatment needs to teach skills to endure, manage, and reduce powerful affects without resorting to self-harm.

BEHAVIORAL DIMENSION

The behavioral dimension consists of overt actions that immediately precede, accompany, and follow acts of self-injury. These are the behaviors that are strongly and recurrently associated with the acts of self-harm. Typical behavioral antecedents include conflicts with family or peers, isolation, failure at an activity, sexual behavior, substance abuse, or eating-disordered behavior. The behavioral dimension also includes actions that prepare for self-injury, such as choosing the physical location, securing it to prevent interruption, and selecting a tool. Other behavioral components include actions that immediately follow self-injury, such as deciding whether or not to provide self-care, disposing of or hiding tools, and communicating with others. The aftermath of self-injury is very important to assess. Some individuals report falling asleep immediately after self-injuring; others return to their usual activities; some remain agitated and seek other forms of release. The behavioral "results" of self-injury provide a great deal of information about why the behavior is repeated.

INTEGRATION OF THE FIVE DIMENSIONS

As I have noted at the beginning of the chapter, the five dimensions of this biopsychosocial model do not function in isolation. They are entirely interrelated and even interdependent. For example, biological vulnerabilities affect the responsiveness of the individual to environmental conditions. A biologically compromised individual will be more negatively affected by aversive experiences in the environment than will one who is constitutionally strong. Conversely, there is evidence that recurrent traumatic experiences have sustained physiological effects, including changes in brain chemistry (van der Kolk et al., 1996). In addition, environmental conditions and physiology have a major impact on cognitions in terms of positivity, negativity, and self-efficacy. Cognitions, in turn, trigger and "refire" emotions, and emotions reciprocally influence future cognitions. Cognitions and emotions precipitate behaviors, which, depending in their results, affect subsequent thoughts and feelings. A tabular summary of the five dimensions is provided in Table 6.1.

CONCLUSION

This chapter has set the stage for Part II on assessment and treatment. In order to conduct a thorough assessment of self-injury, clinicians need to understand in detail the following dimensions of self-injurious acts:

1. Environmental
2. Biological
3. Cognitive
4. Affective
5. Behavioral

This chapter has reviewed these five key dimensions, which influence, trigger, and serve to maintain the behavior, and which must be addressed when providing treatment. The "mix" of the five dimensions is idiosyncratic for each individual; therefore, treatment strategies need to be individualized to meet the needs of each self-injuring client.

TABLE 6.1. Biopsychosocial Model for Self-Injury

Environmental dimension

- Family historical elements (e.g., mental illness, violence, substance abuse, self-injury, suicide in family)
- Client historical elements (e.g., neglect, attachment problems, loss of parent, physical and sexual abuse)
- Invalidating environment within the family
- Family and environmental strengths and assets
- Current aversive environmental elements (e.g., loss, relationship conflict, abuse, peers who self-injure)

Biological dimension

- Serotonin-level dysfunction?
- Endogenous opioid system dysfunction?
- Diminished pain sensitivity?

Cognitive dimension

- Interpretations of environmental elements, especially negative, pessimistic thoughts, judgments, beliefs (e.g., "All my relationships end badly," "No one understands me," "I'm all alone")
- Self-generated cognitions regarding self and self-injury (e.g., "I have to do this," "Only self-injury helps," "I deserve this," "I hate my body," "Now others will understand how much pain I'm in")
- Thoughts, images, flashbacks related to trauma

Affective dimension

- Susceptibility to frequent, intense, sustained emotions
- Negative emotions trigger self-injury, especially anger, anxiety, tension, shame, depression, sadness, contempt, worry
- Emotions and/or dissociation related to thoughts, images, flashbacks from trauma

Behavioral dimension

- Major behavioral antecedents, such as conflicts with others, substance use, isolation
- Preparation for self-injury, such as choosing location, obtaining tool, ensuring privacy
- Aftermath behaviors, such as returning to activities, falling asleep, communicating with others regarding self-injury

Assessment and Treatment
A Stepped-Care Model

INTRODUCTION

Part II, the longest section of this book, concerns assessment and treatment. The present edition of this volume employs a "stepped-care model" in discussing interventions with self-injury. Stepped-care models are being used increasingly in the delivery of mental health services (Bower & Gilbody, 2005; New Zealand Ministry of Health, 2009: Earl, 2010). The principles underlying stepped-care models include the following (after New Zealand Ministry of Health, 2009, p. 5):

- Interventions of different levels of intensity are available to clients.
- Clients' needs are matched with the level of intensity of the intervention.
- Client outcomes are carefully monitored, allowing treatments to be "stepped up" if required.
- Clients usually move through less intensive interventions before receiving more intensive interventions (if necessary).
- Moving up the steps is generally associated with increasing behavioral risk, intensity of intervention, and expense.
- Clear referral pathways should exist between the different levels of intervention.
- Client self-care is emphasized via skills training in order to support independence and manage demand for services.

Figure II.1 presents a stepped-care model for responding to self-injury. This model begins at the baseline (Step O), where no self-injury exists and the preferred intervention is prevention. The next four steps address escalating levels of self-injury. For common, low-lethality self-injury of short duration (with modest or no concomitant problems), interventions are brief in duration and intensity, as shown for Steps 1 and 2. In contrast, for recurrent, chronic, and/or atypical self-injury (with related conditions, such as suicidality, aggression, eating disorders, substance abuse, and risk-taking behaviors), the interventions are complex, multimodal, and intensive, as shown for Steps 3 and 4. Note that the relevant chapters in this book are cited for the interventions at each of these four levels in Figure II.1.

In a stepped-care model, clients and clinicians should be partners. Clients decide on these issues:

- How much treatment they want
- What costs they are willing to pay
- At what frequency
- How much work they are willing to assume during and between sessions
- Whether they want to move up or down a step

In turn, clinicians and other professionals decide on these issues:

- The length, frequency, and duration of interventions
- How many different interventions are offered in combination
- Frequency of contact with clients between sessions
- The degree of training and expertise necessary to provide the intervention(s)
- Staffing patterns necessary to deliver the service(s)
- When to refer clients to other specialists or services

Although this text does not cover all of the interventions included in Figure II.1, it does provide a reasonably comprehensive review of treatments for self-injury. Treatments in Figure II.1 that are not covered in this text are referenced elsewhere with full citations, so that readers can explore them.

Type of Self-Injury/Related Problems		Interventions
Chronic/recurrent/atypical/severe self-injury, with recurrent suicidality, foreign-body ingestion, and other conditions (e.g., aggression, substance abuse, serious eating disorder, risk-taking, failure to self-protect)	**STEP 4:** **Step 3, plus**	• Treatments such as DBT and IMR for multiple self-harm behaviors (Chapter 17) • Residential treatment (Chapter 18) • Supported housing/outreach, case management, day treatment, clubhouse, recovery programs, etc., where indicated
Persistent and/or atypical self-injury, with other conditions (e.g., suicidal ideation and attempts, PTSD symptoms, body alienation, eating disorder, substance abuse)	**STEP 3:** **Step 2, plus**	• Body image work (Chapter 15) • Exposure treatment (Chapter 16) *or* • Cognitive restructuring for PTSD (Chapter 16) • Protective hospitalization/respite services where indicated
Recurrent, common, low-lethality self-injury	**STEP 2:** **Step 1, plus**	• Replacement skills training (Chapter 11) • Cognitive treatment (Chapter 12) • Family therapy (Chapter 13) where indicated • Psychopharmacological treatment (Chapter 14) where indicated
First/early episode of self-injury	**STEP 1**	• Initial responses: Low-key, dispassionate demeanor; respectful curiosity (Chapter 7) • Formal assessment (Chapter 8) • Cognitive-behavioral assessment (Chapter 9) • Contingency management (Chapter 10) • After assessment, if self-injury is deemed to be common/low-lethality, go to Step 2; if self-injury is atypical/severe (Chapters 3 and 9), skip to Step 3
Self-injury education and prevention	**STEP 0**	• Management and prevention of self-injury contagion among youth (Chapters 20, 21) • Education about/prevention of the "choking game" and related phenomena (Chapter 22)

FIGURE II.1. Stepped-care model for treatment of self-injury.

TREATMENT: STEP 1

CHAPTER 7

Initial Therapeutic Responses

The first component in providing Step 1 of the Stepped Care Model (see Figure II.1, p. 75) consists of the initial therapeutic responses. The early clinical responses to self-injury set the stage for the remainder of assessment and treatment. Skillful management at the outset can gain the confidence of the client, comfort family members in a time of intense stress, and correctly delineate the unique features of self-injury. Conversely, mishandling the initial responses to self-injury can have long-term negative repercussions. Misdiagnosis can lead to labeling the behavior as suicidal, resulting in unnecessary psychiatric hospitalizations and related stigmatization. This chapter discusses using language strategically and adopting an appropriate interpersonal demeanor in responding to self-injury.

AVOIDING THE USE OF SUICIDE TERMINOLOGY

Chapter 1 has emphasized the major points of distinction between self-injury and suicide. Consistent with this emphasis, in speaking with clients about their self-injury, it is important to avoid the language of suicide. Unfortunately, many professionals use such terms as "suicide gesture" or "suicide attempt" to refer to self-injury. The use of "suicide gesture" is not only misleading, but generally countertransferential (Maltsberger, 1986) or therapy-interfering (Linehan, 1993a). A "gesture" is a slight movement, a minor act of motion, an insignificant behavior in the grand scheme of things. Professionals use the term "suicide gesture" to convey that a behavior is not a "real suicide attempt" and therefore not deserving of serious alarm. Often an additional implication of the term "gesture" is that the act is "manipulative." My position in this book is that self-injury is neither insignificant nor manipulative. The behavior is important, and as such is deserving of full attention and a concerted therapeutic strategy. Self-injury should not be dismissed or minimized. It is not a mere gesture; it is a significant act.

Although the equally common term "suicide attempt" does not suffer from countertransferential implications, using it in relation to self-injurious behavior often creates confusion. As discussed in Chapters 1 and 2, self-injury is substantially different *from* suicide; yet self-injury is a major risk factor *for* suicide attempts (but not necessarily death by suicide). Good clinical practice suggests that we (1) understand, manage, and treat the two types of behaviors differently, but also (2) carefully cross-monitor them and assess them interdependently. We need to use the terms "self-injury" versus "suicide" accurately in order to assist our clients. This accuracy can be achieved by referring to the details of the method used. Suicide involves such acts as use of a gun, hanging, ingesting pills or poison, and jumping; in contrast, self-injury involves such behaviors as cutting, burning, picking, and hitting. Note the difference in lethality between the two types of behavior. Referring to self-injury as a "suicide attempt" only serves to create a great muddle at a time when clarity is imperative.

Another problematic term commonly used to refer to self-injury is "parasuicide." Coined by Norman Kreitman (1977), it has been employed by many other researchers to refer to a very broad range of self-destructive behaviors. Linehan (1993a), for example, includes behaviors ranging from a scratch on the arm with a paper clip that fails to break the skin, to a high-lethality suicide attempt that fails to end in death only by accident (e.g., a nonfatal self-inflicted gunshot wound to the head). Including such a broad range of self-destructive behaviors under the rubric of a single term is not useful, because it is too heterogeneous. The average clinician finds it baffling to use the same word in referring to such behaviors as modest, low-lethality hair pulling and high-lethality attempts at hanging. Without further clarification, we are inevitably left wondering whether "parasuicide" refers to a low- or high-lethality act. A far more useful way to organize information about self-destructive acts is Pattison and Kahan's (1983) multidimensional schema regarding direct and indirect self-harm, as presented in Chapter 3 (see Figure 3.1). This model offers gradations as to intent, lethality, and frequency. The schema does not co-mingle acts of high lethality with those that have little or no risk of death.

EMPLOYING THE CLIENT'S LANGUAGE STRATEGICALLY

If the language of "suicide gesture," "suicide attempt," and "parasuicide" should be avoided in discussing self-injury, what language *should* be used? It is often very helpful to employ the language of self-injuring clients themselves, with certain exceptions. Most self-injuring persons use behaviorally descriptive language when they speak or write of their self-harm. They will refer to it as "cutting," "scratching," "carving," "burning," "picking," "hitting," and so on. When a therapist responds to a client by using such language, it has distinct advantages. First, it is a joining strategy to use the client's own terminology. It is also respectful of, and empowering to, the client to accept his or her language. The implicit message from the therapist is "I am giving respectful attention to your view of this and using your own language in discussing it."

An additional advantage of mirroring a client's language is that it is a preliminary step in entering that individual's psychological space. This entrance is crucial in coming to understand and assist the person with his or her self-injury. Language that reflects the speech of another is one of the most basic and affirming of empathic behaviors.

However, there are exceptions to this rule. There are times when using the language of self-injuring persons is ill advised. These exceptions involve two types of language: the "minimizing" and the "ultrasubjective." Language of minimization occurs when an individual is performing considerable harm to his or her body and the language does not reflect the damage inflicted.

For example, I worked with a woman in her 30s whose scars were extensive and permanent on both arms. The scars were jagged, random, thick, white keloidic records of 15 years of self-mutilation (the damage went beyond self-injury). Many of her scars came from wounds that should have been sutured at the time of the acts. However, she had cared for the wounds herself, worsening the extent and permanence of her scarring. When this woman first began therapy, she referred to her self-mutilation as "scratching" or "picking." I found this language to be quite minimizing, given the extent of her scars. Moreover, these scars were stigmatizing when noticed by others. People would recoil and avoid her once they had seen the tangled mass of scars on her arms.

Once I had built a positive alliance with the client, I chose to challenge, gently, her use of language. I was careful to avoid shaming or chastising her, but I felt I needed to insert a sense of reality into our dialogue. On one occasion when the time seemed right, I said that in my opinion her "self-harm went way beyond 'scratching' or 'picking.'" Although initially surprised by my comment, she was able to accept my questioning of her use of language. Later, I asked her what words might be more accurate in referring to her self-harm. She suggested that we use "cutting" or "slashing," and I agreed. Her coming to view the extent of the damage more accurately was part of the therapeutic process. She became more motivated to reduce the behavior as she acknowledged the social cost. She began to conceal her scars from others when she was concerned about social repercussions. With those she knew well and felt more comfortable, she took no such precautions.

Another problem with language occurs when clients refer to the behavior in an ultrasubjective way. Most commonly, such idiosyncratic language is used by people who suffer from some form of psychosis.

For example, I worked for a number of years with a man who mutilated himself by punching his face, head, and eyes. (This individual's dilemma is presented at length in Chapter 25.) Years of this self-inflicted abuse resulted in this individual becoming legally blind. His explanations for these acts of self-harm were entirely consistent year after year. His language referring to his self-mutilation was related to a very fixed delusion. He stated that evil spirits took over his body and punished him for his sins; he had no control over the acts of self-punching. In the course of treatment, I often explored his delusional thoughts; however, I never endorsed them and made them my own. I would use his language about spirits from time to time, but always added qualifiers, such as "I know *your view* is that spirits caused this self-assault," or "What, *in your view*, were you being punished for today?" I attempted to walk a narrow path with this client whereby I was respectful of his experience of the world without endorsing or affirming it.

Chapter 25 presents other aspects of responding to delusional thought and language in strategic, therapeutic ways.

THE IMPORTANCE OF INTERPERSONAL DEMEANOR

A second aspect of initially responding to self-injury concerns the importance of interpersonal demeanor. People tend to respond to self-injury with affectively charged behaviors. These include such reactions as

- Intense concern and effusive support
- Anguish and fear
- Recoil, shock, and avoidance
- Condemnation, ridicule, and threats

Most people react to self-injury with positive emotions, such as concern and support. These are responses that convey to the self-injuring person a desire to help and protect. Unfortunately, over time, positive responses from others can become a form of secondary reinforcement for the behavior. The first level of reinforcement for self-injury is the relief obtained from emotional distress. Markedly and rapidly reducing intense emotional discomfort is intensely reinforcing. However, inadvertent social reinforcement can also play an important secondary role. For this reason, even positive reactions of concern and support can be problematic. This is especially the case when the reactions are effusive: The more intense the emotional response, the greater the risk of inadvertent reinforcement.

Of course, many people react to self-injury with behavior that goes beyond concern and support. Hysterical behavior that involves anguish and fear is not uncommon. Consider this example:

A mother with an only child, a 12-year-old daughter, called a therapist. Sobbing on the phone, she said she had just discovered that her daughter had been cutting herself from time to time over a 6-month period. Between gasps for breath, the mother said that she lived for her daughter and didn't know whether she could survive if her daughter killed herself. The clinician tried to comfort the mother, expressing how important her daughter must be to her. Then he asked what the daughter was doing at that moment. The mother said she was outside playing happily. Ascertaining that the daughter was at no immediate risk, the clinician attempted to reassure the mother. Through a series of questions, the clinician discovered that the girl's self-injury consisted of occasional scratches on her wrists and ankles that required no first aid. The clinician then explained to the mother that although self-injury is alarming and needs treatment, the behavior the mother described did not appear to be related to suicide. The mother calmed down markedly in response to this statement. The mother and the clinician made an appointment for the next day. Before hanging up, the therapist gave the mother a phone number for a local psychiatric emergency unit, should any major problem arise in the interim.

In this case, the therapist's job was to calm the mother and provide some brief education about self-injury. Hysterical reactions are rarely helpful in responding to the behavior. They interfere with problem solving and may inadvertently reinforce the behavior in those who find intense reactions in others to be rewarding. Particularly for those who have been ignored or punished frequently, hysterical protective reactions can be quite gratifying.

Another common reaction to self-injury is some combination of recoil, shock, and avoidance. In these circumstances, the people encountering self-injury are overwhelmed by the behavior and feel compelled to leave the emotional field. In these situations, the responders behave in a way that is more protective of themselves than of the self-injuring persons. They may want to help, but find the notion of self-injury to be too upsetting and disorganizing to endure. As a result, they abandon the self-injuring individuals and flee to safer ground. Sometimes even seasoned therapists respond in this manner to self-injury.

A 21-year-old male described his previous therapist's handling of his self-injury: "She never liked to talk about it. If I brought it up—or, worse, if I walked into her office with short sleeves on—her face kind of scrunched up and she looked stressed out. She would start moving around in her chair and breathing like she was real uptight. Then she would make me promise never to do it again and say something like, 'Let's move on to more positive things. . . . '"

Conveying shock, followed by recoil and retreat, is destructive to people who self-injure. Too many of these individuals have encountered multiple losses and rejections in their lives; they do not need additional abandonment experiences. Professionals need to assess why they might be so triggered by self-injury and strive to overcome it. For many, a tendency to be shocked by self-injury fades over time with exposure to, and a greater understanding of, the behavior. If avoidant reactions cannot be neutralized, it is best for clinicians to transfer self-injuring clients elsewhere.

Some individuals go beyond recoil and avoidance to downright hostility. In this case, the excessive affect is the opposite of too much support and empathy. It is punitive and rejecting, as in this example:

A father's reaction to first learning about his daughter's cutting and burning herself was to call her "a stupid idiot." He added, "If you're going to do that kind of sick behavior, you can move out of here and into a mental hospital right now! You know and I know you're just doing it for attention! Get out of my sight!"

It is hard to imagine a less helpful response than this father's, unless violence came into play. It is not surprising that encountering self-injury—particularly when it is unexpected—causes intense emotional reactions in others. The behavior involves tissue damage and blood, which most human beings understandably prefer to avoid. Moreover, the behavior is self-inflicted, which runs counter to typical human expectations regarding self-protection. In addition, the behavior may stir up in others fears of body fragility or fragmentation, and threaten a sense of bodily wholeness or integrity. They may also fear (usually irrationally) that the self-injuring person will attack them.

USING A LOW-KEY, DISPASSIONATE DEMEANOR

The first of several alternative strategic courses of action in responding to self-injury is to use a low-key, dispassionate demeanor. The affect-laden responses cited above are doubly harmful to self-injuring people. First, such responses, be they supportive or condemning, may shame or embarrass a self-injuring person. Emotional reactions in others may make the person less likely to communicate about the behavior in the future. Also, in many cases, the intense reactions may inadvertently reinforce the behavior (i.e., make it more likely to recur). On the one hand, a nurturing, overly solicitous response may be immensely gratifying for people who have been neglected, ignored, or abused. On the other hand, condemnation and recoil may be paradoxically rewarding, especially for adolescents who take some gratification in provoking strong reactions in adults.

For all these reasons, it is clinically advisable to use a calm, dispassionate demeanor in responding to the behavior. Achieving some form of equanimity may take practice, but it has the double advantages of (1) not adding further affect to an already emotionally charged situation, and (2) not inadvertently reinforcing a behavior that the clinician wants very much to see decline and cease.

RESPECTFUL CURIOSITY

Caroline Kettlewell (1999) has suggested another helpful way to respond to self-injury: with "respectful curiosity." She has said that she preferred that response when she was presenting a therapist with information about her cutting (personal communication, 2002). Curiosity conveys an attitude of wanting to know more about the problem, rather than wanting the problem to go away quickly. To be helpful, however, curiosity has to be tempered and respectful. Interest that comes across as prurient or thrill-seeking is aversive (or too reinforcing) for most self-injuring persons. The exception can be in peer groups where contagion is developing, as discussed in Chapter 20.

NONJUDGMENTAL COMPASSION

Another therapeutic response to self-injury is nonjudgmental compassion. Time and again, self-injurers have encountered harsh pejorative judgments related to their self-injury: They are deemed to be mentally ill, impulsive, explosive, dangerous, or the like. When a therapist responds with nonjudgmental compassion, it can be immensely relieving for a self-injuring client. Such a stance positions the therapist to hear the rest of the client's story with some assurance of full disclosure.

A very legitimate question is this: What is the difference between compassion, which is recommended, and effusive concern and support, which are not? Granted, these types of positive responses are not easily differentiated.

The main difference is one that is subtle in tone. Effusive concern and support suggest a certain amount of affective intensity, a yearning to be of assistance, and a desire to protect and intervene quickly. Compassion is more about acceptance, about being with the client in a neutral, nonjudgmental way, with no immediate expectations for change.

An example of this nonjudgmental, compassionate demeanor—which is both hard to describe and hard to achieve—is provided in the following dialogue from an initial therapy session:

> THERAPIST: It's good to hear those details about your life. Could we move now to discussing why you came?
>
> CLIENT: (*looking embarrassed*) Well, I cut myself all the time . . .
>
> THERAPIST: (*low-key demeanor, compassionate tone*) How often do you do it?
>
> CLIENT: Almost every day.
>
> THERAPIST: That is quite frequent. [not minimizing] Where do you tend to cut yourself? [respectful curiosity]
>
> CLIENT: (*even more embarrassed*) Everywhere, I guess.
>
> THERAPIST: I see. Do you have favorite body areas to cut? [respectful curiosity]
>
> CLIENT: Yeah, my arms and legs.
>
> THERAPIST: I see. What do you think cutting does for you?
>
> CLIENT: It gets my feelings out and calms me down.
>
> THERAPIST: Okay. Is it one of the most effective ways you have to deal with your feelings?
>
> CLIENT: (*enthusiastically*) Definitely!
>
> THERAPIST: Well, it's no wonder you do it so often then, is it? [nonjudgmental]
>
> CLIENT: Thanks for understanding. Most people think I'm a jerk or a nut.

This therapy is off to a promising start. The therapist has conveyed to the client that self-injury can be discussed matter-of-factly and compassionately. There is no evidence of excessive empathy, hysteria, shock, recoil, or condemnation. The therapist has even acknowledged nonjudgmentally that self-injury has adaptive features, in that it is effective in managing painful emotions. The client appears to feel understood in a preliminary way. They are now in a position to move on to discussing self-injury, using the client's own language.

CONCLUSION

In summary, in responding to self-injury, it is generally most helpful if clinicians and others do the following:

- Avoid the use of suicide terminology.
- Use the client's own descriptive language.
- Gently challenge language that is minimizing or too idiosyncratic.
- Remain aware of the risks of inadvertently providing secondary reinforcement.
- Employ a low-key, dispassionate demeanor.
- Convey respectful curiosity.
- Be nonjudgmental and compassionate.

CHAPTER 8

Formal Assessment of Self-Injury

JENNIFER J. MUEHLENKAMP

The second component in Step 1 of the stepped-care model (see Figure II.1, p. 75) is the formal assessment of self-injury. This activity allows the clinician or other professional to go beyond intuition and practice-based knowledge to more formal, evidence-based assessment. This chapter begins with a case example that points to the importance of such assessment. Later in the chapter, the use of formal assessment in this case is described, to explicate its utility.

Marissa was a 16-year-old European American female who was a junior at a large public high school. She was a straight-A student and a star athlete on the track team. She came from a middle-class, intact family and had a small but solid group of friends who represented a positive peer group. Despite her successes as a student and athlete, Marissa felt deeply inferior to many of her peers and her younger brother. She became increasingly depressed, but worked hard to mask her distress and was quite successful in doing so. Marissa strove to please her parents, both of whom were very invested in her success as an athlete. For the past month she had been trying to qualify for the state track competition. At the last track meet of the season, Marissa missed qualifying for the state competition by fractions of a second. Later that night, Marissa's mother was awakened by Marissa's soft cries for her mother's help as she stood at the bottom of the stairway to her parents' bedroom with a washcloth wrapped around her forearm, which was covered in numerous superficial cuts. One of these cuts was the letter F (for failure) carved into her wrist. Three days later, many of the cut marks were faint and easily covered by her jewelry as Marissa met with a counselor for the first time.

Marissa represents a growing body of relatively high-functioning, successful adolescents whose inner turmoil and inabilities to cope with intensely negative internal states lead them to engage in self-injury. Empirical studies and anecdotal reports suggest that the number of individuals who self-injure is growing, and numerous mental health professionals are encountering an increasingly diverse clientele of self-injurers. Many who engage in self-injury have difficulty expressing their experiences, fear how their self-injury will be perceived, and thus do not readily disclose their self-injury to health care professionals (Baetens, Claes, Muehlenkamp, Grietens, & Onghena, 2011; Heath, Baxter, Toste, & McLouth, 2010). Given that individuals are more likely to endorse engaging in sensitive and/or shameful behaviors like self-injury on self-report measures than during in-person interviews, having a repertoire of clinically useful and valid questionnaires for screening and assessing self-injury is essential. The purpose of this chapter is to provide a brief review of clinically valid self-report tools to be used as part of a formal initial assessment of self-injury.

Using standardized, validated self-report measures for assessing self-injury is a cost-effective method for obtaining systematic, objective, high-quality information in a reliable format that can enhance service delivery and monitoring of outcomes. Screening for self-injury as part of a formal assessment will assist with initial detection of the behavior, promoting early intervention. As earlier chapters of this book have emphasized, early intervention is important, because single incidents of self-injury can quickly evolve into repetitive behavior. Case conceptualization and treatment planning are enhanced by scales that offer a set of structured questions evaluating the context surrounding the self-injury episode(s) and the potential functions underlying the behavior, since some self-injuring individuals may not have a full understanding of, or be able to articulate, the function of their self-injury. Following up on the information from the self-report measures will assist in forming the therapeutic relationship, particularly if the interventions developed are tailored toward the individual functions the self-injury serves for the client (Muehlenkamp, 2006). In addition, standardized measures often provide norms with which to compare clients' behavior. Having normative comparison data assists clinicians in estimating the severity of their clients' self-injury and can aid the interpretation and application of the empirical literature to the clients' treatment. Last, the data obtained from the formal assessments can also serve as a reliable baseline against which to examine treatment progress; this not only enhances client retention, but also meets the increasing demands for empirically demonstrating treatment effectiveness to third-party agencies. Valid and reliable measurement of self-injury thus forms a critical part of treatment planning and outcome evaluation.

Guidelines for the use of self-report measures in treatment planning and outcome assessment have been established (Newman, Rugh, & Ciarlo, 2004) and adopted by the National Institute of Mental Health. The guidelines include stipulations that the measures be age-appropriate and relevant to the target group; include objective response options for consistent and clear scoring; provide data that are useful to service delivery; be compatible with clinical theories and practices; and meet minimum criteria for psychometric reliability, validity, and sensitivity to treatment-related changes. Although there has recently been a great increase in the number of the scales available for assessing self-injury, many have primarily been developed and used as research tools. Consequently, the self-report scales reviewed below are those that have strong clinical utility (according to our current understanding of self-injury) and have demonstrated reliability and validity within both treatment and community samples.

WHAT NEEDS TO BE ASSESSED?

Descriptive studies of self-injury provide an empirical basis for identifying the dominant characteristics and features to assess (Nock, 2010). These features also coincide with the diagnostic criteria proposed for a "non-suicidal self-injury" disorder in the upcoming *Diagnostic and Statistical Manual of Mental Disorders*, fifth edition (DSM-5; American Psychiatric Association, 2010), and thus they are the necessary pieces of information that should be obtained in assessing self-injury. Questionnaires should evaluate, at a minimum, the presence–absence of self-injury; duration of the behavior; age of onset; methods used to self-injure; perceived severity; and the functions served by the self-injury. Including these items provides a solid foundation for understanding the basic characteristics of a client's self-injury and establishes a baseline to gauge treatment changes upon. These basic data also set the stage for further informal assessment (see Chapter 9, this volume) of the self-injury specific to each individual client. All of the scales reviewed in this chapter provide an adequate evaluation of these features, but some also provide more detailed assessment of other self-injury characteristics that are relevant to individualized treatment planning. Such additional features may include details about the most recent episode; experience of pain during self-injury; strength and frequency of self-injury urges; skills used to avoid self-injury; and potential addictive properties. The decision of whether to utilize a scale that measures these additional domains needs to balance time constraints, desire for comprehensive details, and a clinician's confidence in his or her ability to elicit this information from a less formal assessment process.

REVIEW OF SELF-REPORT SCALES

Functional Assessment of Self-Mutilation

The Functional Assessment of Self-Mutilation (FASM; Lloyd, Kelley, & Hope, 1997) was developed for use with adolescents who are psychiatric inpatients, community high school students, or incarcerated youth. It consists of two main parts. The first part presents clients with a checklist of 11 potential self-injury behaviors and asks clients to indicate which behaviors they have engaged in within the past year. A catch-all "other" item permits clients to write in a behavior not represented in the list. The items on this part of the scale fall into two reliably identified domains of "mild" (e.g., picking at a wound) and "moderate/severe" (e.g., cutting) behavior. Clients also indicate how many times they have engaged in each behavior and whether they have gotten medical treatment for any of them. The second major section of the scale provides a list of 22 statements (plus another catch-all "other" item) describing potential functions underlying the self-injury, which clients rate along a scale ranging from "never" to "often." The scale also has items assessing the impulsive nature of the self-injury (e.g., length of time a client contemplates self-injury before acting); age of onset; whether pain is experienced; whether there has been suicidal intent with any of the self-injury acts; and whether self-injury takes place under the influence of drugs or alcohol.

The FASM has shown strong structural validity within inpatient and community samples of adolescents (Lloyd-Richardson, Perrine, Dierker, & Kelley, 2007). The two major sections of the scale have each demonstrated adequate reliability as well as validity. One limitation of this scale is the limited range of behaviors provided on the checklist. Others are that a number of the behaviors listed are very mild; that some could be easily misinterpreted (e.g., "bit self" could be interpreted as "bit a hangnail"); and that some do not exemplify current definitions of self-injury used in the literature (e.g., hair pulling). In addition, the FASM has not been used in treatment outcome studies, so it is unclear whether it is sensitive to detecting treatment changes. Nor has it been used with adults. However, the FASM is a very cost-effective scale because it is brief (requiring about 5 minutes to complete) and provides a comprehensive screening of the necessary clinical features of self-injury. Furthermore, the scale can provide estimates of the range and importance of different functions for each patient's self-injury, which is good for designing individualized treatment plans. A copy of the FASM can be found in Appendix C of this book.

Ottawa Self-Injury Inventory

Designed specifically for use as a clinical tool, the Ottawa Self-Injury Inventory (OSI; Cloutier & Nixon, 2003) was developed with input from self-injuring adolescents, as well as from psychologists and psychiatrists who work with self-injuring clients. The OSI is unique in that it assesses features of past and present acts of self-injury and thus can provide an estimation of how self-injury behavior has evolved over time from the first episode to current episodes. The scale is among the most comprehensive available: It assesses all the characteristic domains of self-injury, plus it includes subcomponents that evaluate addictive features, motivation to stop engaging in self-injury, effectiveness of the self-injury in achieving reported functions, reasons for continuing self-injury, and the current functions served by recent self-injury acts. Lastly, the OSI also has a couple of items assessing suicidal behavior, including an item as to whether or not the patient has attempted suicide in the past 6 months.

The OSI is still undergoing evaluation of its psychometric properties, but preliminary data suggest that it is reliable over a 2-week time span ($r = .52-.74$ across domains) and that it has validity in adolescent samples (Cloutier & Nixon, 2003). The primary drawbacks to the OSI are that it is a lengthy scale (requiring approximately 20 minutes to complete) and that it is uncertain whether it shows sensitivity to treatment changes. The OSI is available via a free download (*www.insync-group.ca/publications/OSI_clinical_October_20051.pdf*).

Inventory of Statements About Self-Injury

Similar to the FASM, the Inventory of Statements About Self-Injury (ISAS; Klonsky & Glenn, 2009a) consists of two sections that are strongly informed by the theoretical and empirical self-injury literature. The first section evaluates the lifetime frequency and associated features of 12 self-injury behaviors. Included in this section are items inquiring about age of onset, experience of pain, contextual features of the self-injury (e.g., injuring alone or with others), desire to stop self-injuring, and estimated time delay between the self-injury urge and act. A list of 13 potential functions for the client to rate as to relevance for his or her self-injury constitutes the second section. The functions represent a comprehensive list based on the empirical literature; they include affect regulation, self-punishment, interpersonal influence, peer bonding, and sensation seeking.

The ISAS is a newer self-report scale, and its psychometric properties have only been evaluated within one sample of self-injuring undergraduate students so its validity for use with younger adolescents and clinical samples is unknown. Despite this limitation, the ISAS did show strong internal consistency and validity within the self-injuring college student sample. The scale is quick to administer (requiring approximately 5–10 minutes to complete), and it provides a comprehensive assessment of the primary characteristics of self-injury, alongside an evaluation of its functions. Thus it is likely to provide a solid starting point for treatment planning, as well as to set the stage for a more detailed functional analysis of a client's most recent self-injury. The ISAS is available by request from Dr. E. David Klonsky at the University of British Columbia.

Self-Harm Behavior Questionnaire

The Self-Harm Behavior Questionnaire (SHBQ; Gutierrez, Osman, Barrios, & Kopper, 2001) is brief and provides a solid assessment of behaviors across four different sections: self-harm (i.e., self-injury), suicide attempt, suicide ideation, and suicide threat. Each section begins with a dichotomous item asking whether a client has ever engaged in the behavior (e.g., "Have you ever hurt yourself on purpose?"). Follow-up items assess frequency, methods used, age of onset, need for medical severity, age at first and most recent episode, and whether or not the patient told someone of the behavior. For the suicide-related items, an open-ended question assessing precipitants of the behavior (e.g., "What things were going on in your life around the time you tried to kill yourself?") is also included. Although such a question does not appear for the self-injury section, it could be easily added without disrupting the psychometric properties of the scale.

The SHBQ can be completed in about 5 minutes. It has established validity and reliability for use with adolescents and adults across multiple ethnicities, as well as treatment and community samples (Muehlenkamp, Cowles, & Gutierrez, 2010; Gutierrez & Osman, 2008). Studies provide evidence that the SHBQ is effective in differentiating self-injury from suicidal behavior, and clinical cutoff scales are available to assist with suicide risk screening. Limitations of the SHBQ for assessing self-injury are that the scale focuses more heavily on suicidal behavior; that a specific scoring process is required to obtain empirical scale scores (although responses to individual items are easily interpretable); and that it does not directly assess potential functions of self-injury. These limitations are offset by the cost-effectiveness of the scale, because it does provide a quick measurement of both self-injury and suicide, which are known to be associated (see Chapters 1 and 2). In addition, it provides open-ended questions so clients can provide their unique responses, and norms are available for each section separated by gender and age. The full scale is available within the Gutierrez and Osman (2008) text.

Deliberate Self-Harm Inventory

The Deliberate Self-Harm Inventory (DSHI; Gratz, 2001) consists of 17 items reflecting different self-injury behaviors drawn from clinical observations and the empirical literature. Clients indicate whether or not they have engaged in each listed behavior on purpose and without the intent of killing themselves. Additional questions inquiring about the frequency, duration, recency, severity (if the injury required medical attention), and age at onset of the behavior follow each behavioral item. These items can be used individually or combined into two scale scores. One is a dichotomous score that indicates globally whether a patient has ever self-injured, and the second scale provides a continuous summation of the frequency of self-injury across all the behaviors listed.

The DSHI has been widely used in research with college and high school students, as well as some clinical studies of adults with BPD. The scale has strong reliability, including a test–retest reliability of $r = .92$ for the frequency of self-injury behaviors, and the dichotomous scale reliably classifies participants as self-injuring. The validity of the scale is also strong, as both the dichotomous and continuous scores correlate in expected directions with other measures of self-injury/self-harm and psychiatric symptoms. One drawback to the DSHI is that is does not assess potential functions motivating the self-injury. Another is that it may be less sensitive to detecting treatment changes because it assesses lifetime rates of self-injury, although it has been used to assess treatment changes for adults undergoing treatment for BPD (Gratz, Lacroce, & Gunderson, 2006). The fact that the scale can be completed in approximately 5 minutes makes it efficient for detecting self-injury in clients and obtaining a general assessment of the dominant characteristics of the self-injury behavior. A copy of the scale is provided at the end of the Gratz (2001) article.

Alexian Brothers Urge to Self-Injure Scale

Although it is not a comprehensive assessment of self-injury behaviors, the Alexian Brothers Urge to Self-Injure Scale (ABUSI; Washburn, Juzwin, Styer, & Aldridge, 2010) deserves mention, as it is a self-report scale with great clinical utility as a measure of treatment outcomes. The ABUSI is a very brief (5-item) scale that evaluates the frequency, intensity, and duration of the urge to self-injure, along with items that inquire about the level of difficulty resisting self-injury urges and an overall rating of the desire to engage in self-injury in the preceding week.

The ABUSI was developed and validated within a combined sample of adolescent and adult psychiatric patients. In the preliminary study of the

ABUSI's psychometric properties, the scale demonstrated strong reliability and validity. Of particular interest are the findings that scores at admission significantly predicted patients who were readmitted, improved prediction of self-injury frequency at the time of discharge, and showed sensitivity to change in response to treatment (Washburn et al., 2010). Although the ABUSI does not provide an assessment of the characteristic features of self-injury, it appears to be a scale with great clinical utility for monitoring self-injury risk and tracking treatment progress and outcome for self-injury behaviors. A copy of the ABUSI can be found in Appendix C.

STRUCTURED INTERVIEWS

For clinicians who prefer using clinical interviews over self-report questionnaires, there are two strong options from which to choose. The first is the Suicide Attempt Self-Injury Interview (SASII; Linehan, Comtois, Brown, Heard, & Wagner, 2006), which was designed to assess past and current engagement in suicidal and/or nonsuicidal self-injurious behaviors within adult populations. The SASII consists of a combination of open-ended, forced-choice, checklist, and interviewer-rated items that provide a comprehensive assessment of the context surrounding each self-injurious act, as well as the core features (e.g., frequency, function, lethality, intent) of the behavior. The details obtained are a strength of this interview, but they can also make the interview cumbersome and time-intensive; however, a short form is available.

The SASII has been used primarily in clinical treatment settings as part of outcome research with women diagnosed with BPD, and it has demonstrated strong validity as well as interrater reliability. Clinical norms are available for emergency room patients and treatment-seeking women with BPD. A significant strength of the interview is its flexibility, as clinicians can evaluate specific variables of interest (e.g., consequences of self-injury) that will permit identification of individualized treatment targets unique to each client. The SASII, however, is designed to measure past self-injury and is not necessarily valid for use as an evaluation of future risk for suicide or self-injury.

The second option is the Self-Injurious Thoughts and Behaviors Interview (SITBI; Nock, Holmberg, Photos, & Michel, 2007), which is a structured interview that was developed and validated for use with adolescents and young adults from treatment and community populations. This interview evaluates both suicidal and self-injury behaviors across five separate sections: suicidal ideation, suicidal plans, suicidal gestures, suicide attempts, and self-injury. To ease administration and reduce time demand, only those models that are positively endorsed for lifetime presence of the behavior on the initial screening items are administered. Along with evaluating the primary characteristics of self-injury or suicidal behavior, the SITBI inquires about the frequency and strength of thoughts/urges, antecedents to the behavior, experiences of pain, social influences, and impulsiveness, and it has clients estimate the likelihood of a future occurrence of the behavior. Although the interview provides extensive detail, it is relatively quick to administer and can usually be completed within 15 minutes.

The SITBI has shown solid interrater and test–retest reliability, as well as strong construct validity (Nock et al., 2007). Although it has been used in both research and treatment settings, it is unclear whether the SITBI is sensitive to treatment changes. A parent form as well as a short form (which excludes items related to self-injury's functions, to pain experiences, and to peer influences) of the interview are available, providing clinicians with greater flexibility in their assessment based on individualized needs. The SITBI can be obtained from its senior author's website (*www.wjh.harvard. edu/~nock/nocklab/publications.html*).

CASE EXAMPLE: MARISSA'S ASSESSMENT

Comprehensive and accurate evaluation of self-injury is essential for generating useful, individualized case conceptualizations and designing effective interventions for the behavior. Conducting a formal assessment of self-injury is a critical component for responsible treatment, and it can also provide an effective entry into a conversation about a client's self-injury. To facilitate clinically useful and comprehensive assessment, it is strongly recommended that clinicians use one of the brief self-report scales reviewed in this chapter to screen for self-injury in clients as part of the standard intake process. If self-injury is endorsed, clinicians can then use the relevant sections from one of the structured interviews, or one of the more comprehensive self-report questionnaires, to inform the individualized assessment and treatment planning. Once treatment has begun, less formal assessments become appropriate, and the use of functional behavioral analyses for individual instances of self-injury will be relevant. Administering a validated scale of self-injury behavioral frequency or urge ratings (e.g., the ABUSI) periodically through the course of treatment is valuable for monitoring treatment change and is recommended as a standard aspect of practice. Thus formal assessments of self-injury play a vital role in the treatment of this behavior, as can be seen in Marissa's case.

As part of the intake interview during her first therapy session, the counselor asked Marissa whether she had ever hurt herself or had considered suicide. Marissa reported that she had cut herself, which was why her mother had brought her for therapy. The counselor followed up with questions about current suicidal ideation, but failed to inquire about Marissa's intent underlying the cutting. Seeing that the counselor assumed the cutting was suicidal, she honestly denied suicidal ideation and plans, and didn't discuss the cutting any further for fear that the counselor would not understand. The intake continued, and Marissa was diagnosed with depression.

Marissa went to three additional sessions where the counselor focused on treating the depression, and when she was asked whether she had cut herself again, Marissa honestly denied it. Therapy was terminated after the third session, because Marissa's depression appeared to lift and she did not want to continue therapy. Approximately 2 months later, after fighting with a friend and earning a B on an exam, Marissa became extremely distraught and self-deprecating. She began cutting herself again. Her cutting behavior continued in secrecy for over a year and escalated in frequency and severity. Marissa's increasing depression (but not the cutting) became evident to the school counselor, who encouraged Marissa and her mother to try therapy again with a different therapist.

As part of the intake paperwork, the new therapist included a screening scale that inquired about self-injury. Marissa positively endorsed it, reporting that she had cut herself over 50 times in the past year. The counselor saw the positive endorsement on the screening questionnaire, so then included a more comprehensive self-report scale in a small assessment packet that Marissa completed while her mother met with the counselor. Through the questionnaire, Marissa communicated the severity of her cutting (indicating that she probably should have received stitches on one occasion); she endorsed a secondary method of self-injury (banging/intentional bruising); and, for the first time, she was able to express what the self-injury did for her (e.g., release negative emotions, self-punish, communicate distress externally). Marissa also indicated that while the cutting was never suicidal, she did have occasional strong suicidal thoughts and had once contemplated overdosing on pills.

With this detailed information, the counselor was able to proceed with a more in-depth interview of Marissa's self-injury (informed by the SITBI self-injury items). The interview revealed that Marissa experienced very strong urges to self-injure, but was typically able to resist them during the day and engaged in a pattern whereby she cut herself a few times each night to help calm herself and fall asleep. She also reported that she experienced little pain during her self-injury, and that on some occasions she could not resist urges to self-injure, so she kept a sharp tool in her locker at school "just in case." With this detailed information, the counselor began to design a treatment plan in consultation with Marissa. The plan focused specifically on the self-injury by targeting the unique aspects underlying Marissa's behavior. Treatment progress was monitored with weekly assessments of the frequency and severity of self-injury urges, as well as frequency of self-injury episodes.

Marissa's case shows in some detail how using formal assessment tools can facilitate information gathering and enhance clinical planning. If the first counselor had used a self-report measure of self-injury, additional information about the context and functions underlying Marissa's cutting might have been detected at that time. Identifying this additional information might have facilitated a more specific treatment plan (e.g., addressing coping, distress tolerance, self-image) and potentially averted the escalation into repetitive self-injury by targeting the contextual and social-psychological factors motivating the first episode of self-injury.

CONCLUSION

In summary, here are this chapter's main points and recommendations:

- Formal assessment of self-injury is essential to good clinical practice, because it aids detection, enhances case conceptualization for individualized treatment, and permits systematic monitoring of progress.
- For brief and initial clinical assessments of self-injury, I recommend using the Functional Assessment of Self-Mutilation (FASM) or the Alexian Brothers Urge to Self-Injure Scale (ABUSI).
- If a brief initial assessment of the presence of both self-injury and suicide is desired, the Self-Harm Behavior Questionnaire (SHBQ) is recommended.
- The Ottawa Self-Injury Inventory (OSI) is highly recommended for a more thorough clinical or research assessment of self-injury.
- For a more extensive clinical/research assessment of both self-injury and suicide, the Self-Injurious Thoughts and Behaviors Interview (SITBI) is highly recommended.

CHAPTER 9

Cognitive-Behavioral Assessment

The third component of Step 1 in the stepped-care model (see Figure II.1, p. 75) is cognitive-behavioral assessment. This complex activity complements and builds on the formal assessment of self-injury described in Chapter 8. This chapter employs the biopsychosocial formulation discussed in Chapter 6 to demonstrate how to conduct an assessment of self-injury. As described earlier, the biopsychosocial formulation addresses five interrelated dimensions that assist us in understanding and treating self-injury: environmental, biological, cognitive, affective, and behavioral. Assessment begins with the last of these dimensions—behavioral—because it is important to evaluate the specifics of the self-injury at the outset. Then the clinician can begin to identify the conditions that precipitate and maintain the behavior.

The assessment procedures presented here are based on the principles of conducting a thorough behavioral analysis, which involves a three-step process of collecting measurable data and descriptive information regarding (1) the *antecedents* to the behavior, (2) the *behavior* itself, and (3) the *consequences* thereafter (Kazdin, 1994).

ASSESSING THE SELF-INJURY BEHAVIOR

Using a Self-Injury Log

One way to collect accurate information regarding self-injury is to ask clients to complete a Self-Injury Log, as shown in Figure 9.1. Many clients in outpatient treatment are willing and able to complete such a log between

Name: _____

Week of: _____

Category	Monday	Tuesday	Wednesday	Thursday	Friday	Saturday	Sunday
Environmental antecedents							
Biological antecedents							
Cognitive, affective, and behavioral antecedents							
Number of wounds							
Start time of SIB episode							
End time of SIB episode							
Extent of physical damage (length, width; were sutures obtained?); (If yes, how many?)							
Body area(s)							
Pattern to wounds (yes/no; if yes, type)							
Use of tool (yes/no; if yes, type)							
Room or place of SIB							
Alone or with others during SIB?							
Aftermath of SIB (thoughts, feelings, behaviors)							
Aftermath of SIB (biological elements)							
Aftermath of SIB (events in environment)							
Reactions of others to your SIB							
Comments							

FIGURE 9.1. Self-Injury Log. SIB, self-injuring behavior.

weekly psychotherapy sessions. Clients living in supported housing and residential programs can also use logs quite productively. Such clients may require and benefit from being prompted or assisted by members of their support staff.

The information generated from the use of the log is far more reliable than recall alone. My experience is that adults who are motivated to stop self-injuring are quite reliable about remembering to complete the log and bring it to sessions. In contrast, adolescent clients can be highly variable; some lose the log, forget to complete it, or fail to bring it to sessions. For clients who tend to forget to complete their logs, the therapist can ask for a homework update by e-mail one to two times per week between sessions. Or the therapist can offer to provide one to two prompts betweens sessions. Permission to make this brief contact should be obtained in advance from the clients. When clients *still* forget their homework, the best course of action is to ask them to complete the grid in the session from memory as best they can. The clinician may need to assist clients in this process with suggestions and clarifying questions.

It should be emphasized to clients that it is far more helpful if they complete the log themselves on a daily basis between sessions. When clients have been able to do so, they should receive considerable acknowledgment and praise for making this important contribution to the treatment process. The reasons for failing to complete the log should be pursued in detail. Some clients are worried that other members of their households will discover the log. Other clients may need time to recover from the intensity of a psychotherapy session by not thinking about challenging problems for a few days. In trying to obtain the most accurate information possible, clients should be addressed compassionately but persistently in this area.

I almost always review the Self-Injury Log with clients early in a session. I begin with the number of wounds, the length of episodes, and the extent of physical damage. First and foremost, I want to know the amount and extent of physical harm done to the body. Later I move to antecedents and consequences of the behavior.

It is important to ask routinely whether there are behaviors that the client has *omitted* from the log. Some clients will write down the more typical forms of self-injury, such as arm and body cutting, but will leave out atypical forms, such as wounds to the breasts or genitals. I have found that asking about additional behaviors may elicit important information about self-injury that clients are too embarrassed to acknowledge in writing.

Another important detail is to ask clients to put zeros in the row for number of wounds when there has been no self-injury. Writing "0" serves to make explicit the fact that the client has not self-injured on that day. It can be quite reinforcing for clients to be able to look at a row of zeros over the course of a week as visible evidence of having successfully resisted self-injury.

Definitions for the Self-Injury Log

The following are definitions and related explanations for the various items contained on the Self-Injury Log. Even if the therapist chooses not to use a Self-Injury Log, the categories should be reviewed informally as part of a thorough assessment.

Baseline Frequency of Wounds and Episodes

Collecting baseline data regarding self-injury involves counting both the number of wounds and the duration of episodes. Accurate information can only come from the client. No therapist, counselor, or significant other can be privy to all of the details pertaining to self-injury.

WOUNDS

A "wound" is defined as each discrete instance of tissue damage. A wound can be a 2-inch scratch, a 10-inch cut, a single cigarette burn, or a self-inflicted tattoo.

EPISODES

An "episode" is defined as a time period during which an individual is involved in relatively uninterrupted self-injury. A single episode of self-injury can result in multiple wounds.

    The client is asked to count the number of wounds that are inflicted during an episode and to estimate the start and end time of the episode. The following example includes both types of baseline data:

After a bad day at work, Jaime has a habit of coming home and retreating to his bedroom. He often removes an X-ACTO knife from his art supplies and makes a series of cuts on his left arm. Jaime states that he cuts until he feels relief. Sometimes he cuts himself 2 or 3 times and feels better. Other times it takes 8 or 10 cuts. The time period that Jaime cuts varies from about 10 minutes to half an hour. Therefore, in terms of baseline data for Jaime, a single *episode* lasts from 10 to 30 minutes and results in from 2 to 10 *wounds*.

    Collecting baseline data of this type can be complicated. Some configurations of wounds are hard to count; some episodes are ambiguous as to when they start and end. The following case vignette includes both types of ambiguity:

Nikki's pattern of self-injuring involved making cuts on her forearms that resembled the grids on graph paper. Episodes of cutting sometimes took 3–4 hours. During her lengthier episodes, she often "took a break" from cutting to eat or do an errand. Several hours later she resumed executing the grid-like pattern on her arm. In such instances, it was difficult to determine whether the behavior represented single or multiple episodes. In Nikki's view, an episode began when she started incising her arm, and ended when she completed the entire design of the grid. The therapist accepted this definition of an episode.

    The number of wounds also was difficult to determine. Quite often, several days after Nikki had cut the grid-like designs into her arm, she would excoriate the wounds. This involved scraping a blade over the length of her arm and reopening the wounds considerably. It was essentially impossible to quantify the number of wounds in such an episode. After such instances, Nikki tended to write "many" in the Self-Injury Log.

Although precise counts are preferable, they are not necessary. The goal is to obtain accurate information about the general frequency of self-injury and the length of episodes. The client should be encouraged to be as clear as possible, but there is no need for extreme precision. The "Comments" row in the Self-Injury Log is provided to deal with ambiguous circumstances. In this space, the client can provide brief details that explain ambiguities in defining an episode or number of wounds. The blank reverse side of the Self-Injury Log can also be used to record additional information.

The start time of a self-injury episode is an important detail in the life of a self-injuring person, because it can provide crucial information about antecedents to the behavior. It can also provide important opportunities to interrupt the habit of self-injury and to practice replacement behaviors.

I am not aware of any empirical studies regarding the times of day when people self-injure. In my clinical experience, there appears to be considerable variation. Some people begin inflicting self-harm as soon as they wake up in the morning. Others hurt themselves at any time of day when stressful events occur or unpleasant feelings emerge. Some prefer self-injuring immediately after they get home from school or work—when they have their homes to themselves. The majority of people with whom I have worked report harming themselves in the evenings, often right before going to sleep.

Why is bedtime the preferred time of day for so many people who self-injure? Clients provide many different explanations. One is that they tend to reflect on the events of the day at the time of its conclusion. Unfortunately, many self-injuring people tend to put a negative spin on daily events—and they do so day after day. These individuals tend to view a day as series of failures, rejections, or embarrassments; self-injury provides some solace for them before bedtime.

For others, bedtime has the obvious association with sexuality. As people prepare to retire, they are likely to think of other experiences they have had in bedrooms. If individuals are trauma survivors who have been abused in bedroom contexts, they may be especially likely to have a series of mental images or even flashbacks. Many people report having been abused at night when others in their household were asleep. For these people, the time of day when they enter the bedroom and prepare for sleep is fraught with danger and painful memories.

For other individuals, the hour of sleep symbolizes a time of vulnerability and loss of control. Sleep is a time when one is not alert—when one's defenses are down and sense organs are quiescent. For those who are able to feel safe and secure in the world, sleep is a time of renewal and rest. In contrast, for those who feel chronically unsafe and vulnerable, nighttime is a period to be endured until the light of day returns.

Hannah often discussed her night terrors in therapy. She felt a need to speak again and again about the memory of the sound of her father's footsteps coming down the hall around midnight, when he got home from his night job. Sometimes he came into her room and molested her; other times he went to her mother's room and left Hannah undisturbed. For Hannah as a child, midnight was the most terrifying time of the day. Twenty years later, it still was.

Extent of Physical Damage

"Extent of physical damage" is defined as the amount of tissue damage or disfigurement associated with a self-injurious act or episode. Amount of physical damage is one of the most important elements in a behavioral analysis of self-injury. When clients are completing the Self-Injury Log, the key detail is whether a self-injury required medical intervention, such as suturing. Clients are not expected to do a medical assessment of their self-injury, but they can write down the dimensions of the wounds and whether sutures were obtained. The extent of physical damage conveys crucial information about the following:

1. The level of risk presented by the individual, and whether or not the individual may need emergency medical treatment, psychiatric assessment, and protective intervention
2. Whether the individual's level of distress is relatively stable or escalating
3. Possible diagnoses

As noted in Chapter 6, the large majority (90% or more) of self-injuring acts result in modest physical damage. The large majority of persons who harm themselves recurrently in low-lethality ways cut themselves, excoriate their wounds, or hit themselves. They also exercise a level of control over what they do to their bodies. Granted, they are in considerable distress and act in alarming ways by hurting their bodies. Nonetheless, they have a modicum of control over their acts, in that their assaults do not require suturing or other medical intervention, and do not result in extensive permanent scarring.

An additional feature of self-injurious behavior is that self-injurers are somewhat selective about the areas of the body that they assault. Most commonly, they cut their arms and legs and may then pick at their wounds as they are healing (excoriation). These are body parts that can be hidden with long sleeves or pants, indicating an awareness of the social repercussions of the behavior.

However, some individuals—the minority—also perform acts of self-harm on their bodies that require suturing and/or are permanently disfiguring. These forms of self-harm differ from the self-injury scenario and suggest a level of dyscontrol that is alarming. When people cut themselves more deeply, burn themselves extensively, or cause other forms of significant scarring, they *are* mutilating their bodies. The scars are there for a lifetime unless they are removed through cosmetic surgery (and, even then, restoration tends to be only partially effective). Self-inflicted burns also tend to cause permanent scarring. For example, most cigarette burns on the skin leave reddish-blue, circular scars that are unsightly and disfiguring.

When physical damage is more serious, protective intervention may be necessary, such as obtaining medical treatment and utilizing a psychiatric inpatient unit, hospital diversion program, or respite service. The general rule of thumb as to what defines "serious" is the need for suturing or other professional medical intervention. Another rule of thumb is that inflicting many cuts or burns during a single episode suggests considerable emotional agitation and distress. For example, a client once cut both of her arms over 40 times within a 2-hour period. She did not do a level of damage that required suturing, but the sheer volume of cuts suggested that a psychiatric assessment at an emergency mental health unit was in order.

Extent of physical damage can also provide important information about escalation of psychological distress. For example, if an individual usually scratches an arm with a paper clip, barely breaking the skin, but then shifts to using a razor blade and inflicting deeper cuts, this is an important development. The level of physical damage may still be modest, but the increased damage suggests a greater level of distress. This modest increase in physical damage should be explored in detail as part of the behavioral analysis.

When individuals self-inflict massive trauma or disfigurement, they are usually in a floridly psychotic or an acute manic state. In these cases, the individuals have passed over from self-injury into self-mutilation. Examples of these behaviors are among the most unpleasant in the annals of human-kind; they include self-enucleation, autocastration, autocannibalism, and self-amputation. Preventing extreme acts of this type is discussed in Chap-ter 25.

Body Area

"Body area" is defined as the location on the body where the self-injury is inflicted. Body area or topography is an especially important piece of infor-mation. The two most common areas assaulted are arms and legs. Often the arms are selected because of easy accessibility. A person holding a blade or hot object in one hand can very conveniently harm the other wrist or fore-arm. It takes no great contortion or physical discomfort to reach this body area. In addition, self-injuring individuals often state that they harm the arms or legs because the wounds can be hidden under clothing.

The wrist and forearm may also be popular because cutting the wrists has long had connotations of suicide. Although the position of this book and many others (e.g., Ross & McKay, 1979; Favazza, 1987; Walsh & Rosen, 1988; Alderman, 1997; Conterio & Lader, 1998) is that wrist cutting is rarely likely to result in death, the behavior can convey a message of desperation. Self-injuring individuals often wish to communicate to others that they are in considerable psychic pain. Although their message may include implica-tions of suicide, the actual risk to life is modest. Therefore, cutting the wrists can have considerable communicative utility, with the additional advantage of posing little or no risk to life.

Although some generalizations can be made about many self-injuring people, it is nonetheless crucial to assess each individual afresh. Each per-son should be asked why he or she selects a particular body area for self-harm. A few brief examples of the types of highly individualized responses are provided below:

Twenty-five-year-old Sarah almost always cut her forearms. Her explanation was that she loved to look at the blue veins on her arms. She said that only on her arms was the blood under the skin visible in that transparent way. She got "a rush" when, under the pressure of the blade, "all that blue turns to red."

Twenty-two-year-old Gina said that she preferred to cut her abdomen because she could still wear short sleeves and shorts in the summer. She added that she would "never get caught dead in a bathing suit," so her abdomen was the place for her.

Seventeen-year-old Joel had been cutting for about 6 months. To date he had cut his right and left calves exclusively. Asked why he chose these two body areas so consistently, Joel, a born comic, said in an exaggerated Shakespearean voice, "Doctor, I regret to say, yet again, 'I do not know!'" Cajoled to say more, Joel eventually explained that he liked to lift weights at the gym and he didn't want his "lifting buddies asking a lot of stupid questions"—so he left his arms alone. Joel added that he always wore sweat pants to cover his legs.

For most clients, the body areas selected involve a combination of symbolic meaning and practical utility. The therapist should seek to learn these idiosyncratic aspects for each individual. In so doing, the therapist begins to learn important information about the client's relationship with his or her own body. For many individuals, body image may become a central focus in treatment, as explored in the chapters on body alienation and trauma resolution (Chapters 15 and 16).

It should be noted that clients who select a body area in part for purposes of concealment are showing a level of control that others do not. Although cutting or burning oneself may seem like a completely out-of-control act, this may not be true for those who take great care to injure a body area covered by clothing. Despite their anguish and pain, such clients are nevertheless exercising a substantial level of control in keeping subsequent social repercussions in mind. Such "future planning" is a good prognostic sign. For others, the self-injury can be much more impulsive, with little regard for social consequences. Consider this example:

Anne stated, "When I have one of my bad cutting times, I just let it rip. When I'm really out of control, I cut any part of my body. Sometimes I've cut my face and scalp. Sometimes I've cut my left breast and pubic area. Afterwards, I'm freaked out at all the damage and the blood around, but at the time I'm doing it, there's no stopping the helter-skelter."

An important detail in the assessment of self-injury occurs when a client shifts to self-injuring a new body area. Such a change usually indicates a psychological shift in the client. Sometimes the alteration can suggest an exacerbation of distress, requiring psychiatric emergency assessment. For example, when a client shifts to harming face, eyes, breasts, or genitals, it often should be considered an emergency requiring immediate psychiatric assessment (explained immediately below). In other cases, the shift is essentially parallel in nature—for example, when a client moves from arms to legs, or from left bicep to right. As stated before, the key information can be found in the details, which should be sought with persistence.

ESPECIALLY ALARMING BODY AREAS

In my experience, injury to any one of four areas of the body is cause for special concern. These are face, eyes, breasts (in females), and genitals (in either gender). Harming the face is a very ominous sign, suggesting a profound lack of regard for personal attractiveness and social repercussions. Cutting or otherwise harming the face may convey the message "I hate how I look, and I hate myself." It also conveys "I don't care if I'm excluded from many social contexts." Harming the face thus suggests an alarming level of both psychological distress and social disconnectedness.

Harming the eyes is even worse. Eyesight is fundamental to daily life. To run the risk of reducing or eliminating sight is an extreme act. Eye tissue is fragile, and its healing abilities are only modest. Permanent damage is easy to inflict.

Harming the breasts and/or genitals is cause for concern for different reasons. These parts of the body usually remain hidden from public view, so social repercussions for the injuries may be less of an issue. Nonetheless, the symbolic meaning of breast or genital self-harm, and the level of distress it implies, is cause for special alarm. Breasts and genitals are sensitive regions with nerve endings that are very responsive to stimulation and pain. To harm these areas deliberately, the person has to have somehow "turned off" the usual physiological pain responses (Bohus, Limberger, et al., 2000; Russ et al., 1992, 1994). Intense distress or dissociation may neutralize pain responses, enabling people to harm these body locations. There is also the symbolic significance of harming these areas. Extreme distress about sexuality is usually indicated. Psychotic decompensation or primitive trauma reenactment may be involved in such self-injury. The link between psychosis and major self-injury is discussed in Chapter 25; the topic of trauma and self-injury is reviewed in Chapters 15 and 16.

In general, when persons injure the face, eyes, breasts, or genitals, an emergency psychiatric evaluation should be considered. The level of distress accompanying such behavior is often considerable, meriting protective intervention and close supervision.

VISUAL INSPECTION

A final question about assessing body areas is whether or not the therapist chooses to look at wounds. Seeing wounds for oneself often provides far more information than hearing verbal descriptions. Therefore, I routinely ask to see wounds, while emphasizing that it is entirely up to the client to grant or deny the request. If clients are approached politely and respectfully, in my experience they rarely say "no." I justify the request by explaining that seeing the wounds may be helpful in understanding and helping the individual. Obvious exceptions to my asking to look at the wounds occur in the circumstances when the body areas are beyond the bounds of modesty— that is, breasts, thighs, genitals, or abdomen.

However, I do *not* go as far as Levenkron (1998), who often provides first-aid-like attention to his clients' wounds. He has written that he applies ointment and bandages to the wounds of clients who cut, and that he believes these clients benefit psychologically from this intervention. He has speculated that his physical attentions to the wounds may even be crucial in successful treatment (personal communication, 2000).

Each therapist must define his or her own limits. I am not comfortable in administering to clients physically. I am a therapist who rarely physically touches clients, out of a sense of caution and respect. The main exception to this rule occurs when I sometimes hug a client goodbye at the termination of an extended, multiyear treatment. Some may find this formality too aloof. Others may deem it common sense in a litigious age. I believe that many clients—especially those who have histories of physical and/or sexual abuse—are relieved to be in a treatment where there is no physical contact.

Pattern of Wounds

"Pattern of wounds" is defined as the visual arrangement of wounds inflicted during a single episode. Self-injuring people often inflict more than one wound on their bodies during an episode. In such cases, it is useful to ascertain whether the wounds are organized into some sort of pattern. Multiple-wound episodes can be said to fall into four general categories: (1) random or disorganized, (2) organized, (3) symbolic, and (4) verbal/numerical. In my experience the majority of wounds inflicted by self-injuring people are either random or organized. The use of symbols, words, or numbers is much rarer. Many people inflict wounds that have no discernible pattern. For example, an individual may inflict five wounds during a single episode, confined to a single body area, the forearm. Although the wounds are clustered in a common area, they are neither parallel nor at right angles nor otherwise patterned. They display no discernible design. Therefore, this configuration can be considered random.

A second especially common type of self-injury is one that reflects a modest type of organization. For example, a person may inflict four cuts on the forearm that have been precisely executed in parallel fashion. They are the same length and width. Such precision in execution is usually no accident. To create such a design, the individual has to have been focused and taking considerable care to inflict the self-harm "in just the right amount, in just the right way." Thus it is often the case that an individual who inflicts an organized pattern may be in greater control of his or her actions than an individual who inflicts random, disorganized wounds. The latter type of self-injury suggests some type of ritual, or at least a precise, focused process. The former type indicates a more random "Let's see where this takes us" experience. Either way, if the presence or absence of a pattern to the self-injury wound is scrutinized, valuable information can be obtained.

Ironically, wounds that involve symbols or words/numbers tend to be associated with less control and greater level of disturbance. That is to say, although symbols and words require greater attention to detail than simple, nonrepresentational patterns, they tend to occur in people who are significantly distressed. There are probably many exceptions to this observation, but I share here what I have observed about these types of wounds.

People who inflict symbols on their bodies tend to use such markings as crosses, stars, lightning bolts, flowers, and tears. They may execute the designs with sharp blades, producing patterned scars, or use needles and ink to create crude self-inflicted tattoos. I have never encountered a self-injuring client who showed great craftsmanship in the creation of a design on his or her skin. The large majority of self-injuring persons I have met who make symbols on their bodies have been adolescents. It may well be rare for adults to make such designs on their bodies, except for persons in institutions, such as psychiatric hospitals or correctional facilities.

When therapists encounter self-injurious symbols on clients' bodies, they should inquire in detail and with "respectful curiosity" (see Chapter 7) about their meanings. I like to ask a client how he or she selected that specific symbol among all the possible options, how it came out, how he or she likes it now that it's healing, and especially what that symbol means to him or her. Self-injuring people can provide some poignant and startling explanations for these symbolic designs.

Justin was a 14-year-old boy who carved a star onto his lower neck and another on his forearm. Asked why he chose a star design for his body, he initially replied with the not entirely unexpected "I don't know." Encouraged to say more, he explained that he and his girlfriend had each carved stars on their bodies, and that they had done so together. He said that the stars pointed to their love for each other in an otherwise "shitty, fucked-up world."

Keekee had many symbols, words, and numbers on her body, mostly in the form of self-inflicted tattoos. The designs included multiple inverted crosses, tears (identifiable only with her assistance), the words "hate" and "LOVE," and the numbers 666. Keekee stated that she was a satanist and was proud of it and wanted the world to know. Then again, she said, she didn't really care what anyone else thought. "It's my body and I'll do what I want with it. Bodies eventually rot, anyway!"

Keekee is an especially interesting example because she presented with both symbols and words. Words are a special and relatively rare category of self-inflicted injury. It is quite telling when someone feels a need to give a word such emphasis as to carve, tattoo, or burn it into the skin. We all encounter thousands of words every day via conversation, advertisements, radio, television, the Internet, letters, phone calls, texts, mail, and so on. To take from these thousands of words a single one and inflict it on one's body is a dramatic and significant act. In some cases the self-injuring person inscribes the name of a beloved one in order to convey passion or commitment. In others the inscription is designed to impress someone they are pursuing or attempting to regain. Sometimes the name or word is carved to express grief, rage, or both.

Using a cigarette, Beth burned the word "MOM" into the back of one hand and "HATE" into the back of the other. Asked about her intentions, Beth said, in the sardonic tone she used when she wasn't upset, "Actually, it's multipurpose! It means 'I hate Mom,' but it also means 'Mom hates me!' or 'Mom equals hate,' or 'Hate equals Mom!' And that's just a few of the possibilities!"

Beth had great rage and deep sadness in relation to her mother because of years of sexual abuse and her mother's recurrent failure to protect her. Beth's feelings for her mother were so overwhelmingly complex and painful that she felt the words "Mom" and "hate" deserved to be permanently burned into her skin. No other form of verbal expression was powerful, vivid, and dramatic enough to convey the depth and rawness of her feelings. Beth once said that she would have liked to burn "love" into her body as well, then added with bitterness, "I don't really have the word in my vocabulary."

Some of those who inscribe words into their bodies are experiencing a psychotic process. These are individuals who may be descending into psychological disorganization and decompensation. For these persons, the inscription of words may be a desperate attempt to hold onto some centrally important concept or sense of identity. Here are two examples:

Cecily had been convinced since her early teens that she would die before her 20th birthday. At times she felt she would die from a physical illness such as cancer, even though she showed no evidence of the disease. At other times she said she was likely to kill herself because of all the pain in her life. As she approached age 20, she became increasingly agitated and frightened. Once again, she began to hear voices calling her "bitch" and "slut." The voices also instructed her with the single-word command "Die!" One morning she took a shard of glass and carved her birth date into her upper arm, including month, day, and year. Cecily stated that this act symbolically helped her to accept that she might survive her 20th birthday and live beyond it—which she, in fact, did.

Sidney had an especially severe case of schizophrenia with serious, persistent symptoms that seldom remitted. Almost every day involved hours of intrusive auditory hallucinations. He also suffered from persecutory delusions involving devils taking over his body and "causing" self-destructive acts. When Sidney's psychosis exacerbated, he became mute. During these times he occasionally cut or scratched a word into his body, such as "No" or "Yes" or "Gone." In these cases, the best his caregivers could deduce was that he was desperately holding onto language in his state of deterioration. By inscribing a word into his body, he seemed to be striving to retain his capacity as a speaking human subject.

Use of a Tool

"Use of a tool" is defined as a person's using an implement other than his or her own body to inflict self-harm. As with other details of self-injury, the use of a tool or implement conveys a great deal of information regarding the person's state of mind and level of disturbance. It is very informative to ask whether or not a tool is used, and if so, what type. Details about the recurrent use of the same implement, the cleaning of the implement, where it was obtained, and where it is stored when not in use can be quite illuminating.

In general, self-injuring persons who do *not* use a tool are suffering from a more primitive level of disturbance. Persons who hit themselves with their fists, gouge themselves with their fingernails, or bite themselves with their teeth are often in more impulsive, explosive states than those who use an implement. People experiencing psychotic decompensation or those with significant intellectual disability often hurt themselves repetitively by using only their fists, fingers, or teeth. The absence of a tool can point to problems of biological origin that must be diagnosed and addressed.

However, I have also worked with clients who have never used tools but have been very high-functioning. These were individuals who had families and successful careers, yet they picked their bodies frequently, resulting in multiple small wounds in diverse areas. A special challenge for these individuals in trying to stop self-injuring was that they couldn't discard their "tools"; their fingers were always with them. They especially struggled during the summer months, as they had more skin exposed. Their level of disturbance was not substantial, but their recovery was prolonged and involved numerous relapses.

Persons who employ razor blades, small knives, or burning cigarettes are generally in more precise control of the damage they inflict. The same is true for those who use paper clips, pocket knives, and the hot metallic ends of butane lighters. Still, there are so many exceptions to this rule of thumb that it can be considered no more than tentative. The examples provided below are "exceptions to the rule" about the use of tools, in three different ways: (1) non-use of a tool due to environmental factors; (2) non-use of a tool, with only precise, modest damage inflicted; and (3) use of a tool in an impulsive, out-of-control way.

Gustav had a long history of cutting himself. It was his only mode of self-harm when he was living in the community. However, when he was hospitalized for mania or suicidal impulses, he sometimes resorted to hitting himself. Gustav stated that in the hospital there was tight security, and blades were unavailable to him. He did not prefer to hit himself, but when the tension built up, "something had to give."

Tina used only her fingers to extract hair from her head. For several months, her hair pulling resulted in multiple bald spots that were disfiguring. Tina never used a tool to extract hair or to harm herself in any other way.

Angela, an eighth-grade student in regular education, became so enraged in class one day that she took sharp-pointed scissors from her desk and began assaulting her legs with high-arcing blows. The tips of the scissors penetrated her clothing and made wounds in her thighs that required suturing. Angela ended up hospitalized for her self-harm.

The *type* of tool also conveys important information about the mindset of the self-injurer or the environment in which he or she lives. For example, use of a very sharp X-ACTO knife suggests a different state of mind than employing a burning cigarette does. Use of a paper clip to inflict superficial scratches is very different from employing the tip of a meat cleaver to inflict the very same wounds. A paper clip has little potential to inflict massive self-harm at a later date, whereas the cleaver has considerable potential. Questions about the selection of a particular tool can provide all kinds of amplifications that aid the treatment and move it to a different level of specificity.

Room or Place of the Self-Injury

"Room or place of the self-injury" is defined as the physical space in which the self-injury occurs. Most people perform acts of self-injury indoors. The most common location reported is within a person's private space, usually a bedroom. Those who share a bedroom with a sibling, roommate, spouse, or partner may select a bathroom as an alternative private space to self-injure. Others choose a basement or garage as a preferred location. The key issue for most persons is finding a space where they are unlikely to be interrupted during the self-injury episode.

Whereas most individuals prefer privacy, others do not care and take few precautions to prevent discovery during the episode of self-injury. Obtaining information regarding place is important, because it provides some information about a client's social connectedness. In some cases, a self-injuring person may do little to prevent discovery because he or she has ceased caring what others think. Other people may prefer to be discovered; their behavior has a communicative function, and these individuals want the interpersonal message to be delivered.

It is useful to ask self-injuring persons *where* they self-injure and *why* they selected that location. Often the explanation is a matter of pragmatics, but the place may have other significance, as evidenced in the following two vignettes:

Stacy said, "I usually cut myself at school, which is why I don't cut myself much during the summer. I hate school. All the pressure about grades, all the cliques, all the worrying about what to wear, the loud jokes, the stupid, loud guys trying to outdo each other with their sarcastic putdowns. Most days it feels like the most negative pressure pot in the world. I go into the girls' room, lock the door in my favorite stall (can you believe I have a favorite?!), and cut away. I get really upset if somebody's in my stall. How dare they! I wait until they come out and give them a really dirty look."

Joseph preferred to harm himself outside, usually deep in the woods. He stated, "I usually burn or scratch myself behind my family's barn. I go far away where it's peaceful and quiet. When I hurt myself, I get quiet inside, just like it is on the outside. Then I tend to feel good for a while. It's my one peaceful place."

Social Context

"Social context" is defined as whether a person self-injures alone or with other persons. This detail often says a great deal about the conditions that maintain the individual's self-injurious behavior. The social context of self-injury can be viewed as occurring within six categories:

1. Persons who self-injure alone and keep it secret from all others
2. Persons who self-injure alone and disclose it to a few others
3. Persons who self-injure alone and disclose it to most others
4. Persons who self-injure with others and keep it secret from all others
5. Persons who self-injure with others and disclose it to a few others
6. Persons who self-injure with others and disclose it to most others

The majority of people appear to fall into category 2. These are individuals for whom the self-injury has primarily a tension-reducing function; they are concerned about the social repercussions of disclosing the behavior and are very selective to whom they disclose. They also have some normative social ties and are not part of a social network that endorses self-harm. They may be adolescents or adults. They tend to have some close friends or intimates who know about their self-injury and attempt to help them overcome it.

As the list above suggests, there are many other variations. Some people keep their self-injuring behavior secret from all others all the time. Hyman (1999) discusses examples of such individuals in her book *Women Living with Self-Injury*. She provides examples of self-injuring women who have concealed their acts from all others for years, including spouses or partners with whom they reside.

For others, the behavior pattern of self-injury is the opposite: Their self-injury only occurs with others, and they choose to disclose this group behavior fully to many other persons who do not self-injure. Persons in categories 4, 5, and 6 tend to participate in active social contagion episodes (discussed at length in Chapter 20).

There is no need to discuss each of the six categories, because the content is self-evident. Suffice it to say that the therapist should assess for social context as an important variable in the self-injury behavior of any individual.

ANTECEDENTS TO THE SELF-INJURY

Having completed the assessment of the details of self-injury, the clinician now turns to the antecedents of the behavior. Once again, the biopsychosocial model includes five dimensions: environmental, biological, cognitive, affective, and behavioral.

Environmental Antecedents

"Environmental antecedents" are defined as events or activities in the environment of the self-injurer that trigger an episode. Some individuals are consistently triggered by external events; others self-injure primarily in response to internal psychological conditions. It is crucially important to determine what, if any, events set the self-injuring sequence in motion. Once identified, these events can be employed as opportunities to practice healthier behaviors in place of the self-injury. External events that clients commonly identify as precipitating self-injury include these:

- Loss or threatened loss of a relationship
- Interpersonal conflict
- Performance pressure
- Frustration about unmet needs
- Social isolation
- Seemingly neutral events that trigger associations with trauma

Loss

It has been noted for decades in the literature on self-injury that loss is a frequent precipitant to self-harm. Loss can take many forms, ranging from the complete and permanent (such as death of a loved one) to the nuanced and subtle (such as an almost imperceptible slight in a relationship). Authors have noted that the histories of self-injuring persons include high rates of parental death, marital separation, or divorce (e.g., Walsh & Rosen, 1988), as well as of adoption (Walsh & Doerfler, 2009). Self-injuring individuals have also experienced high rates of foster home placements, psychiatric hospitalizations, and residential placements, all of which involve multiple moves and relationship disruptions (Walsh & Rosen, 1988). Researchers on self-injury have cited histories of physical and sexual abuse as associated factors (Walsh & Rosen, 1988; Shapiro & Dominiak, 1992; Favazza, 1998). In these cases, the loss takes the form of psychological abandonment and recurrent victimization.

Linehan (1993a) has noted that persons with a diagnosis of BPD may be easily triggered into episodes of emotional dysregulation and may be slow to return to baseline. For these persons, relatively modest forms of loss, such as a disdainful look or a person's failure to return a phone call or text promptly, can be experienced as a deliberate affront or terrifying rejection.

More recently, self-injury has emerged as a major problem in psychologically healthier populations, especially middle school, high school, and college students (see Chapter 4). Often these individuals do *not* have the histories of significant loss and trauma previously reported to be associated with self-injury. They may have not experienced the death of or separation from a significant other, and may have no history of physical or sexual abuse trauma. Nonetheless, these healthier, less traumatized individuals may be exquisitely sensitive to interpersonal slights and use self-injury repeatedly to deal with their psychological pain. In some cases it may be difficult to understand why a seemingly innocuous event is experienced as grievously hurtful, but the old truism applies: "Pain is pain." If a client experiences the playful taunting of peers as an overwhelming humiliation, then it must be responded to with a sense of empathy that is congruent with the client's level of discomfort. The key deficiency in the psychological functioning of these individuals is that they lack self-soothing skills to deal with perceived loss; hence they use self-injury.

Interpersonal Conflict

Many self-injuring persons report harming themselves immediately after a disagreement with a partner, peer, or parent. Their response to this conflict is often an intense rage and a desire to attack. The sequence for these persons can resemble the following:

> Interpersonal conflict → Cognitive interpretation of slight or unfairness → Affective response of rage (or other intense emotion) → Decision to act on rage → Decision to self-injure → Self-injurious behavior

When a client and therapist are able to identify a pattern such as the one above, the therapeutic course can be fairly direct. The client can be helped to reduce the occurrence of self-injury by (1) learning more effective interpersonal negotiation skills (thereby reducing the potential for interpersonal conflict), and (2) learning more effective affect management skills related to anger (thereby reducing the affective dysregulation). Of course, clearly identifying the goals for treatment does not mean that they are easy to accomplish.

Performance Pressure

Other clients cite pressures related to performance as key precipitants to self-injury. Among the most common forms of external pressure related to self-injury are academic demands in middle school, high school, college, or graduate school. Other examples include deadlines or productivity demands at work, athletic competition, preparation for a prom or other big social event, and the like. Individuals who self-injure in response to performance pressure often have perfectionistic expectations for themselves. Uncovering irrational, unhelpful expectations related to performance can lead to productive work in treatment designed to reduce such self-imposed pressure.

Frustration about Unmet Needs

Frustration about unmet needs does not entail loss per se. Rather, it involves expectations that are not fulfilled. One of the most common complaints of adolescents is that they are misunderstood. They convey what they want and subsequently discover that they have not received what they want. This may result in frustration and rage that are subsequently relieved via self-injury. An effective behavior analysis attempts to identify recurrent sources of frustration that precede self-injury. Once again, skills can be targeted to assist clients in becoming more effective in getting what they want and in dealing with frustration when they do not. Cognitive restructuring becomes necessary when the desired goals are unrealistic, grandiose, or based on entitled misconceptions.

Social Isolation

Aloneness is a trigger to self-injury for some clients. These are people who work hard to avoid time alone and become desperately agitated when confronted with isolation. Although this is not the most common pattern, it can be found fairly often in trauma survivors. Such individuals may fear being attacked when alone and take solace in having others around to protect them or at least distract them.

Seemingly Neutral Events

Some individuals are triggered into self-injury by events that seem utterly innocuous to others. A good behavioral analysis of self-injury can identify precipitants that no therapist would expect to find. In such cases, neutral events may have been paired with traumatic circumstances in the past, resulting in conditioned responses to benign antecedents. Here are two examples:

Reanne approached all elevators with great caution. She would scan the entire area to avoid being alone on an elevator with a man. If a man approached the elevator while she was waiting, she would look preoccupied and wait for the next one. However, if a man entered an elevator after she had already traveled a floor or two toward her destination, she would experience great anxiety. Not infrequently, she would cut her body afterward. Reanne stated, "Too many memories of being alone with my father invade my consciousness and need to be cut out."

Beth, described earlier in this chapter, hated it when men made an upward motion with their heads, indicating direction. When she encountered such behavior out in the world, she usually hurt herself within 24 hours. Upward head motions in men reminded her quite powerfully of her abusive father's head gestures from her childhood. These movements indicated her father's ultimatum that they were to go upstairs to have sex. Years later, if Beth saw such a motion in a restaurant or store, she usually would have to leave. She preferred one-story buildings where men were less likely to make such head motions. She was not reactive to similar gestures made by women.

Biological Antecedents

"Biological antecedents" can be both chronic physical problems or vulnerabilities and more immediate physical conditions. As discussed in Chapter 6, a thorough assessment considers biological vulnerabilities that may predispose an individual to self-injury. These can include forms of mental illness thought to have a strong biological component, such as depression, BPD, bipolar disorder, and schizophrenia. Behavioral assessment involves identifying the warning signs associated with such mental illness, in order to work toward the goal of preventing and managing relapse. Many clients cycle in and out of episodes of intense anxiety, sadness, rage, mania, or psychotic decompensation. Once clients are able to acknowledge that they have such vulnerabilities, they can strive to avoid relapse by avoiding or managing key triggers. Some of these triggers are biological. Short-term triggers include fatigue, insomnia, over- or undereating, excessive exercise, and abuse of alcohol or drugs. Other common, more immediate biological triggers include failure to follow prescribed psychotropic medication regimens or abuse of these psychotropic drugs.

Also discussed in Chapter 6 are specific biological vulnerabilities that research has linked to self-injury. These include limbic system dysfunction, diminished serotonin levels, endogenous opioid system factors, and reduced sensitivity to physical pain. Clients with recurrent self-injury should be assessed for the following;

- Emotional dysregulation (which may respond to anticonvulsant medications such as Tegretol or mood stabilizers such as Depakote)
- Depression, anxiety, and impulsive aggression (which may respond to an SSRI or a selective norepinephrine reuptake inhibitor)
- "Addiction" to the release of endogenous opioids associated with self-injury (which may respond to naltrexone)
- Diminished sensitivity to physical pain (for which there is no known pharmacological treatment)

Each of these areas of dysfunction can be an important biological contributor to the recurrence of self-injury. Awareness of these elements allows them to be targeted for treatment, along with environmental and psychological contributors.

Cognitive Antecedents

"Cognitive antecedents" are defined as thoughts and beliefs that trigger episodes of self-injury. In Beck's (2005, 2011) cognitive model, the types of cognitions that precede self-injury include the following:

- Interpretations of external events
- Automatic thoughts
- Intermediate beliefs
- Core beliefs
- Cognitions and other mental activity related to trauma

In performing a behavioral analysis of self-injury, assessing cognitions is centrally important. What people think and believe about their experiences in the world and their internal experiences has much to do with the recurrent pattern of self-injury. Interpretations of events, automatic thoughts, intermediate and core beliefs, and trauma-related cognitions often occur right before acts of self-injury.

Interpretations of Events

The environmental antecedents to self-injury have been discussed earlier. It should be noted here that whatever the external events, it is a person's *interpretation* of them that determines their power and influence. Assessing the interpretation of an event that precedes self-injury adds a client's subjective world to his or her observable world. Some people encounter devastating losses and interpret them benignly; others run into modest challenges and view them as catastrophic. The cognitive mindset of the self-injuring individual determines a great deal about the nature of the coping responses (i.e., positive vs. negative). Unfortunately, many such individuals suffer from the negative cognitive triad characteristic of depression, which involves persistent pessimism about self, world, and future (Rush & Nowels, 1994; Beck, 2005, 2011). The following is an example of an inaccurate, pessimistic interpretation that preceded an act of self-harm:

Liz was at school when she noticed her friends clustering at the side of the dining hall. She perceived them to be looking at her and laughing. Liz assumed that they were ridiculing what she was wearing, as well as her weight. Embarrassed and enraged, Liz left school early, went home, and excoriated several wounds she had inflicted earlier in the week. Only the next day did Liz discover that her friends' conversation had had nothing to do with her.

Assessing interpretations of events and identifying gross distortions are important parts of cognitive assessment.

Automatic Thoughts

"Automatic thoughts" are the most immediate form of thought; they are situation-specific (Beck, 2011). An example of an automatic thought that preceded a client's self-injury is "What my boyfriend said was so unfair, I must cut myself right now!"

Many thoughts become so routinized as to become automatic. A simple analogy is the process of learning to drive a car. At first, driving requires a great deal of self-instruction. Beginning drivers talk to themselves, using self-instructions such as "Okay, now put on the brake," or "Next, put on the left blinker." Eventually these explicit self-instructions fade because the thoughts have become automatic. The thoughts are still operational in some semiconscious manner, but they do not require full attention.

For some individuals, self-injury is so frequent that the thoughts that precede the acts have become automatic. Thoughts such as "This is too much to bear," "I need to find my blade," or "Only cutting will do the job" become so commonplace as to be essentially out of consciousness.

The task for the clinician assessing self-injury is to bring such automatic cognitions back into conscious awareness. Persistent, respectful questioning can identify thoughts that support and immediately precede a self-injuring episode. Recovering these out-of-awareness cognitions is a necessary component of behavior analysis, as in this example:

THERAPIST: So tell me what you were thinking just before you burned your leg.

CLIENT: I wasn't thinking anything. It just happened.

THERAPIST: Well, maybe there were some steps that happened so fast, you weren't aware of them.

CLIENT: I don't think so.

THERAPIST: You mentioned that you hung up the phone feeling frustrated after talking to your boyfriend.

CLIENT: (*sarcastically*) Don't I always?

THERAPIST: Did anything pass through your mind before you hurt yourself?

CLIENT: No, I just did it.

THERAPIST: Let's break it down into small steps. As you were walking from the phone to your room, did you have anything on your mind at all about your boyfriend?

CLIENT: Now that you mention it, I was thinking, "He's going to break up with me again."

THERAPIST: And what did you think about that?

CLIENT: I guess I thought it sucked and he sucked and life sucks, and that I might as well hurt myself, because what's the use?

Intermediate Beliefs

"Intermediate beliefs" include attitudes, rules, and assumptions that are fundamental to an individual's thought process (Beck, 2005, 2011).

Intermediate beliefs serve as linkages between automatic thoughts and core beliefs. Examples of intermediate beliefs that precede self-injury include (1) the attitude "I deserve this pain," (2) the rule "Cutting myself relieves distress better than anything else," and (3) the assumption "It will always be this way."

Core Beliefs

"Core beliefs" are persistent convictions about self, world, and future. As Beck (2011) has indicated, core beliefs tend to be global, firmly held, and not easily revised. They are often derived from patterns of affirmation and support (or lack thereof) that individuals experienced in childhood. An example of a core belief shared by a chronically self-injuring client is "I'm an unlovable loser."

Many self-injuring persons are prone to excessively negative self-evaluations. Linehan (1993a) considers this problem to be so central to treating BPD that she includes being "nonjudgmental" as one of six components of mindfulness training. For many self-injuring individuals, their thoughts involve recurrent, exaggerated self-criticism. These self-statements may be chronic, pessimistic, and brutally self-denigrating.

One useful way to elicit such negative judgments is to ask clients to share "favorite ways of putting themselves down." Many clients respond immediately with an extensive list of critical self-statements. The rapidity with which they rattle off these negative thoughts and judgments points to the frequency of their occurrence and the conviction with which they are held. The following excerpt from a transcript of a skills training group illustrates the sharing of "favorite" negative core beliefs:

> GROUP LEADER: Since we're talking about being judgmental today, I'm wondering if any of you have favorite ways of putting yourselves down? (*Four of seven members nod enthusiastically or say things like "Oh, yeah!"*) Okay, well, these may be important. Who would be willing to share one of these putdowns?
>
> MEMBER 1: (*with conviction and disgust*) I call myself a baby.
>
> GROUP LEADER: A baby? What do you mean by that?
>
> MEMBER 1: Because I'm immature, can't do anything. I'm anxious all the time. I just can't handle anything.
>
> GROUP LEADER: All those putdowns sound like quite a burden to be carrying around. Remember those, okay? Who else would be willing to share theirs?

MEMBER 2: I'm always saying to myself how fat, ugly, and stupid-looking I am!

MEMBER 3: (*to Member 2*) You think *you're* fat? Look at me. I'm a pig, plus I also call myself a loser.

MEMBER 4: My favorite way of putting myself down is to say, "You're a burden to society. You don't deserve to live!"

GROUP LEADER: Well, I guess we have some excellent examples of being judgmental here. Let's get to work on the skill of letting go of these judgments.

Cognitions and Other Forms of Mental Activity Related to Trauma

"Trauma-related cognitions" are thoughts, images, flashbacks, memories, and dreams derived from trauma that precede acts of self-harm. These various forms of mental activity are especially challenging, because clients often experience them as being entirely out of their control. Persons with trauma histories report experiencing flashbacks at any time during waking hours and may also report intrusive trauma-linked nightmares during sleep. It is no wonder that trauma survivors feel anguished that their histories may revisit them at any moment. Also complicating the picture is that these mental activities can take so many forms, including visual images, tactile sensations, odors, sounds, flashback dialogues, and so on.

Assessing these forms of cognitive antecedents to self-injury has to be done skillfully, because a client has to be ready to do detailed disclosure work related to trauma. Knowing when to proceed with trauma resolution work is discussed in Chapter 16. If the client is not ready, probing for details may be too much for him or her to handle, and may in fact cause the self-injury to worsen. If the clinician notices any escalating pattern of self-harm in the client, he or she should evaluate whether the behavioral analysis is inadvertently playing a role in the exacerbation. Retreating from such probing may be necessary until the client has acquired the skills necessary to discuss trauma in detail. In such cases, the clinician may have to confine analysis of cognitive antecedents to interpretations of events, automatic self-statements, and intermediate and core beliefs related to self-injury.

This topic of cognitive antecedents to self-injury is discussed in considerably more detail in Chapter 12, which is devoted to cognitive treatment.

Affective Antecedents

"Affective antecedents" are the emotions experienced prior to self-injury. In some cases, these emotions can build for an extended period of time, even several days; in others, the emotions flash in an instant. For most persons, the primary function of self-injury is to reduce the intensity of these painful emotions. Brown (1998) has provided a thorough review of reports that link negative emotions with self-injury. Almost any conceivable negative emotion has been identified as precipitating self-injury, but the primary ones noted by Brown are these:

- Anxiety, tension, or panic
- Anger
- Sadness or depression
- Shame
- Guilt
- Frustration
- Contempt

I have also heard self-injuring persons refer to fear, worry, embarrassment, disgust, and excitement as preceding their self-harm, although these are not cited in the literature.

A smaller proportion of people self-injure in order to rid themselves of feeling too *little* emotion. These are the individuals who report feeling "dead," "empty," "like a robot," or "like a zombie." The self-injuring is comforting for these people because it restores a sense of being alive, as in this example:

A client stated, "Yesterday when I cut, I was feeling nothing. I was feeling absolutely dead inside. I went to the mirror to see if I still looked the same. I thought I might have turned into a machine or something. But there I was—same old shitty me. When I cut myself, I felt so much better. The blood really helped. I looked down at my arm and saw the blood and realized I was still alive, even though I felt nothing."

Identifying the emotions that precede self-injury is important, because the primary motivation for the behavior is reducing unpleasant feelings. Sometimes clients have difficulty identifying specific emotions. The best they can do is to indicate that they are experiencing an intense generalized discomfort. For these persons, a list of emotions such as that provided by Linehan (1993b, pp. 139–152) can be helpful. For younger clients or those with intellectual challenges, a chart with faces and accompanying emotion names can facilitate identifying key emotional antecedents.

Another important consideration is to evaluate whether particular forms of self-injury are tied to specific emotions. For example, some clients tend to cut themselves when they are anxious but burn themselves when they are enraged. For others, the emotional antecedents to cutting versus burning are the exact opposite. An important question can be "Are there specific emotions tied to specific forms of self-injury for you?" A relevant follow-up question is "Is this link consistent, or does it vary over time?"

Behavioral Antecedents

"Behavioral antecedents" are defined as observable actions by a self-injuring person that trigger or are associated with episodes of self-injury. These behaviors are key elements in the sequence that culminates in self-injury. For example, some people self-injure only when they are high on marijuana or intoxicated on alcohol. Some tend to cut or burn themselves only after they have made the decision to stop taking their medication, and the psychotropic effects have worn off. Some self-injure after they have consumed a great deal of food and are thinking judgmentally and feeling disgusted with themselves. Still others self-injure immediately after they have behaved in a way that embarrasses them. One client I knew tended to self-injure after masturbating. He found himself unable to resist the impulse to masturbate, but immediately afterward became extremely judgmental and felt shame and disgust about the behavior. The self-injury served to punish him and his body for the "evils" of his masturbation behavior.

Whereas all of these behavioral antecedents have thoughts and feelings that accompany them, the behaviors themselves can be the key element that triggers the self-injury. In many cases, if the therapist does not know the specific behavioral antecedents, the cognitive and affective antecedents will not come to light. Thus it is important for the therapist to learn what the client was *doing* right before self-injury

> THERAPIST: What were you doing right before you opened those wounds?
>
> CLIENT: Lots of stuff. I was racing around.
>
> THERAPIST: Okay, but was there anything you did that seemed to get you going in the direction of hurting yourself?
>
> CLIENT: Hmm (*thinking*). Well, I was getting pretty uptight, so I smoked some grass.
>
> THERAPIST: Do you think that smoking grass plays a role in your hurting yourself?
>
> CLIENT: I don't think so. They both do the same thing for me. They chill me out.
>
> THERAPIST: Well, how often do you think you smoke grass right before you cut yourself or pick at your wounds?

CLIENT: I guess most of the time, actually.

THERAPIST: What do you make of that connection?

CLIENT: I think being stoned makes me brave enough to do it.

THERAPIST: Well, do you want to keep doing it?

CLIENT: That's the big question, isn't it?

CONSEQUENCES OR AFTERMATH OF THE SELF-INJURY

The consequences or aftermath of self-injury can be discussed in terms of the following components:

- Specifics of the psychological relief
- Presence–absence of self-care after the self-injury
- Presence–absence of excoriation after the self-injury
- Presence–absence of communication regarding the self-injury
- Demeanor of the client describing the self-injury
- Social reinforcement

Specifics of the Psychological Relief

The term "specifics of the psychological relief" refers to the alleviation of affective discomfort provided by the self-injury. Although it has been stated repeatedly in this book that the prime reason for self-injury is reduction of affective distress, this element of behavioral analysis should go beyond that insight. The question for this part of assessment is this: What specific type of psychological relief does the self-injury provide? It is helpful if the client can describe exactly how he or she feels after self-injury. The type of relief provided is key, because the positive replacement behaviors to be sought in treatment should "echo" or "mimic" this type of relief. For example, if the client says that self-injury produces feelings of deep relaxation, then self-soothing activities that produce similar feelings should be taught. If the client says that self-injury produces peaceful sleep, then sleep induction techniques may be helpful. If the client says that the self-injury reduces anger to manageable proportions, then a focus on anger management is key. Behavioral analysis must move from the general concept of obtaining relief to the specific details of the *type* of relief.

A helpful question related to analyzing the aftermath of self-injury is this: "After you have self-injured, where in your body do you feel relief?" This question can yield some unexpected answers, as shown in this dialogue with a 22-year-old female client:

THERAPIST: What sort of relief does cutting yourself provide?

CLIENT: It stops the pain.

THERAPIST: Do you mean psychological pain?

CLIENT: Sort of. Different kinds of pain, I guess.

THERAPIST: What are the different kinds?

CLIENT: Well, some of it's physical.

THERAPIST: Where do you feel this physical pain in your body?

CLIENT: (*noticeably uncomfortable*) Right up the middle of it.

THERAPIST: Starting where?

CLIENT: (*pointing*) Down there.

THERAPIST: Are you pointing to your genitals?

CLIENT: (*embarrassed*) Yes.

THERAPIST: Are you saying that you have pain in your genitals, and that cutting your arms relieves that?

CLIENT: (*showing some relief*) Yes.

This dialogue led to a disclosure of sexual abuse that involved her father's digitally penetrating her vagina. This abuse—which had occurred about 10 years earlier and lasted for 2 years—caused her not only great shame and rage, but also considerable physical pain. Years later, when she experienced pain in her genitals as a trauma-related symptom, she cut herself. Cutting immediately relieved both the physical pain and the emotions of shame and rage related to the abuse.

Presence–Absence of Self-Care after Self-Injury

"Presence–absence of self-care after self-injury" refers to whether or not the client cares for wounds after acts of self-harm. Many clients take at least basic precautions to ensure that their wounds do not become infected. They keep the wounds clean and may apply an antiseptic salve and bandage, if necessary. Therapists should be reassured when clients take care to prevent their wounds from becoming infected.

However, other clients provide little self-care to wounds or may even deliberately attempt to induce infection. For these individuals, the lack of care to wounds after self-injury may represent an extension of the self-harm episode, as in this example:

Naomi, described in Chapter 5, was a 16-year-old who had a 3-year history of cutting her wrists, arms and legs. On one occasion when she was especially agitated, she pierced one of her nipples. She did this without sterilizing the needle she employed to make the hole. In addition, she made no attempt to treat her nipple with antiseptic salve after the piercing. Eventually, her piercing came to the attention of the nurse in the group home where she resided. The nurse discovered that Naomi had developed an infection in her nipple due to the absence of self-care.

There are multiple aspects to the self-injury episode in a case such as Naomi's: (1) failure to use sterile procedures, (2) harming a body area deemed atypical and alarming, and (3) failure to use self-care after the self-injury. These details, in combination, point to an intense level of distress that requires assessment for psychiatric hospitalization/diversion.

Presence–Absence of Excoriation after the Self-Injury

"Presence–absence of excoriation after the self-injury" refers to whether or not the client deliberately reopens wounds after self-injury. Failure to care for wounds is a passive form of self-injury; excoriation is an active form. There may be symbolic meanings for clients who reopen the same wound time after time. What is striking is that self-injuring people always have the option of moving on to a different, unharmed body area (even if it is only centimeters away); yet some reopen the same wounds repeatedly. In such cases, the therapist needs to explore the meaning of these repetitions. Is the message one of unfinished business, unresolved probings, or the need to go deeper? The answer is different for each individual and always important to assess.

Presence–Absence of Communication Regarding the Self-Injury

"Presence–absence of communication regarding the self-injury" refers to whether or not the individual chooses to inform others of the self-injury after the act. This detail is an important one in determining whether the behavior is essentially intrapersonally motivated, or (at least in part) is intended to have an interpersonal communicative function. As stated above in the section on social context, the majority of self-injuring persons harm themselves when alone but disclose the self-harm to a small number of people thereafter. For adolescents, these confidants are usually peers. Eventually, the parents or caregivers of these adolescents tend to find out about the self-injury, but the disclosure is usually delayed and/or quasi-accidental. For adults, the confidants are friends, partners, or psychological caregivers.

For all but the most secretive of self-injuring persons, the behavior has a communicative function. First and foremost, the behavior may be driven by internal psychological distress, but it may also be intended secondarily to speak to others. The job of the therapist is to discover (1) the intended recipient of the self-injurious message, and (2) the content of the message. An example of two such communicative functions of self-injury is provided in the following vignette:

Amelia's message in the form of self-injury was delivered with aggressiveness. Her pattern was to cut jagged wounds into both arms, using razor blades. Afterward, Amelia made no attempt to conceal the wounds. Rather, she wore short-sleeved shirts at home and school. The message to her parents was that she was in intense emotional pain. When her parents ignored the wounds, dismissing her as "just doing it for attention," Amelia cut deeper and more often. Amelia's message to her parents was one of rageful unhappiness and an appeal for help.

Amelia's self-injury had a different communicative function at school, where she had been belittled and ridiculed for years. Asked why she made no attempt to conceal her wounds at school, she stated that she didn't care if they called her "freak" or "psycho." Amelia was beyond social connectedness in her school setting. The exhibition of her wounds conveyed a defiant and vengeful message.

Often the intended recipient of the self-injurious message is someone in the day-to-day life of the client. However, a therapist can also become the intended recipient. In such cases, the therapist may be unintentionally reinforcing the behavior. When this occurs, the therapist needs to perform behavioral analysis on his or her own actions.

Inge disclosed in therapy that she sometimes cut herself right before coming for a session. She stated that the therapist appeared to like talking about self-injury, and she wanted to make sure she "wasn't boring." In response to this disclosure, the therapist indicated that he liked talking about many issues with Inge, not just self-injury. He also deliberately muted his response to Inge's discussion of self-injury for several sessions thereafter.

Demeanor of the Client Describing the Self-Injury

"Demeanor of the client describing the self-injury" refers to the behavior of the self-injuring person when describing or exhibiting the wounds. This demeanor conveys a great deal of information about the client's motivation to stop, or at least reduce, the frequency of the behavior. Some clients express remorse that they have lapsed into self-injury again; others are bland about having committed the act, considering it a routine and entirely unavoidable action; still others are openly defiant of external disapproval, clearly indicating a commitment to continuing. The best advice for the clinician is to put aside assumptions and listen to each self-injuring person with great care. Asking the client how he or she feels about a particular wound or episode can be quite illuminating. The following is an example of an unexpected disclosure from a self-injuring person:

Betsy was a 13-year-old who had been self-injuring for 6 months. In the course of the second interview, the therapist asked to see the wounds on her arm. She complied quite agreeably. After she rolled up the long sleeve on her left arm, two types of scars became visible: a series of five or six finely executed parallel scars on the forearm, and four or five random, jagged, discolored wounds inside her elbow. The therapist commented that there seemed to be two types of wounds on her arm. She responded, "When I'm really nervous I cut myself, but when I'm really angry, I gouge myself with my fingernails."

As Betsy was saying these words, the therapist noticed her looking at her wounds with a beatific smile on her face. Curious about this seemingly incongruous response, the therapist asked her what she thought of when she looked at her scars. She said, "To me, they're beautiful. They remind of everything I've learned from all the pain in my life."

Social Reinforcement

"Social reinforcement" refers to behavior on the part of others that increases the likelihood of self-injury's recurring. Any sort of attentional response to self-injury may reinforce the behavior. Social reinforcement can be intentional or unintentional. If a peer says to a self-injuring adolescent, "Oh, those cuts look so cool!", the social reinforcement is direct and intentional. However, unintentional reinforcement can be just as powerful, such as when people are very supportive or condemning of self-injurious acts. This is why my recommendation in Chapter 7 is to use a low-key, dispassionate demeanor in responding to self-injury. The strategy is to be compassionate, but to try to avoid inadvertent social reinforcement.

It is important to emphasize that obtaining social reinforcement is rarely the primary motivation for self-injury. However, the social responses of others can be important *secondary* motivators. Almost all self-injurious behavior requires some measure of psychological distress. People do not self-injure "just to get attention." Although this argument is frequently proposed, it is specious. People may self-injure because it meets their internal psychological needs *and* it is socially reinforced, but they are unlikely to self-injure for the interpersonal "rewards" alone. There are too many other methods available to "get attention from others" to justify self-injury as a means to that end.

A thorough analysis of self-injury focuses on the reactions of everyone in the person's environment, including peers, partners, spouses, fellow students, coworkers, siblings, parents, teachers, supervisors, other therapists, and so on. Those who inadvertently reinforce the behavior may need to become part of the treatment; they need to be educated in the basic management of self-injury, as presented in Chapter 7. They need to become allies in the treatment if the effort to reduce and terminate self-injury is to be successful.

PRIORITIZING ELEMENTS WITHIN THE ASSESSMENT

The first step in performing an assessment of self-injury is to ask the client to complete the Self-Injury Log between sessions for multiple weeks. This step in the assessment process considers the entire field of environmental, biological, and psychological events associated with self-injury. It takes a broad approach and does not initially assign priority to any particular events.

A second step involves asking the client to complete a Brief Self-Injury Log, as shown in Figure 9.2. This log is a concise version of the full log in Figure 9.1, but it adds the component of prioritization. I ask clients to shift

Name: _____

Dimension	Antecedents	SIB events	Aftermath
Environmental			
Biological			
Cognitive			
Affective			
Behavioral			

Rank-order in each column the item that had the strongest role in producing or reinforcing the self-injury: 1 = most important; 2 = very important; 3 = moderately important; 4 = somewhat important; 5 = least important.

FIGURE 9.2. Brief Self-Injury Log.

to using the Brief Self-Injury Log only after a thorough assessment has been conducted and a reliable baseline has been obtained. Although individual practice varies widely, it is not unusual to switch to using the Brief Self-Injury Log after 8–10 sessions.

The language used in the Brief Self-Injury Log is identical to that used in the full log, in that it refers to antecedents, events associated with self-injury, and aftermath. For younger or more intellectually challenged clients, the language can be changed to something simpler, such as "triggers," "behaviors," and "results."

The brief log allows the client and clinician to prioritize components on a scale of 1–5. This prioritization can be done by the client alone, the clinician alone, or both in collaboration. At the outset, a collaborative approach is generally the recommended course. Later the client can assume sole responsibility for its completion. Use of the Brief Self-Injury Log ensures that treatment focuses initially on the primary elements that precipitate self-injury. Later the treatment moves to less important items that are nonetheless contributors.

Figure 9.3 shows how the Brief Self-Injury Log has been completed for a hypothetical case. In this case, under "Antecedents" the client has identified the top two priorities as (1) fighting with a peer in school and (2) feeling sad, empty, and panicked. Treatment therefore might well target reducing peer conflicts and improving social skills, as well as teaching emotion regulation and self-soothing skills.

In a similar vein, under "SIB Events" the client has prioritized (1) the excitement of anticipating self-injury and (2) the insistent thought of "I have to do this." Treatment might thus prioritize learning to endure or reduce these anticipatory feelings and cognitively restructuring the maladaptive thought.

Under "Aftermath" the client has prioritized (1) the feelings of calmness and relief and (2) the thought "I deserved that!" Treatment would prioritize teaching the client alternative self-soothing skills and restructuring thoughts regarding self-punishment and self-blame.

This simple assessment tool can be used on a continuing basis. It is dropped only when the client has ceased self-injuring for extended periods. When a relapse occurs, the clinician must decide whether to reinstitute the full or brief version of the log as the preferred assessment tool.

CONCLUSION

In summary, in the assessment of self-injury, it is generally most helpful if clinicians and others do the following:

Name: <u>16-year-old female</u>

Dimension	Antecedents	SIB events	Aftermath
Environmental	Fight with a peer at school 1	Looked for blade hidden in bedroom 4	No consequences at first; alone in bedroom 5
Biological	Already overtired; not high 5	Still overtired; headache starting 5	Headache gone; slept better later 4
Cognitive	"I'm all alone; I have no friends." 3	"I have to do this!" 2	"I deserved that! Phew!" 2
Affective	Felt sad, empty, panicked 2	Excited, feelings of anticipation 1	Felt much calmer; obtained relief 1
Behavioral	Retreated to bedroom; intentionally isolated self 4	Cut forearm four times, causing tissue damage without need for first aid 3	Washed cuts; applied Band-Aid; later was able to do homework 3

Rank-order in each column the item that had the strongest role in producing or reinforcing the self-injury: 1 = most important; 2 = very important; 3 = moderately important; 4 = somewhat important; 5 = least important.

FIGURE 9.3. Example of a completed Brief Self-Injury Log.

- Use a Self-Injury Log to collect information systematically, if possible.
- Be especially attentive to extent of physical damage and body area(s) affected.
- Identify idiosyncratic details about the self-injury, such as number of wounds, use of patterns or symbols, use of a tool, and physical location.
- Identify recurrent environmental, cognitive, affective, and behavioral antecedents to the self-injury.
- Identify consequences of the self-injury, such as emotional relief.
- Be alert for social reinforcers in the environment.
- With the client's assistance, identify the most important variables in triggering and maintaining the self-injury, and target these in treatment.

CHAPTER 10

Contingency Management

After a baseline assessment has been obtained, the first level of intervention in treating self-injury is "contingency management"—that is, either the informal or systematic dispensing of reinforcement in relation to self-injury. Managing informal reinforcement of self-injury has already been discussed in Chapter 7, where I have recommended employing a low-key, dispassionate demeanor along with respectful curiosity in responding to self-injury. As a treatment intervention, formal contingency management is useful in reducing the frequency of self-injury, but it is unlikely to eliminate the behavior. One advantage of contingency management is that it can be used with clients who are unmotivated to stop self-injuring. In these instances, the focus is on analyzing and modifying the environmental conditions that support the behavior.

Oddly, sometimes the mere activity of collecting baseline data in preparation for contingency management can result in a reduction or extinction of the behavior. This has been referred to as the "reactivity effect" (O'Leary & Wilson, 1987, p. 27). Consider this example:

Several years ago I worked with a client who had multiple problems with self-harm behaviors. She frequently lacerated her arms, legs, and abdomen. In addition, she was involved in daily hair pulling (trichotillomania), which produced multiple disfiguring bald spots on her head and related wounds from persistent skin picking on her scalp. This client also presented with a variety of indirect forms of self-harm, such as medication discontinuance, risk-taking behavior, and peer relationships in which she was exploited and disrespected. Having conducted an assessment of her forms of direct and indirect self-harm, I asked her which of these problems she wanted to address first, and she said the hair pulling. She explained that it caused her the most embarrassment socially, and therefore she wanted to stop it.

Given this preference, we began collecting baseline data regarding her hair pulling. I employed the Keuthen, Stein, and Christenson (2001) protocol for charting daily hair removal. This involved asking the client to count as precisely as possible and record on a simple chart the number of hairs she removed from her head each day. Despite being quite disorganized in many aspects of her daily life, the client was remarkably consistent in responding to this request. Over a 3-week period, she never failed to record the number of hairs she had removed. The counts ranged from 0 to 360 hairs per day, with a mean of about 185.

At the conclusion of this period, the client announced to a surprised therapist that she was no longer removing her hair. She explained that the data collection had been so annoying and time-consuming that it was "no longer worth the trouble." This cessation of hair pulling continued for months afterward and, to my knowledge, has not recurred. Also worth noting is that there was no evidence that her other self-destructive behaviors increased during the hair-pulling data collection period.

Why was the act of data collection effective in eliminating this client's hair-pulling behavior? There are several possible answers:

1. The data collection was aversive, and she stopped the hair pulling because of negative reinforcement.
2. The data collection was a recurrent, time-consuming activity that was both different and dramatic enough to interrupt a chronic pattern.
3. The client was already motivated to stop the behavior, and the data collection might have distracted her from hair pulling or allowed her to self-soothe in other ways; the counting itself might have been somewhat self-soothing.
4. There might have been other factors beyond my knowledge that influenced her, such as additional pressure from peers regarding her appearance.

I experienced a similar reactivity effect in doing baseline data collection with a 17-year-old male who presented with encopresis. Although this behavior was a form of *indirect* self-harm for this young man, rather than self-injury, the case is still relevant as an example of the therapeutic effect of assessment per se. In this case, the data collection was informal (as opposed to quantitative) and involved only one session—which made the result especially surprising. This young man, despite having an IQ of 140, had an extensive problem with soiling himself and either walking about with feces in his pants for extended periods of time or storing his soiled underwear in family bureaus, closets, school lockers, or the like. Not surprisingly, this behavior caused him to be shunned in any setting where it occurred. It also caused some mild tissue damage to his buttocks.

I conducted my preliminary assessment interview of the youth with his parents present. The assessment consisted of asking the client a series of very detailed questions about the soiling behavior. The progression of questions included the following:

"How often do you store soiled underwear in your parents' house?"

"How often do you store soiled underwear on school property?"

"How do you decide when to walk about with feces in your pants, as opposed to using the toilet?"

"Please describe the physical sensation of having feces in your pants. Is it uncomfortable? Pleasant? Neutral?"

"Are you aware of the feces all the time or every so often?"

"Are you aware of any odor?"

"Does the looseness or firmness of the stool affect whether you decide to keep the feces on your person?"

"Are there types of feces you prefer?"

I continued in this vein for 40 minutes or more, careful to employ a low-key, dispassionate demeanor. I believe I came across as nonjudgmental and respectful, as well as intensely curious. That the client was becoming ever more uncomfortable was quite evident during this series of questions. I noticed him increasingly squirming in his seat and beginning to sweat on his forehead. I wanted to spare him discomfort, but also felt that completing the assessment was important. He had suffered from his encopresis problem for years and had spent months in psychiatric hospitals because of it. What was remarkable about the interview was that after its conclusion, he never soiled himself again.

Although many other explanations for this cessation are possible, I believe that the assessment process played a key role. Somehow, the detailed questioning interrupted a chronic, self-destructive pattern. Clinicians therefore should be alert to the possibility of a reactivity effect derived from baseline data collection—and although dramatic cessation of self-harm behaviors during the assessment process is rare, subtler changes in behavior are quite common.

CONTINGENCY MANAGEMENT CONTRACTS

The far more typical experience is for baseline data collection to yield valuable information but no immediate therapeutic effect. Baseline data can be used to construct simple contingency management contracts designed to reduce the frequency of the self-injury. I find that generally at least 4–5 weeks are necessary to collect adequate baseline data. However, for clients who self-injure infrequently, such as every 3 months, a much more extended time period may be needed. For clients who self-injure very infrequently (e.g., every 6 months), behavioral contracting is unlikely to be helpful. In such cases, reducing the frequency of the behavior is more likely to require cognitive restructuring and replacement skills training than contingency management. The baseline frequency is just too modest to target reduction as a primary treatment goal.

For clients with a high rate of self-injury, a baseline of a few weeks can be quite adequate. As described in Chapter 9, the therapist and client should begin by using a Self-Injury Log. After detailed baseline data have been obtained, they can shift to using the Brief Self-Injury Log. The client and the therapist are then in a good position to construct a simple Self-Protection Contract. I prefer the term "Self-Protection Contract" to "Self-Injury Contract" because it is worded positively. Moreover, the same contract can be used later to target other self-destructive and self-defeating behaviors.

The basic principle in using a Self-Protection Contract is for the client to commit to *reducing* the frequency of the behavior. The goal need not be extinction of the behavior at the outset. Note that I am not talking about "contracting for safety," which is a very different strategy that is discussed below. A Self-Protection Contract should have at least the following elements:

1. Quantitative baseline data
2. A clearly stated, measurable goal
3. Identification of needed replacement skills
4. Identification of a reward if the goal is reached
5. A "hold harmless" statement if the goal is not reached
6. Commitment statement involving signature, witness, date, and time period

An example of a simple Self-Protection Contract for a 33-year-old recurrently self-injuring female client is provided in Figure 10.1. A blank version of this contract is provided in Figure 10.2.

Note that the contract depicted in Figure 10.1 is very individualized, using recent baseline data and a measurable goal. The contract identifies self-soothing and distraction skills that the client has previously noted as useful in fending off self-injury. In addition, the contract is a written document that makes the commitment of the client and therapist both formal and concrete. It is also a short-term agreement (1 week) that rewards the client if she is successful and holds the client harmless if she is not. Why is it important to hold the client harmless? A client who is punished for disclosing self-injury may choose to hide self-harm thereafter. This risk is discussed more extensively in the section below on contracting for safety.

Baseline data (frequency of self-injury): My rate of self-injury over the past 4 weeks has been an average of 3 episodes per week with 3 to 8 cuts per episode.

Goal (reduced frequency of self-injury): I agree to attempt to reduce the frequency of my cutting over the coming week to 1 time per week with 2 to 3 cuts per episode.

Skills to be used in place of self-injury: In order to do so, I commit to using the following self-soothing or distraction skills when I feel angry or anxious:

1. Listening to music
2. Patting my cat
3. Calling my friend Sam
4. Listening to my relaxation tape

Reward for reaching goal: If I am able to fulfill this contract, I will treat myself to a new haircut. If I am not able to fulfill the contract, there is no penalty.

Commitment:

Signature: _____

Witness (therapist, counselor, etc.): _____

Date: _____

For the time period of _____ to _____

FIGURE 10.1. Example of a completed Self-Protection Contract for a 33-year-old female.

Another example of a Self-Protection Contract was used with an adolescent client residing in a group home (see Figure 10.3). This 16-year-old male had been in residential treatment for 3 months. He was placed in the program because of violence toward others, destruction of property, and recurrent self-injury (burning, cutting, self-inflicted tattoos). Other contracts and treatment strategies were used to target his aggression, and the residential staff developed the contract in Figure 10.3 with him to address his recurrent self-injury. This client was quite adept at obtaining tools and self-injuring despite close staff supervision.

In this case the goal was more ambitious (only one episode of self-injury), because the client had been in treatment for 3 months and had learned and practiced many replacement skills. All the other elements of the Self-Protection Contract are the same as those in Figure 10.1, including the

Baseline data (frequency of self-injury):

Goal (reduced frequency of self-injury):

Skills to be used in place of self-injury:

1.

2.

3.

4.

Reward for reaching goal:

Commitment:

Signature: _____

Witness (therapist, counselor, etc.): _____

Date: _____

For the time period of _____ to _____

FIGURE 10.2. Self-Protection Contract.

"hold harmless" provision—which is unusual in most residential treatment settings. Note that Chapter 18 of this volume provides a detailed discussion of such residential treatment.

CONTRACTING FOR SAFETY WITH SELF-INJURY

A common question is whether to use contracting for safety in responding to self-injury. This strategy usually takes the form of obtaining commitment from a client to refrain from self-injuring for a given period of time, such as a day or week. Using Safety Contracts for self-injury is a common strategy in

Baseline data: My rate of self-injury over the past 3 months has been 3 episodes per week with 2 to 4 burns or 4 to 6 cuts per episode (no tattoos).

Goal: I agree to attempt to reduce the frequency of my self-injury over the coming week to 1 episode.

Skills: In order to do so, I commit to using the following self-soothing or distraction skills when I feel angry or depressed

1. Lifting weights
2. Talking with my residential counselor, Jim
3. Practicing deep breathing
4. Listening to nonviolent music

Reward: If I am able to fulfill this contract, I will be eligible for a pass from the program without staff supervision. (I must also be on the proper level in the program.) If I am not able to fulfill the contract, I will not be dropped a level unless my level of self-harm requires medical intervention.

Commitment: [same as in Figure 10.1]

FIGURE 10.3. Example of a completed Self-Protection Contract for a 16-year-old male.

many settings, such as outpatient clinics, psychiatric emergency rooms, and group homes. The purposes of Safety Contracts are generally (1) to attempt to prevent the behavior from recurring, and (2) to protect the professional from liability should subsequent self-harm occur. As noted by Shea (1999), Safety Contracts may *not* do a very good job of accomplishing either purpose. There is little empirical evidence that Safety Contracts serve a deterrent function. Moreover, the protection against liability by having employed a Safety Contract is at best modest (Shea, 1999).

In fact, I generally recommend *against* using Safety Contracts as a strategy to deal with self-injury, because they often have more risks than benefits. The main risk is that contracting for safety often drives the behavior underground by fostering dishonesty. For the most part, clients are unable to stop self-injuring until they have acquired effective replacement skills. Asking them to forgo the behavior before they have incorporated these skills into their repertoire is requesting the near-impossible. The expectation (or demand) is that they endure their usual intense level of emotional distress (or emptiness) without using their preferred management technique. This is generally asking far too much.

Therapists have a tendency to place extensive pressure on clients to stop self-injuring. They may communicate this pressure by offering effusive praise when a client does not self-injure or by expressing disappointment, dismay, frustration, or condemnation when the client has self-injured. Clients react to such pressure by feeling misunderstood, resentful, and like failures; they learn very quickly how to solicit praise and avoid condemnation. They may attempt to please a therapist (or other professional) by saying that they have not self-injured when, in fact, they have. When this kind of deception occurs, the therapeutic alliance is seriously compromised. Clients have learned to avoid negative responses from the therapist, but at the cost of providing accurate information. The therapy may not recover from this setback. A therapy based on misinformation cannot proceed productively.

Another result of therapists' inappropriately using Safety Contracts is that clients drop out of therapy, feeling that they have failed their therapists (and themselves) by not meeting the therapist's expectations. The last thing most self-injuring clients need is another experience with failure. When clients prematurely drop out of therapy, they may be even less likely to seek out treatment in the future. Thus multiple adverse effects can be the result of "forbidding" self-injury too early in treatment.

My general rule of thumb is this: *Do not ask self-injuring clients to give up the behavior before they are ready, unless the behavior involves extensive tissue damage or alarming body areas.* In these cases, Safety Contracts are beside the point. Protective intervention involving inpatient psychiatric care or residential respite services is necessary.

This is not to say that the use of Safety Contracts is *never* indicated. Sometimes clients *ask* to use Safety Contracts, saying that they are helpful in fending off self-injury. When clients makes this request, I am usually willing to develop a Safety Contract with them, making sure to incorporate the features they prefer.

Shea (1999) has provided an invaluable review of safety contracting with suicidal individuals. A number of his suggestions are useful in designing Safety Contracts regarding self-injury as well. He indicates that if a clinician is going to use safety contracting, it should be viewed primarily as an assessment tool as opposed to a preventive intervention. He also suggests that a clinician wishing to develop a valid Safety Contract should look for good eye contact, genuine affect, and a natural and unhesitant tone of voice from the client.

According to Shea, an effective Safety Contract often concludes with a firm handshake and the signing of a formal, written document. Any signs of hesitancy, ambivalence, or deceit should result in the clinician's starting over or abandoning the pursuit of a Safety Contract in favor of other strategies.

One client who used a Safety Contract productively with me was a 29-year-old woman with a long history of self-injury. She requested that I develop a Safety Contract with her, saying that it had previously helped in other therapy. She wrote the Safety Contract shown in Figure 10.4, which I agreed to witness and sign.

Although this contract did not include all the elements I like to see in a Self-Protection Contract, I still accepted it because the client wanted to design her own vehicle. The client subsequently stated that the contract was quite helpful in decreasing her self-injury. She reported that when she had impulses to cut, she gently reminded herself that she had promised herself and me that she would not do so. This prompt was effective in helping her postpone or altogether avoid self-harm. Over time, Safety Contracts, in combination with replacement skills, enabled her to give up self-injury permanently.

With most populations, the most effective contingency management procedure is informal social reinforcement. Many self-injuring clients come from backgrounds of abuse and neglect. They are not used to warm, empathic attention and positive feedback. My strategy is to extend the majority of social reinforcement not on the *absence* of self-injury, but on the *presence* of clients' use of healthy cognitive restructuring techniques and replacement skills. These key areas of treatment are the foci of the next two chapters.

I, _____, have been cutting myself about 2 or 3 times per month recently and want to stop. I realize that cutting indicates disrespect for myself and my body. I want to learn to respect and love myself for who I am. I promise not to cut myself over the next week. I will report on my progress at my next therapy appointment on Wednesday.

Signed: _____   Date: _____

Witness: _____   Time period: _____ to _____

FIGURE 10.4. Safety Contract.

CONCLUSION

In summary, in the contingency management of self-injury, it is generally most helpful if clinicians and others do these things:

- Collect baseline data regarding the frequency of self-injury for several weeks.
- Use Self-Protection Contracts that have clearly stated measurable goals, identify replacement skills to be employed, and specify any rewards to be obtained.
- Include a "hold harmless" statement if the goal is not reached, in order to foster full disclosure.
- Employ a formal commitment statement involving signature, witness, date, and time period.

TREATMENT: STEP 2

CHAPTER 11

Replacement Skills Training

When treatment moves to Step 2 in the stepped-care model (see Figure II.1, p. 75), the interventions become more complex and assertive, because the self-injury to be addressed is more prolonged and challenging. Step 2 interventions are for individuals whose self-injury has not remitted in response to the informal response described in Chapter 7, the assessment strategies reviewed in Chapters 8 and 9, and the contingency management reviewed in Chapter 10. Individuals requiring Step 2 interventions are presenting with common, low-lethality self-injury that is recurrent, thereby requiring more comprehensive, targeted treatment.

The first component of Step 2 in treating self-injury is teaching replacement skills. The therapist's role is to assist the client in identifying skills that will be a good match for that individual, and to convey a sense of urgency about learning and using the skills. The client's role is to select skills carefully with the therapist and to practice them over and over again. Early in treatment, after the assessment has been completed, the therapist and client discuss skill options repeatedly and practice them together during sessions. Once some useful, relevant skills have been identified, the emphasis shifts to the client's using the skills in his or her real-world living environments. Skills need to be practiced at home, school, work, and social settings. Over time the client finds that some skills are not particularly helpful, whereas others are especially effective. The client frequently revises his or her roster of skills as some skills fade in importance and others take prominence. The goal is for the client to develop a core set of skills that can be counted on when really needed.

147

It would be nice to be able to say that considerable empirical support has emerged regarding the effectiveness of a skills training approach to treating self-injury. The reality is that the literature is still in its infancy regarding the effectiveness of skills training. Linehan et al. (1991) and Miller et al. (2007) have demonstrated the effectiveness of dialectical behavior therapy (DBT) in treating self-injury, among other problems. Linehan et al.'s study of adult women with a diagnosis of BPD found that participants receiving DBT had significantly fewer "parasuicidal acts" during the treatment period than participants receiving a "treatment-as-usual" (TAU) control. (In this study, "parasuicide" referred to both suicide attempts and low-lethality self-injury.) Linehan et al. reported that the parasuicidal behavior of participants receiving DBT declined from 100 to about 37% during the 1-year treatment protocol. In contrast, this behavior in the TAU participants declined from 100 to 63%. Thus a statistically significant, positive treatment effect was demonstrated for the participants receiving DBT, although more than a third were still presenting with parasuicidal behavior at the conclusion of treatment.

Comtois (2002) presented a review of interventions designed to reduce parasuicidal behavior. Her conclusion was that only four psychosocial studies have shown a positive impact on parasuicide. One was the previously cited DBT study; another was a study of cognitive-behavioral therapy conducted in England; and the other two were home visit models provided in England and Belgium (where the presenting problems were more suicidal than self-injurious). The DBT and cognitive-behavioral therapy studies shared a focus on problem solving and compliance with treatment protocol. Given this dearth of outcome studies, the field clearly needs much more in the way of empirical research regarding the treatment of self-injury via skills training approaches.

In the meantime, this chapter presents a skills training approach that has been found anecdotally to be helpful in treating self-injury. A skills training approach seems likely to be helpful, in that other skills training interventions have been found to be effective in treating such problems as youth suicidal behavior (Miller, Rathus, Linehan, Wetzler, & Leigh, 1997) and substance abuse (Marlatt & Vandenbos, 1997; Marlatt, 2012).

BEGINNING REPLACEMENT SKILLS TRAINING

Early in treatment, the client especially needs to practice skills when he or she is relatively calm and focused. This rehearsal will enable the client to use the skills at other times when emotional distress is high. The therapist needs to remind the client, "You can't learn to ride a bicycle away from a tornado."

SELECTING THE RIGHT SKILLS

If clients select the right skills and practice them diligently, they are very likely to get better; conversely, if they practice halfheartedly or not at all, their problems with self-injury are likely to continue. This is not to say that individuals cannot recover through other means that do not involve treatment (see Shaw, 2002), but learning replacement skills is the most direct route.

If clients are going to overcome self-injury, they need to acquire skills that manage their emotional distress (or emptiness) *at least as effectively* as self-harm behaviors. Initially, clients may be understandably skeptical that anything will work as well as cutting, burning, excoriation, or whatever their preferred methods may be. The therapist's role is to emphasize how many others have been helped by these skills. The therapist needs to repeat a basic mantra: "Replacement skills have worked for many others, and they will work for you if you find the right skills and practice, practice, practice." (Regarding the crucial importance of practice, see Linehan, 1993b; Segal, Williams, & Teasdale, 2002; and Miller et al., 2007.)

NINE TYPES OF REPLACEMENT SKILLS

Numerous resources review different types of skills that can be used to deal with emotional distress (e.g., Nhat Hanh, 1975, 1991; Davis, Eshelman, & McKay, 1982; Kabat-Zinn, 1990; Levey & Levey, 1991, 1999; Linehan, 1993b; Alderman, 1997; Conterio & Lader, 1998; Segal et al., 2002; Miller et al., 2007). Although there are myriad possibilities, I have found nine different types of skills to be especially useful in treating self-injury. I am not claiming that these are uniquely effective, only stating that they have repeatedly worked with clients. The nine skills are as follows:

1. Negative replacement behaviors
2. Mindful breathing skills
3. Visualization techniques
4. Physical exercise
5. Writing
6. Artistic expression
7. Playing or listening to music
8. Communicating with others
9. Diversion techniques

These are discussed in the order presented.

Negative Replacement Behaviors

A controversial set of skills that some individuals use to fend off impulses to self-injure consists of behaviors that resemble self-injury. Conterio and Lader (personal communication, 2000) have argued against using what they call "negative replacement behaviors," because they believe that such activities are too fraught with associations to self-injury. They contend that negative replacement behaviors are likely to trigger relapse, because they maintain the client's focus on, or preoccupation with, self-harm. They recommend that therapists avoid—or even forbid clients from using—such techniques. Although their concerns are understandable, I have found that many clients use such replacement behaviors productively, at least in the short term. I would certainly agree that no individual should depend on negative replacement behaviors exclusively to eliminate self-injury. However, some clients use negative replacement behaviors early in treatment, because they represent such familiar territory and serve an important *transitional* function. Here are some examples of negative replacement behaviors:

- Marking one's body with a red-colored marker rather than cutting or burning (symbolic representation of wounding, but without tissue damage)
- Applying BenGay or other topical stimulants to a previously self-injured body area (tactile sensation, but without tissue damage)
- Snapping a rubber band on the area of an arm or leg that is usually cut or burned (tactile sensation and a stinging discomfort, but without tissue damage)
- Briefly applying ice or portable cool packs to body areas usually assaulted (physical stimulation and discomfort, but without tissue damage)
- Holding a frozen orange in the hand (same as applying ice/cool packs)
- Applying a temporary tattoo to a portion of the body and scratching it off with a finger nail (tactile stimulation of the area usually harmed, but without tissue damage)
- Gently stroking a previously assaulted body area with a soft cosmetics brush or other soft implement (soothing that which was previously harmed)
- Drawing a picture depicting the self-injury of a body area (visual cues representing self-injury, but without tissue damage)
- Writing about the act of self-injuring in great detail, from start to finish of an episode, without implementing the scenario (beginning

of a transition to verbal mastery, while distancing the client from the immediacy of self-harm)

- Dictating a self-injury sequence into a recording device (verbal mastery and distancing)

Note that these strategies include tactile, visual, and auditory options. For some clients, self-injury is primarily tactile; for others, it is a more visual or even self-instructional experience. I believe that for most it is a combination. In choosing such skills, clients need to select an option that intuitively feels right for them.

The assumption with all of these examples is that the act of self-injury is symbolically represented, but that no tissue damage is inflicted. The client experiences something that resembles the act of self-harm, but remains sufficiently in control to go through the sequence without harming the body. The advantage of these techniques is that for some clients the activities seem vivid and "real" enough to take the place of actual self-harm. The disadvantage is that the behaviors may cue actual self-injury, because the replacement behaviors are so similar to the real thing. Using negative replacement skills may seem a bit like suggesting to a person recovering from alcoholism that he or she enter a bar and order a soda water as part of becoming sober. For some clients, the stimulus cues can be too triggering. Nonetheless, other clients report that negative replacement behaviors have played a key role in helping them make the transition away from self-injury. Consider this example:

As described in Chapter 9, Nikki's pattern of self-injury was to incise precisely executed grid designs on her forearms. She conceived of a replacement behavior that she used to fend off impulses to self-harm. From her art supplies she took three sheets of construction paper. She colored the first sheet deep red; the second, yellow and orange; and the third, skin tone. She then stapled the three sheets together at the corners. Using her X-ACTO knife, Nikki cut a grid pattern into the layers of paper. The resulting design was identical to what she had previously incised into her arms. She reported that this technique helped her avoid self-injuring several times before she moved on to other replacement skills.

Nikki's experience is not atypical. Clients often find that using behaviors that resemble self-injury may be useful transitionally, but they are not likely to use these techniques for extended periods of time successfully.

Mindful Breathing Skills

Mindful breathing skills are often the most important in learning to give up self-injury. The term "mindful" requires some explanation. Mindfulness skills have increasingly been identified as playing an important role in the empirically validated treatments of diverse disorders. Kabat-Zinn (1990) has reported using mindfulness skills in treating chronic illness, physical pain, and psychological stress. Linehan and colleagues consider mindfulness a "core component" of DBT for individuals diagnosed with BPD (Linehan et al., 1991; Linehan, 1993a, 1993b; Miller et al., 2007). Segal et al. (2002) and Williams, Teasdale, Segal, and Kabat-Zinn (2007) assign mindfulness training a central role in their treatment of recurrent depression. Hayes (2004) has gone so far as to identify mindfulness as central to the new "third wave" of behavior therapy. There are also extensive writings about mindfulness that have a philosophical and religious orientation, such as those by the Buddhist monk Thich Nhat Hanh (1975, 1991).

When I present the term "mindfulness" to clients, I generally keep the discussion simple, because most clients are interested in practical results as opposed to philosophical discussions. The explanation that I provide is that "mindfulness" refers to full, calm awareness in the present moment (Nhat Hanh, 1975; Linehan, 1993b). I also explain that mindfulness is about doing one activity *at a time*. Multitasking is the opposite of mindfulness, as are reminiscing and anticipating. Nhat Hanh has written:

> While we practice conscious breathing, our thinking will slow down, and we can give ourselves a real rest. Most of the time, we think too much, and mindful breathing helps us to be calm, relaxed and peaceful. It helps us stop thinking so much and stop being possessed by sorrows of the past and worries about the future. (1991, p. 8)

I explain that learning mindfulness is generally a good match for self-injuring clients, because they experience the opposite of mindfulness so frequently. Rather than calm, they are frequently intensely distressed; rather than focused, they are often confused and distracted. All too frequently, the lives of self-injuring individuals are dominated by emotional lability and cognitive disjointedness. Clients learn to be mindful in order to calm themselves and solve problems more effectively.

Although any activity can be done mindfully (e.g., eating, walking, doing the dishes, mowing the lawn), mindful breathing skills are particularly recommended, for many reasons:

- They are easy to learn.
- They enable individuals to calm themselves physically by reducing heart and respiration rates; they also lower blood pressure.
- They can be practiced and used at almost any time.
- There is no cost or need for equipment.

- There are no side effects.
- The skills require no assistance or participation from others.
- With a modest amount of practice, they produce very quick results.

Some clients, particularly adolescents, express distrust or discomfort when first presented with mindful breathing skills. They label these activities as "weird" or "strange" and indicate no intention of trying them. Other clients state at the outset that they have tried breathing skills before and the skills did not work. It is important to be patient with dubious clients and to assure them that if they *practice* breathing, they will be surprised by the results. I sometimes say to skeptics, "The first step in using breathing skills is being convinced they will *not* work." I tell them of many clients who have stated that mindful breathing skills did not work for them, only to acknowledge 3 months later how useful they had become.

It is often productive for therapists to refer to their own use of mindful breathing skills in order to encourage clients. When therapists indicate that mindful breathing is a "living skill" that anyone can use and not just some therapeutic technique, clients may become more receptive. I sometimes share this story with clients:

"Several years ago, I was driving south along the California coast. It was a beautiful but frightening ride, with miles of road along cliffs that dropped off hundreds of feet to the ocean. There were no guardrails on many sections of road, and it was clear that even a slight mistake could result in a catastrophic accident and death. Although I am not normally a nervous driver, I became increasingly fearful. My forehead began sweating, and my hands gripped the steering wheel more and more tightly. My driving slowed to about 15 miles per hour as I negotiated hairpin turns on the edge of the ocean. Fortunately, there were no cars behind me.

"One thing and one thing only got me through this driving experience. As I realized how stressed I was becoming, I began deliberately using my mindful breathing skills while I was driving. Within several minutes I calmed down, and I was then able to drive with much less fear and improved concentration."

I conclude this story by asking clients whether they ever feel afraid or have too much emotion.

I tell many other stories about former clients who have successfully used mindful breathing skills during sports competitions, when taking exams, talking with an intimidating boss, having an argument with a partner, and (most important) as an alternative to self-injuring. Here is one example of a story that clients appreciate:

A 15-year-old male came into therapy because he had been cutting himself about every 2 weeks for a year. This young man was an excellent high school baseball player. He was the star pitcher, even though he was one of the youngest players on the team. One area of his life he really wanted to work on was dealing with stress during competition. Very frequently, if he made a bad pitch that was hit hard, he would become furious with himself and launch into a series of self-denigrating judgments, such as "You're an idiot! You don't belong on the field. You're going to lose the game for the team."

This client learned mindful breathing as part of treatment. He practiced diligently every evening before going to bed. He found the skill so useful that he began deliberately slowing his breathing while on the mound. He also focused on his breathing while sitting on the bench between innings, as an alternative to making negative judgments about himself. Use of breathing skills enabled this client to experience much less stress on the baseball field. It also helped him give up self-injury within about 8 months.

Teaching Mindful Breathing

It is particularly important to teach and practice mindful breathing skills *in vivo* with clients. Descriptions are not as effective as demonstrations. Practicing *together* teaches the skills in a specific, vivid way and models for a client how to overcome any sense of awkwardness or skepticism. If the therapist is willing to look "weird" or "strange," why not the client?

Early in treatment, I begin the practice of mindful breathing with these basic instructions:

> "Let's begin by sitting in a chair or on a cushion in a balanced way. Find a comfortable alignment. The spine should be straight but not rigid. Try not to lean right or left. If you are in a chair, it is recommended that you place your feet flat on the floor. Place your hands and arms on your legs or the arms of the chair. It is best to sit rather than lie down, because people tend to fall asleep when reclining; mindfulness is about being both calm and alert.
>
> "Bring your attention gently to your breathing. Notice the physical sensations of your abdomen and chest expanding and contracting with each breath. . . . Notice the air entering and leaving your mouth, nose, and throat. . . . Become aware of the basic rhythm of the body and the breath.
>
> "When you experience distractions such as thoughts, feelings, worries, anticipations, and the like, gently return your attention to your breathing. Distractions are inevitable, but they can be reduced with practice."

After providing these basic instructions, I like to teach three different types of mindful breathing within the first month or two of treatment. The pace of instruction depends on the client's readiness to learn and willingness to practice. Some clients learn all three breathing techniques within the first few weeks. Others need much more time.

I should emphasize that there is no empirical support for the specific breathing exercises selected. They are comfortable for me to teach, and I find that many clients respond to them. Clinicians should feel free to select other breathing exercises that they prefer. Following are the three types of breathing.

"I AM HERE. . . . I AM CALM"

The instructions for the first type of breathing are as follows: "This breathing exercise needs some explanation. 'I am here' is shorthand for the longer sentence 'I am here in the present moment without judgment.' 'I am here in the present moment' means 'I am not thinking about the past, and I am also not anticipating the future; I'm just residing in the present moment.' 'Without judgment' means 'I am suspending judgment right now about myself and others. I am taking a complete break from criticizing myself and other people.' With this exercise, as you breathe in, you say to yourself, 'I am here.' As you breathe out, you say, 'I am calm.'"

Comment: For whatever reason, this breathing exercise is the all-time favorite of clients at my agency, The Bridge. I believe people like it because it conveys the essence of mindfulness in a brief, concise way. It is complex enough to hold a client's attention and meaningful enough to foster conviction.

1 THROUGH 10 EXHALE BREATHING

Here are the instructions for the second type of breathing:

> "As you breathe in, say nothing inside your mind; as you breathe out, say '1.' Next, as you breathe in, say nothing again, and as you breathe out, say '2.' Continue in this manner up to 10, counting only on the exhalations. When you reach 10, return to 1. If you lose count or go beyond 10, return to 1 and start over."

Comment: This breathing exercise has a good balance of complexity and parsimony. It is complex enough to require attention; however, it is still quite simple and easily remembered. The counting aspect of this breathing dispels any concerns clients may have that mindful breathing will be weird, strange, or cult-like. There are no religious mantras or foreign words to learn; it is just counting. It should be noted, though, that this form of breathing has been practiced for 2,500 years by serious meditators (Rosenberg, 1998).

"LETTING GO OF . . . " BREATHING

The third breathing technique is a modification of one presented by Nhat Hanh (1975). The instructions for it are as follows:

> "As you breathe in, say inside your mind, 'Mindfully breathing.' As you breathe out, say inside your mind: 'Letting go of X. . . . ' Here X represents whatever feeling or thoughts you'd like to have less of, such as anxiety, tension, anger, judgments, or perfectionism. The X selected should be something that is powerful in the moment or is known to be a key antecedent to self-injury. As you breathe out, imagine the feeling or thought leaving your body as you become more and more relaxed. You can select one thing to 'let go of' and say that recurrently, or you can let go of a series of different feelings or thoughts. Thus the first time you might say, 'Mindfully breathing, letting go of anxiety,' and the second time, 'Mindfully breathing, letting go of judgments,' and so on. After doing this exercise for several minutes, people tend to move naturally toward simply saying, 'Mindfully breathing' on the in breath, and 'Letting go' on the out breath."

Comment: The idea is not to "drive out" or forbid any thoughts or feelings, but rather to notice them and then let them pass. This exercise can be done quite successfully in groups, with staff members and clients taking turns saying out loud, "Mindfully breathing, letting go of X." This activity builds a sense of group cohesion and conveys the message that everyone has feelings and judgments they'd like to have less of; such an experience can be quite "normalizing" for clients who view their distress as unique or extreme. If a group has clients who are particularly anxious about speaking in front of others or disclosing personal feelings, the members can be told that they can say "pass" when it comes to their turn.

One disadvantage to this technique is that it is complex and requires good verbal skills. With some developmentally disabled clients, I've reduced the exercise to saying the word "breathing" on the in-breath, and saying only "X" on the out-breath (thus eliminating the words "mindfully" and "letting go of," for the sake of simplicity).

There are many other mindful breathing techniques that work well with clients. Appendix A is a Breathing Manual with diverse examples for teaching mindfulness skills. Please consult it for other techniques not presented here.

Some clients are particularly inspired by the link between mindful breathing and meditation. All of the world's great religions have meditative or contemplative traditions, including Buddhism, Christianity, Islam, and Judaism. For clients who respond to the spiritual aspects of mindful breathing and meditation, there are many helpful resources, including Sekida (1985), Nhat Hanh (1975, 1991), Bayda (2002), Fontana (2001), and Rosenberg (1998). However, I should emphasize one more time that mindful breathing can be taught in a completely secular manner that requires no reference to philosophical or religious traditions. The therapist's strategy is to understand the client's mindset and to proceed in a manner that is consistent with the client's attitudes and beliefs.

Tips for Mindful Breathing Practice

In teaching mindful breathing skills, the therapist also needs to monitor the frequency and length of practice, the physical location, and the results obtained. In order for mindful breathing to become a useful skill, most people need to practice the behavior at least three times per week. A Mindful Breathing Tracking Card (see Figure 11.1) can be a useful way to monitor practice.

The length of practice is very important. Many clients may try the behavior for a minute or so and declare that it does not work. They are correct that 2–3 minutes of mindful breathing are unlikely to produce a deep sense of calm and enhanced alertness. Clients generally need to practice mindful breathing each time for 10 minutes or more in order for it to become a useful skill. Segal et al.'s (2002) mindfulness-based cognitive therapy for depression requires that clients practice breathing for 40 minutes multiple times per week. Although I find this expectation too demanding for many clients (especially adolescents), I do think that a goal of 10–20 minutes is appropriate. In order for mindful breathing to work, clients need to move beyond the highly distractible first few minutes of mindful breathing into the calmness that emerges after 10 or more minutes. Clients need time to work up to more extended mindful breathing practice. Many can reach 15–20 minutes within a month or so. After several months of practice, the skill becomes increasingly effective and can be used in periods of high emotional arousal.

The physical location for the practice is also an important detail. Clients need to select a quiet place in their homes or elsewhere where they are

Name: _____

Week of: _____

	Mon.	Tues.	Wed.	Thurs.	Fri.	Sat.	Sun.
*Type of breathing							
Location							
Length of practice **Subjective units of distress (SUDs 0–10)							

*Type of breathing: "I am here . . . I am calm"

Counting 1 through 10 when breathing out

"Letting go of X . . . " breathing

Other

**Note: 0 = the most relaxed you've ever been; 10 = the most distressed you've ever been; 5 is in the middle. Please rate yourself at both start and finish of the mindful breathing practice.

FIGURE 11.1. Mindful Breathing Tracking Card.

unlikely to be disturbed. Clients who live in chaotic environments may need to seek out a library, prayer room, meditation center, or quiet outdoor location. They should use either a comfortable chair or meditation cushions. It is unwise to practice lying down, for reasons previously stated. However, once mindful breathing has been well learned, it can be used quite productively as a sleep induction technique for those with insomnia.

Another detail is whether the eyes should be open or closed. My opinion is that it does not matter. Some individuals prefer having their eyes open, because they feel safer this way and are less likely to doze off. Others prefer having their eyes closed because they are better able to concentrate without visual stimuli. Clients should decide which is the more comfortable practice for them. In general, if they decide to keep their eyes open, it is useful to cast their eyes down at the floor to minimize distractions.

It is also useful to monitor effectiveness with the client. I find a useful technique is to teach clients the concept of "subjective units of distress," or SUDs (Wolpe, 1969). Clients can record on their Mindful Breathing Tracking Card how they are feeling immediately before and after breathing practice. Tracking breathing with SUDs involves teaching clients that 0 represents the most relaxed they have ever been in their lives and 10 the most distressed, with 5 approximately in the middle. Most clients report substantial reduction in SUDs after 10 or more minutes of mindful breathing.

For those who consistently report no change—or, even worse, an escalation of SUDs—it may be best to look toward other replacement behaviors. I encountered one client who consistently became more anxious while practicing mindful breathing. Initially, her only explanation was "Breathing just doesn't work for me." Having heard this many times before, I plodded on, urging her to keep trying. Then she disclosed the following:

> "Breathing never works for me. It just makes things worse. Whenever I practice breathing, I *hear* my breath, and it just reminds me of my abuser breathing hard in my ear while he raped me. I hear his breath all over again, and everything comes back. Breathing will never work for me, and now you know why."

Humbled by my misguided persistent attempts to teach her breathing, I apologized for my insensitivity, and we moved on to other replacement skills (as well as trauma resolution work later in treatment).

Visualization Techniques

Visualization techniques involve identifying pleasant, relaxing scenes and retrieving them *vividly* as a self-soothing strategy (Schwartz, 1995). Some clients experience the world in predominantly visual terms and respond especially well to techniques of this type. They will say quite clearly, "Visualization works better for me than any other skill."

Through years of practice with clients, I have come to believe that the most effective way to use visualization exercises is to help clients develop their own. This can be done simply by suggesting that clients draw on their own experiences to retrieve an especially calming place or scene in their lives. Then the instruction is for the client to develop a visualization *using all five senses* so that the visualization is as vivid and specific as possible. Developing the scene can be done in writing, via voice recording on a smart phone, or just retained in memory.

For example, I once worked with a client who had a significant problem with self-injury multiple times per week. However, I noticed that she never self-harmed on days when she had access to grooming or riding horses. Not surprisingly, this client identified being with horses as her most relaxing experience. When I introduced the idea of a using a calming visualization, she immediately selected the experience of grooming her favorite horse. In her mind's eye, this client imagined seeing the horse, smelling and tasting the barn, feeling the brush groom his coat, and hearing him swish his tail and move about.

Another client with developmental disabilities chose the visualization of praying in church where she was most at peace with the world. And a third client who had problems with schizophrenia and related self-harm developed/retrieved a visualization from childhood at the seashore, using all five senses.

Visualization can be combined with mindful breathing. Some clients get themselves settled and breathe mindfully for several minutes before retrieving a pleasant scene. Mindful breathing that focuses on counting or "letting go" can get stale over time, and visualization can provide a fresh focus.

Rarely, clients develop scenes that are not soothing but counterproductive. For example, I discovered that one client was imagining scenes of violence—which he stated he found quite soothing. I questioned the appropriateness of these scenes and shaped him in the direction of more prosocial content (e.g., listening to guitar music in a cafe). Pastoral scenes would not have worked for this client; he had never been out of the city. The point is that it is important to monitor the scenes clients are using, lest they go astray into negative or destructive content.

Physical Exercise or Movement

Nock (2010) has shown that physical exercise can be quite useful in fending off urges to self-injure. Some clients prefer vigorous physical activity as one of their replacement skills. Adolescents, in particular, are understandably bored by too much sedentary activity. The affectively intense feeling states that dominate the lives of self-injuring people often include significant bursts of adrenaline. Clients may need the assistance of physical activity to bring the intensity of the adrenaline response back within typical limits. The full range of physical exercise options does not need a thorough review here. Suffice it to say that clients can use such activities as walking, running, playing basketball, swimming, kayaking, martial arts, lifting weights, and so on as replacement skills. Some clients use atypical forms of "exercise" as a replacement skill. For example, one client likes to vacuum her house when she feels agitated. She finds that the physical movement calms her; the noise distracts her from emotional pain; and after the completion of the vacuuming, she feels a modest sense of accomplishment.

It is important that the preferred mode of exercise be accessible when the client becomes distressed. If the client selects swimming as a replacement skill but the pool is not open during evening hours, an alternative mode of exercise should be selected as a backup.

One recommendation is to avoid violent forms of physical exercise, such as boxing or psychodrama activities that express aggressive impulses. The goal of treatment is to arrive at better forms of impulse control. Violent activities are too close to self-inflicted aggression and should be avoided.

Another pitfall that therapists should be aware of is that clients may exercise in a self-destructive manner. Some individuals push themselves beyond ordinary levels of endurance and cause physical injury repeatedly. Not infrequently these are individuals for whom excessive physical exercise is related to an eating disorder; they may restrict their eating, induce vomiting, and exercise compulsively. Eating disorders have been found to be strongly associated with self-injury in a number of empirical studies (Walsh, 1987; Favazza, 1989; Warren et al., 1998; Favaro & Santonastaso, 1998, 2000; Rodriguez-Srednicki, 2001; Paul et al., 2002). Therefore, before encouraging exercise as a replacement behavior, the therapist should be careful to assess whether the behavior is within typical limits. Clients who repeatedly report exercise-related injuries may be using exercise in the service of self-destructiveness. The therapist and client can monitor the healthiness of the exercise selected by agreeing to an amount of time and frequency per week.

One form of physical movement that can be useful is "walking meditation." This involves walking very slowly and deliberately while concentrating on the breath. Specific instructions for walking meditation are provided in the Breathing Manual in Appendix A.

Writing

Writing about the sequence of self-injury has previously been discussed under negative replacement behaviors. There are many other forms of writing that do not have self-injury content and assist individuals in fending off self-harm. Most typically this involves some type of journaling about day-to-day experience. Verbal expression is important because it provides a bedrock for mastery of overwhelming emotions. If a client can begin to distance him- or herself from the immediacy of an experience and write about it, it is a key step in moving toward expressing discomfort rather than acting on it.

Conterio and Lader (1998) have placed more emphasis on writing assignments in the treatment of self-injury than any other authors have. In their treatment program, they require 15 written assignments in sequential order. Their assignments include such topics as an autobiography, a self-appraisal, discussion of the most influential female and male in one's life, the emotions surrounding self-injury, anger, nurturing oneself, saying good-bye to self-injury, and future plans. I have not used this sequence myself in treatment; however, Conterio and Lader report considerable success in their program in reducing and eliminating self-injury. Their writing activities serve as a cornerstone of their treatment approach. Clinicians would do well to read the Conterio and Lader (1998) volume and to consider using some or all of the writing assignments in their own treatment, if it is a good match for their clientele.

I have not used these assignments myself, in part because many of my clients lack adequate verbal skills or organizational abilities. I think that the structure and time-limited nature of Conterio and Lader's inpatient unit make the completion of such assignments more practical than for many other client situations. However, for clients who are verbally adept enough, the Conterio and Lader approach deserves serious consideration.

Artistic Expression

Many clients use art as an effective replacement behavior. They do not need to be technically accomplished in order to use artistic expression productively. A client's willingness to use art when triggers occur is the only necessary feature. The therapist should first ask whether the client is artistically inclined, and then should have the client use his or her preferred medium during a session to assess its utility. The therapist may want to have a variety of art materials in the office in order for clients to try the skill *in vivo*. This does not mean that the therapist becomes an art therapist, but rather that artistic expression is practiced as a possible replacement skill.

I worked with one client who was a talented sculptress. When she experienced key antecedents to self-injury, she chose consistently to work with clay. The physical, visceral sensation of manipulating the clay was very soothing for her. Sometimes she did uncanny self-portraits; at other times she created tortured, twisted, anguished abstract figures that were painful to behold. As she experienced cues that had in the past triggered self-injury, she routinely got out her art supplies and began sculpting. She found that if she worked for 30 minutes to an hour, the more intense urges to self-injure would pass. She could then return to other activities. When art failed to work for this client, she knew that she was especially distressed and needed to contact her therapist or friends for support, structure, and assistance.

Another client used art quite differently. Early in treatment, she experienced high levels of stress on a daily basis. When she returned home from work, she developed a ritual of either practicing mindful breathing or drawing in a free-form manner. She found both behaviors to be quite soothing and meditative. Each day she selected one or the other, depending on her mood or intuition. If she felt more agitated or "antsy," she tended to select the activity of drawing; if she felt more morose or contemplative, she did mindful breathing. This simple skill set was transforming for the client. Her self-injury dropped off to zero, and she experienced the added benefit of improving her artwork through all the practice.

Playing or Listening to Music

Music is a key replacement skill for many individuals. In general, active participation is better than passive listening. Although one can listen to music quite mindfully, with full attention and concentration, playing an instrument is a more engaged, participatory skill. I have encountered only a few self-injuring clients who were accomplished musicians. One was a cello player who used playing as a form of expression and emotional regulation. On multiple occasions she was able to defer self-injuring by playing. However, music for her was also an arena of self-imposed perfectionistic demands, so playing "poorly" sometimes made her feel worse.

Most clients I have encountered use music as a replacement skill via listening. Listening to music can be problematic as a replacement skill, because it tends to be done with partial attention. "Half-listening" to music is likely to have little effect on emotional distress. Clients can learn to listen to music mindfully by focusing deliberately and intensively on various aspects of the music (melody, specific instruments, dynamics, cadence, vocals, beat, harmony, etc.). Adolescents often prefer listening to music to almost any other replacement skill. I urge them to develop more active, participatory skills such as mindful breathing, visualization, or creating art.

It is important to monitor music selection with adolescents. Some clients choose aggressive, violent music that makes them feel angrier or more agitated. Others listen to music that is maudlin and sad, thereby amplifying their feelings of depression and isolation. It is useful to teach adolescents that music either can serve as a trigger for self-injury or can be used as a self-soothing skill. They can develop separate playlists on their music devices that are helpful and soothing.

Listening to music is often more of a diversion technique than a true self-soothing skill. It can be very productive, but should be monitored closely so that it does not become a way of avoiding more active, engaged skills practice.

Communicating with Others

Communicating with others is obviously a useful alternative to self-injury, but it should be structured as to specifics. Details need to be identified as to who the others are, as well as their availability, judgment, influence, supportiveness, and patience. If possible, these others should be trained in replacement skills, as discussed in a later section on engaging family members in treatment. The content of the talk is important as well. Too much aimless venting without a shift to skills practice is counterproductive. Some forms of communication can be clearly conducive to self-injury, as in this example:

One client, when she was depressed and inclined to cut herself, would call a "friend" who would belittle her. As soon as he heard her voice on the phone, he would begin mocking her as a "psycho" who was "so needy, stupid, and incompetent." This demeaning talk would go on for half an hour or more as the client became ever more depressed and hopeless. In her case, calling the male friend was not a replacement skill, but part of her self-injuring sequence. During the assessment process, she identified these phone calls as a key antecedent that she needed to avoid. As an alternative, we developed a list of five nurturing people she should call in a prescribed order related to their likely availability and judgment.

The greatest assets are friends or family members who understand what triggers the client's self-injury and will talk him or her through and beyond the urges to self-harm. These people can be at least as useful as clinicians, because they are more available and likely to remain engaged for years. It is useful to bring these significant others into sessions when the client agrees and to use them as coaches and allies. They can be taught reinforcement principles regarding which behaviors they should especially reward and which ones they should place on extinction. They can also be very helpful in reducing any cues that they themselves provide to the self-injury sequence. Of course, friends and family members are not just ancillary therapists; their main role is to provide care and support, with no specific strategic goals in mind.

One client who used communication with others particularly well was a 42-year-old female. With her best friend, who was of similar age, she could share almost anything. Her friend knew extensive details about the client's abuse history, related self-injury, divorce, and so on. When the client had strong urges to cut herself, she frequently called her friend and described the emotions she was experiencing. This friend had had her own challenges and was able to empathize with and support the client. She also had a black sense of humor that was excellent in diffusing tension and panic. Over time, the client had shared the skills she had learned in therapy, and the friend would prompt her. Although I never met this friend, I considered her my co-therapist. She provided hours of support and good judgment that went way beyond my psychotherapeutic influence.

For clients who have very limited social skills and few or no social supports, hotlines can provide useful guidance. Many hotlines have the distinct advantage of being available 24 hours a day. Some hotlines are much better than others at tolerating what they call "frequent" or "regular" callers. Hotline staff can consider recurrent callers a distraction from their main business, which is to save those in life-threatening crises. Staff members on other hotlines (e.g., the Samaritans hotline) are quite willing to talk with the same callers several times per week and view it as consistent with their mission or "befriending" role. For more isolated clients, the therapist should locate a hotline that is receptive to regular callers and suggest it as a resource. For some clients, the sound of a human voice is far more soothing than texting or e-mail.

Therapists should assess whether clients frequent chat rooms or watch videos on YouTube that focus on self-injury. More often than not, such venues involve sharing of lurid details (about the methods of self-injury, the extent of wounds, the amount of blood, the length of scars, etc.). A competitive one-upsmanship atmosphere can flourish in these sites that is clearly triggering. Occasionally, I have heard clients talk about a small chat room where several individuals help each other with recovery. The therapist should assess whether a chat room is a potential help or is part of the problem.

Diversion Techniques

Diversion techniques are means of deflecting attention from thoughts, plans, and urges to self-injure. This is a very idiosyncratic category of replacement skills. I have had clients who watch TV, pet their cat, groom their dog, play solitaire, clean the house, play video games, wash the car, make brownies, read a book, knit, or quilt. I even had one who reviewed new tax laws as a diversion!

Clients need to have multiple diversion techniques in their repertoires, because what works in one situation will be irrelevant in another. The main point that needs to be made about diversion techniques is that they are *not* high-order replacement skills. They really serve to temporize and fend off problems rather than to solve them. Diversion techniques generally do not have a major self-soothing function; they do not really compete with self-injury in terms of potential relief from affective distress or emptiness. Therefore, clients should be encouraged to have replacement skills other than this set. The limitations of diversion techniques are well indicated in this example:

Scott, age 16, was not about to try mindful breathing or visualization. He called them "psychobabble" and laughed uproariously whenever they were suggested. Scott was only willing to use diversion techniques. He agreed to play video games, text a friend, or shoot basketball when he started to feel like burning or cutting himself. He also decided to listen to music, primarily very vigorous alternative rock. The problem with these activities for Scott was that he already did them quite frequently. They were so familiar that he could do them and still think about self-injury.

Because his rate of self-injury was in no way declining, Scott decided to try a new diversion technique: walking to the mall, which was over 2 miles away from his home. This technique was modestly more successful, perhaps because it involved physical exercise and was novel enough to distract him. He found looking at people and passing cars sufficiently engaging to redirect his thoughts from themes of self-injury. However, Scott's treatment needed to move beyond diversion techniques in order for him to make real improvement.

Generally clients rely on diversion techniques before they have learned the new skills of negative replacement behaviors, mindful breathing, visualization, writing, artistic expression, and communicating with others. In order for clients to reduce and eliminate self-injury, they need to learn to calm themselves and to focus. Diversion techniques do not teach either element in a truly transformative way.

TRACKING THE USE OF SKILLS AS REPLACEMENT BEHAVIORS

Now that skills have been selected, practiced, and employed in the real world, it is important in treatment to monitor their use. In Chapter 9 (see Figure 9.2), a Brief Self-Injury Log has been introduced to track the five types of antecedents and consequences for self-injury. This same format can now be used to monitor the use of skills as replacements for self-injury. Like Figure 9.2 in Chapter 9, the Brief Skills Practice Log in Figure 11.2 tracks the environmental, biological, cognitive, affective, and behavioral dimensions of self-injury. However, now the emphasis shifts to which skills are utilized in the place of self-injury. Please refer to the end of Chapter 9 for the case example that is again employed here, with a new focus on replacement behaviors.

As the completed log in Figure 11.3 shows, the 16-year-old client used two main replacement skills in place of self-injuring: She did mindful breathing in the school library and communicated with her guidance counselor. These skills, along with some cognitive self-instruction ("I have to calm down"), helped her avoid cutting. These behaviors were reinforced in that she obtained a sense of relief and rewarded herself by saying, "Phew, I actually didn't cut myself!"

This simple assessment tool should be reviewed with clients early in each session. Clients should continue to complete this form on a weekly

Name: _____

Dimension	Antecedents	Skills employed	Aftermath
Environmental			
Biological			
Cognitive			
Affective			
Behavioral			

FIGURE 11.2. Brief Skills Practice Log.

Name: <u>16-year-old female</u>

Dimension	Antecedents	Skills employed	Aftermath
Environmental	Argument with friend at school	Distanced from friend	No further contact with friend
Biological	Already overtired; not high; had a headache	Still overtired, but didn't smoke grass	Headache gone; slept better later
Cognitive	"I'm all alone; I have no friends"	"I have to calm down!"	"Phew! I actually didn't cut myself!"
Affective	Felt sad, empty, panicked	Very anxious; wanted to cut, wanted to avoid it	Felt much calmer; obtained relief
Behavioral	Decided not to do the usual cutting	Did mindful breathing in school library; talked with guidance counselor; returned to class one period later	Talked with friend about the conflict later; friend reassured me that we're still friends

FIGURE 11.3. Example of a completed Brief Skills Practice Log.

basis until skills are used so automatically that they no longer need to be monitored. Deciding to discontinue formal skills monitoring should be considered a "graduation" that can be celebrated in the therapy.

When a relapse of self-injury occurs, the clinician should ask the client to temporarily complete both a Brief Self-Injury Log and a Brief Skills Practice Log. When the acts of self-injury cease for several weeks, the completion of the Brief Self-Injury Log can be discontinued.

USING E-MAIL TO SUPPORT SKILLS

I find that e-mail serves as a useful support in assisting clients to learn and employ skills. When clients have access to e-mail accounts, I either ask them to contact me between sessions or obtain permission to contact them (the former is preferred). I use e-mail to support practice and to exchange feedback between sessions. E-mail is far less intrusive than phone calls or texting for both parties. It permits a reasonably prompt response without interrupting one's daily life. In prompting clients to practice their skills, the therapist needs to strike the right balance. Clients do not want to feel nagged or coerced, but they do want to feel supported. A therapist can ask whether a client would like a reminder about skills practice every few days. Or, better yet, the client agrees to provide the therapist with updates about homework. What happens most frequently over time is that the therapist and client exchange one to two e-mails between sessions. The client briefly describes situations in his or her life and indicates which skills have been tapped as coping measures. In turn, the therapist offers support, provides reinforcement, and makes suggestions for improvements in using the skills. It is very important for the therapist to emphasize skill acquisition and practice in e-mails, rather than detailed discussion of life situations; these should be saved for therapy sessions. The therapist particularly wants to avoid reinforcing any venting or complaining that does not lead to skills practice. Of course, it is important that the clinician notify the client when he or she will be electronically unavailable. Also, the client should be advised not to expect immediate responses from the therapist.

SIGNIFICANT OTHERS AS TREATMENT ALLIES

Treatment often involves significant others. It is very helpful when family members or friends actively practice skills with clients. The skills to be learned are generally "living skills" that almost anyone can use productively. For example, many family members report using mindful breathing skills themselves, although they originally learned them to support the clients. Significant others can also play the important role of prompting clients to practice and reminding the clients to use skills when they are distressed. Skills practice gives families a new arena for positive interaction and shifts their attention away from a problem focus. With adolescent clients, however, parents need to be judicious with their prompts; too many reminders can be counterproductive, producing an aversion to practice.

CONCLUSION

In summary, when clinicians and others are teaching replacement skills to self-injuring clients, it is generally most helpful to do the following:

- Select skills with the client that are relevant, appealing, developmentally appropriate, and effective.
- Draw from the nine categories of replacement skills.
- Downplay reliance on negative replacement skills, because these run the risk of triggering episodes.
- Draw up and monitor a very specific practice schedule.
- Use the Brief Skills Practice Log when possible.
- Prompt and monitor practice via e-mail or assistance from significant others.
- Reinforce the clients enthusiastically for ongoing skills practice.

CHAPTER 12

Cognitive Treatment

The second dimension of Step 2 in the stepped-care model (see Figure II.1, p. 75) is cognitive treatment. This component targets the thoughts, assumptions, rules, attitudes, and core beliefs that support self-injury. As discussed in Chapter 6, thoughts constitute one of the five key determinants of self-injury, along with environmental, biological, affective, and behavioral elements. Thoughts, in their myriad forms, play a fundamental role in the onset and continuation of self-injury. Cognitive processes always precede the emotions and behaviors associated with cutting, excoriation, self-burning, self-hitting, and so on. Cognitions need to be identified collaboratively with the client and targeted in order for treatment to be comprehensive and successful.

Cognitive therapies are among the most empirically supported available. They have the advantage of having undergone considerable replication. Cognitive treatment is structured, sequential, reasonably standardized, and sometimes manualized. It is also fairly simple, direct, and easy to learn. Moreover, it is often short-term and cost-effective.

Cognitive therapy has been documented to be effective in treating diverse problems, including depression and suicidality (Beck et al., 1979; Freeman & Reinecke, 1993), anxiety (Clark, 1986), eating disorders (Garner, Vitousek, & Pike, 1997; Wilson, Fairburn, & Agras, 1997), trichotillomania (Rothbaum & Ninan, 1999; Keuthen et al., 2001), personality disorders (Beck, Freeman, Davis, & Associates, 2003), PTSD (Foa & Rothbaum, 1998; Rothbaum, Meadows, Resick, & Foy, 2000; Mueser, Rosenberg, & Rosenberg, 2009), and schizophrenia (Kingdon & Turkington, 2005; Penn, Waldheter, Perkins, Mueser, & Lieberman, 2005).

Judith S. Beck (2005, 2011) has provided a concise summary of the conceptualization on which cognitive therapy is based. A brief version of her diagrammatic presentation of the cognitive model is presented in Figure 12.1. In doing a cognitive assessment of self-injury, the therapist generally starts at the bottom of the sequence and moves up. At the outset, the clinician analyzes the self-injury behavior itself, along with the emotions and physiological responses that precede and follow it. This aspect of assessment is discussed in Chapter 9. Next, the analysis considers the automatic thoughts, followed by intermediate beliefs, and ending with core beliefs. These terms require some explication.

AUTOMATIC THOUGHTS

"Automatic thoughts" are the actual words or images that go through a person's mind. They are the most immediate form of thought and are situation-specific (Beck, 2011). This form of thinking can be so fleeting and routinized that it becomes "automatic"; hence the terminology. As noted in Chapter 9, an example of an automatic thought is the self-instruction that occurs when one is driving a car, such as "I need to put on my left blinker now." This type of thought becomes so familiar and habitual that it often occurs out of conscious awareness.

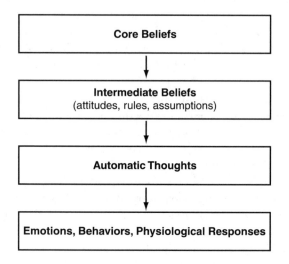

FIGURE 12.1. Cognitive model.

INTERMEDIATE BELIEFS

"Intermediate beliefs" consist of attitudes, rules, and assumptions (Beck, 2011). These aspects of cognition serve as connections or linkages between automatic thoughts and core beliefs. To continue with the example of driving, an attitude might be "It is important to drive safely." A related rule might be "Always put on the blinker before turning." And an assumption would be "If I drive safely, I am unlikely to get into an accident."

CORE BELIEFS

"Core beliefs" are the most fundamental and pervasively influential form of thinking. They tend to be global, firmly held, not easily subject to revision, and "overgeneralized" (Beck, 2011). Core beliefs are often fundamental convictions about the cognitive triad of self, world, and future (Beck et al., 1979; Rush & Nowels, 1994). Beck (2011) has suggested that counterproductive core beliefs tend to fall into the two basic categories of *incompetence* (e.g., "I'm stupid, a loser") and *unlovability* (e.g., "I have no friends"). An example of a core belief related to driving would be "I am a competent person (and therefore likely to be a good driver)."

Not surprisingly, when the conceptual model described above is employed in working with self-injuring clients, the cognitions identified are often pejorative. Evidence is emerging that self-derogation and self-criticism play an important role in self-injury (Glassman, Weierich, Hooley, Deliberto, & Nock, 2007). When a thorough cognitive analysis is performed with these clients, complex layers of negative, pessimistic core beliefs, attitudes, rules, assumptions, and automatic thoughts often emerge. Provided in Figure 12.2 are examples of such thoughts and beliefs associated with self-injury; again, Beck's cognitive model is used.

In beginning to work on the cognitive antecedents and consequences that support self-injury, the therapist has to start with education by showing the client Figure 12.1 and explaining the content. Most clients will easily understand the material, but for a few it can be too complex. The illustrative examples of cognitions should be tailored to the client's individual situation. Thus clients who do not drive may need an example such as brushing teeth, getting dressed, cooking, or feeding the cat. Once familiar nonthreatening examples of cognitions have been discussed (e.g., driving a car), examples related to self-injury can be identified, as shown in Figure 12.2.

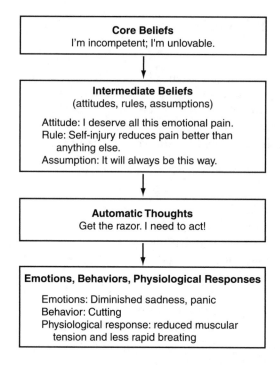

FIGURE 12.2. An example of the cognitive model for a self-injuring person.

In addition, the therapist needs to explain the following aspects of cognitive treatment to the client:

- Thoughts are important in maintaining self-injury; they precede feelings and behavior.
- Thoughts are multilayered and complex; they take time and work to understand.
- The therapist and client will employ "collaborative empiricism" as a method of proceeding in treatment (Beck, 2005, 2011; Mueser et al., 2009).
- Thoughts occur in the present (i.e., automatic thoughts), but are also derived from long-term personal history (i.e., core beliefs).
- Thoughts are not facts (Beck, 2011; Mueser et al., 2009), but they may be fueled by influential, powerful opinions.
- Dysfunctional thoughts that support self-injury can be altered and need to be changed over the course of treatment.
- The therapist will *not* challenge the client's thoughts cavalierly or

label them as wrong or incorrect; the client will *not* hear "It's all in your head" (Linehan, 1993a).

• Thoughts will be discussed in terms of whether they assist or hinder a client in reaching his or her goals.

Empathy, warmth, support, and validation are centrally important parts of cognitive therapy. If the client doesn't feel understood and supported, the therapy is unlikely to work and should be improved. The client is urged to communicate any deficiencies in this area to the therapist.

The assessment of thoughts that support self-injury occurs as part of the behavioral analysis. Eliciting automatic thoughts takes persistent, respectful questioning, given that clients often initially report that the self-injury "just happened." In addition to the example presented in the section on cognitive antecedents in Chapter 9, the following excerpt demonstrates the process of identifying automatic thoughts (and related core beliefs) tied to self-injury:

THERAPIST: So tell me about hitting yourself with the wooden coat hanger. What led up to that?

CLIENT: Sam had just called and put me down, and I was feeling so low and useless.

THERAPIST: That must have been painful.

CLIENT: It was. I was just feeling so tired and hopeless and alone.

THERAPIST: How did hitting yourself affect those feelings?

CLIENT: It made me feel better and then worse.

THERAPIST: Explain, please.

CLIENT: At first I felt so much better. It got the anger and the sadness out. Now it was on the outside instead of inside. I looked at the welts on my back in the mirror, and it was such a relief.

THERAPIST: I can see why you are drawn to hitting yourself, given that it provides so much relief.

CLIENT: Yes.

THERAPIST: But you said it also made you feel worse. What do you mean?

CLIENT: Afterward I regretted doing it. I just felt, "You're such a loser. There you go hitting yourself again. That's not going to help anything."

THERAPIST: Good. I'm glad to see you starting to challenge the behavior of striking yourself. What were you thinking right *before* you hit yourself . . . right after you hung up the phone?

CLIENT: It wasn't good. I was thinking, "What a piece of shit! No one loves me, and no one ever will."

THERAPIST: Okay, those sound like the core beliefs we've talked about. What were you thinking *immediately* after you got off the phone?

CLIENT: I was thinking, "You're such a piece of shit! You should be whipped and struck until it hurts."

THERAPIST: Wow, what a sequence of thoughts. You must have been in a lot of emotional pain.

CLIENT: I was.

THERAPIST: Let's look very specifically at the automatic thought in this situation, which appears to be "I should be whipped and struck until it hurts."

CLIENT: (*sarcastically*) Oh, that sounds like fun!

THERAPIST: (*mirroring*) Yes, doesn't it? I can see why you come here! It's so light-hearted!

In this sequence, the therapist is careful to provide a lot of empathy and support. The dialogue has produced a lot of helpful information. Core beliefs are referenced when the client states, "No one loves me, and no one ever will." But beyond that are the cognitions that immediately preceded the self-flagellation—the automatic thought of "I should be whipped and struck until it hurts."

USING A FIVE-STEP PROCESS IN TARGETING DYSFUNCTIONAL THOUGHTS

Although there are many cognitive treatment strategies to address dysfunctional thoughts, one that I find to be especially clear and practical is the five-step model provided by Mueser and colleagues (2009). I was intensively trained in this model during 2010–2011. Although the five steps were developed originally for clients with PTSD, many cognitive therapists now use them with any client who suffers from cognitive distortions and self-deprecation. I describe the five-step process here within the context of treating those who self-injure. For a full discussion of the five steps with reproducible forms, see Mueser et al.'s (2009) book-length presentation.

Step 1: Identifying the Situation

The first step involves the client's identifying a situation that recently led to self-injury. In demonstrating the five steps, I refer to the same individual throughout, whom I call Sara. In this instance, the client identified and wrote down the following precipitating situation on her Five-Step Worksheet. (A blank version of this worksheet is provided as Figure 12.3.) Sara's words are presented below in italics.

Ask yourself, "What happened that made me upset?" Write down a brief description of the situation.

Situation: *My boyfriend and I had a fight on the phone, and he hung up on me.*
Right afterward I cut myself six times on my arm.

Note that throughout the five steps, it is crucially important that the therapist *elicit the situations, thoughts, and feelings from the client,* rather than suggesting them. Evidence suggests that it is far more effective when the client uses his or her own words, as opposed to words provided by the therapist (Mueser et al., 2009). The use of the Socratic method (i.e., active, open-ended questioning) is very important in this treatment. Thus, in eliciting the situation with which to start the five steps, the therapist would say, "What situation would you like to concentrate on regarding self-injuring during the past week?" as opposed to "Let's talk about that situation with your boyfriend."

Step 2: Identifying the Feeling(s)

The second step focuses on the emotion(s) triggered by the situation. Mueser et al.'s approach targets four categories of emotions that occur most commonly in distressed clients. However, other emotions can be targeted if they predominate. Below is the example from Sara, who had just had a difficult phone call with her boyfriend, culminating in cutting.

Circle your strongest **feeling(s):**

* Fear/Anxiety   Sadness/Depression   Guilt/Shame   Anger

In this case, Sara circled (1) fear/anxiety, (2) sadness/depression, and (3) anger. The asterisk indicates that the client identified fear as the strongest of the three emotions. Clients often identify more than one intense emotion as emanating from an upsetting situation. In facilitating the five steps, the therapist should ask the client *why* he or she selected the specific emotions, and which are strongest. These questions lead the way to the next step of identifying thoughts.

Step 3: Identifying the Underlying Thoughts

For this step, Mueser and colleagues direct the therapist to inquire: "Ask yourself, 'What am I thinking that is leading me to feel this way?'" As with

1. Situation

Ask yourself, "What happened that made me upset?" Write down a brief description of the situation.

Situation: _____

_____

_____

2. Feeling

Circle your strongest **feeling(s):**

    Fear/Anxiety   Sadness/Depression   Guilt/Shame   Anger

3. Thought

Ask yourself, "What am I thinking that is leading me to feel this way?" You may identify more than one thought related to the feeling. Write down your thoughts below, and circle the thought most strongly related to the feeling.

Thoughts: _____

_____

_____

Are these thoughts **Common Styles of Thinking?** If yes, circle which one(s).

All-or-Nothing	Emotional Reasoning
Overgeneralizing	Overestimation of Risk
Must/Should/Never	Self-Blame
Catastrophizing	Mental Filter

Belief rating: How accurate is the thought? _____ (0 = definitely untrue, 100 = definitely true)

Distress rating: How upsetting is the thought? _____ (0 = not upsetting, 100 = extremely upsetting)

4. Evaluate Your Thought

Ask yourself, "What evidence do I have for this thought?" "Is there another way to look at this situation?" "How would someone else think about this situation?" Write down the answers that *do* support your thought and the answers that *do not* support your thought.

(cont.)

FIGURE 12.3. Five-Step Worksheet.

Adapted from Mueser, Rosenberg, and Rosenberg (2009). Copyright 2009 by the American Psychological Association. Reprinted with permission in Walsh (Guilford Press, 2012). Permission to photocopy this figure is granted to purchasers of this book for personal use only (see copyright page for details). Purchasers may download a larger version of this figure from the book's page on The Guilford Press website.

Things that DO support my thought: _____

_____

_____

Things that DO NOT support my thought: _____

_____

_____

5. Take Action!

Considering all the evidence FOR and AGAINST your thought, now how accurate do you believe your thought is?

Belief rating: _____ (0 = definitely not accurate, 100 = definitely accurate)

Does the evidence completely support the thought? Is your belief as strong as before? (Step 3)

   ☐ **YES,** the evidence *does* support my thought; my belief is just as strong as before.

   ☐ **NO,** the evidence does *not* completely support my thought; my belief is lower than before.

If the evidence does NOT completely support your thought, come up with a new thought that is supported by the evidence. These thoughts are usually more balanced and helpful. Write your new, more helpful thought in the space below. And remember, when you think of this upsetting situation in the future, replace your unhelpful automatic thought with your new, more accurate thought.

New Thought: _____

_____

_____

Belief rating: How accurate is the new thought? _____ (0 = definitely not accurate, 100 = definitely accurate)

Distress rating: How upsetting is the new thought? _____ (0 = not upsetting, 100 = extremely upsetting)

If the evidence DOES support your thought, decide what you need to do next in order to deal with the situation. Ask yourself, "Do I need to get more information about what to do?" "Do I need to get some help?" "Do I need to take steps to make sure I am safe?" Write down the steps of your action plan for dealing with the upsetting situation.

1. _____
2. _____
3. _____
4. _____

FIGURE 12.3. *(cont.)*

emotions, clients often identify more than one related thought. Clients are then directed to write down their thoughts on the Five-Step Worksheet (see Figure 12.3) and "to circle the thought most strongly related to the feeling" (Mueser et al., 2009, p. 341). Here is what Sara wrote:

Thoughts: *I thought—here we go again, another breakup. I am such a loser.*

[After some reflection, Sara teared up. The therapist encouraged her to say more, whereupon she added and wrote:] *It's just like when my mother left when I was 9.*

There must be something wrong with me that everyone leaves me.

Common Styles of Thinking

An additional component of Step 3 is identifying whether the thoughts just identified represent "Common Styles of Thinking" (Mueser et al., 2009). These are essentially refinements of the early work of Albert Ellis, the pioneer in identifying irrational thought patterns that trigger emotional pain (e.g., Ellis, 1962). Mueser's five steps employ eight common styles of irrational or ineffective types of thinking. These are provided below with examples from clinical practice, including (but not limited to) the current example of Sara:

- All-or-nothing—for example, "Either he loves everything about me, or we can't continue dating."
- Overgeneralizing – for example, "My mother left me when I was 9; therefore, everyone else will leave me for the rest of my life."
- Must/should/never – for example, "I must have done something wrong for my mother to leave me." Or "Given my history of sexual abuse, I should avoid all sexual relationships."
- Catastrophizing—for example, "He just hung up on me. The relationship is clearly over." Or "I relapsed a little on my cutting; it's only going to get worse and never stop."
- Emotional reasoning—for example, "I believe this so deeply, it must be true." Or "I'm so angry, he must have meant to hurt me intentionally."
- Overestimation of risk—for example, "All relationships end in heartache and pain; there's no point in trying." Or "I have a cough, so it must be cancer."
- Inaccurate or excessive self-blame----for example, "I should have done something to stop the abuse; it went on too long; I must have wanted it to happen."
- Mental filter—for example, "One detail went wrong with the project; therefore, the whole thing should be destroyed." Or "I got a promotion at work, but my raise wasn't at the highest level; therefore, I'm a failure."

The display below shows how Sara identified which common styles applied to her current thought process.

Are these thoughts **Common Styles of Thinking?** If yes, circle which one(s).

All-or-Nothing	Emotional Reasoning
⟨Overgeneralizing⟩	Overestimation of Risk
⟨Must/Should/Never⟩	⟨Self-Blame⟩
Catastrophizing	Mental Filter

For these Common Styles, the client circled (quite accurately): Overgeneralizing ("Here we go again, I'm such a loser"); Must/Should/Never ("There must be something wrong with me"); and Self-Blame ("There must be something wrong with me; everyone leaves me, including my mother"). And she could easily have added Mental Filter and Emotional Reasoning ("I'm such a loser").

Belief and Distress Ratings

The final aspects of Step 3 involve asking a client to rate his or her levels of belief and distress related to the thoughts just identified. This requires that the client select which of the various thoughts is most important, stressful, and directly related to ineffective behavior such as self-injury. In Sara's case, she selected this as the most important thought: "It's just like when my mother left when I was 9. There must be something wrong with me that everyone leaves me." Note that this thought is in all likelihood a core belief.

Sara then rated her belief in this thought and the related level of distress as shown below, using the simple scales that end Step 3 of Figure 12.3:

Belief rating: How accurate is the thought? _100_ (0 = definitely untrue, 100 = definitely true)

Distress rating: How upsetting is the thought? _70_ (0 = not upsetting, 100 = extremely upsetting)

Sara explained her belief rating of 100 by saying, "I've thought this way for many years," and "I really do believe there's not much to like about me." She added that the distress rating was "only a 70 because I'm so used to that thought; it's not as upsetting as it used to be when I was a kid, because it's so familiar."

Step 4: Evaluating the Thought

Step 4 is the heart of the five steps. Here the client examines the evidence for and against the key thought. As noted above, it is especially important that the therapist use the Socratic method in assisting the client with the evaluation of thoughts. Clients are much more likely to "own" and believe in evidence they have identified themselves. Even though therapists intend to be supportive and helpful in providing their own "accurate" evidence, this practice actually impedes progress. Clients need to believe in the evidence both for and against their thoughts in order to modify the thoughts meaningfully. One way to teach clients to objectively evaluate their thoughts is to explain the "evidence" should meet the standard either of (1) "evidence in a court of law" or (2) "scientific evidence" (Mueser et al. 2009). Deeply held opinion or ingrained belief does not suffice. Mueser et al. (2009, p. 128; see Step 4 of Figure 12.3) directs client to do the following:

4. Evaluate Your Thought

Ask yourself, "What evidence do I have for this thought?" "Is there another way to look at this situation?" "How would someone else think about this situation?" Write down the answers that *do* support your thought and the answers that *do not* support your thought.

In completing Step 4, Sara wrote (again, it is important for the client to be actively writing down the material):

Things that DO support my thought: *A lot of people have left me in my life.* [Prodded to be more specific, as is required with "evidence," she said:] *My mother left me. I've had three boyfriends leave me.* [Prodded again to be more specific, she stated and wrote:] *Well, for two it was mutual.*

Things that DO NOT support my thought: *One angry phone call does not mean the relationship with my boyfriend is over. We've had arguments before and stayed together. He does say he loves me sometimes.* [Encouraged to link this evidence with the more fundamental thought about her mother leaving, Sara then said and wrote:] *My mother left me when I was 9 because she was a junkie. She had that problem before I was born, and she still struggles with it today. Maybe it wasn't my fault she left; she's had a lot of issues.* [After writing this, the client wept and then noticeably calmed.]

In facilitating Step 4, the therapist needs to elicit the evidence even-handedly. For the exercise to be credible, both sides of the dilemma need to be heard. Fortunately, because self-denigration is so common among people who self-injure, *the evidence almost always falls in the therapeutic direction*. That is to say, in the large majority of instances, thoughts are found to be inaccurate—often profoundly so.

Step 5: Taking Action

In the fifth and final step, the client reaches a conclusion about the evidence just weighed. Having considered the evidence pro and con, the client is asked to rate his or her belief in the thought again. Sara provided this rating:

Belief rating: How accurate is the thought? *30*   (0 = definitely untrue, 100 = definitely true)

Sara explained the drop in rating from the previous 100 to 30 as follows: "It helped to look at the real evidence. I like this process. Just because I believed something since I was a kid, that doesn't mean it's true."

The client then indicates in a check box whether the evidence completely supports the thought or does not. In Sara's case, she checked the latter:

☐ **YES,** the evidence *does* support my thought; my belief is just as strong as before.

☒ **NO,** the evidence does *not* completely support my thought; my belief is lower than before.

When the evidence does not completely support the thought, the client is then encouraged to create a new thought that is more accurate, balanced, and helpful. After some serious deliberation, Sara wrote down a new thought. It is very common that developing a new thought is challenging and stressful for clients. The new thought is often so foreign to their ingrained way of thinking that it initially feels false, contrived, or even "disloyal." Nonetheless, Sara was able to develop new cognitions:

New Thought: *My boyfriend may not leave me, but even if he does, it has nothing to do with my mother. It's not my fault she left. I wish I could have helped her more, but I was the kid and she was supposed to be the parent. Boyfriends and mothers are different.*

The concluding action is to rate the belief and distress related to this new thought on the same 0–100 scales as in Step 3. Sara responded:

Belief rating: How accurate is the thought? _80_____ (0 = definitely untrue, 100 = definitely true)

Distress rating: How upsetting is the thought? _20_____ (0 = not upsetting, 100 = extremely upsetting)

Sara said that she believed the new thought to be "pretty accurate," but that she would "need some time to get used to it." She added that if she firmly came to believe this thought, she would have a lot less distress; therefore, she gave it the low rating of 20.

This session concluded with the development of an "action plan" (Mueser et al., 2009). The action plan returned to the original Step 1 situation, where a fight with her boyfriend led Sara to cut herself. The therapist and Sara collaboratively identified arguments with the boyfriend as significant triggers for episodes of self-injury. Sara recognized that these conflicts in the present were linked to core beliefs from her past about her mother's abandonment. As part of her action plan, she agreed to do the five steps immediately after disagreements with her boyfriend. This homework was provided as an important alternative to self-injury. By doing the five steps, Sara became aware that self-punishment via self-injury was linked to self-blame about her mother's leaving many years before. She then became committed to unlearning this link and living with more accurate and helpful thoughts about herself, her past, and her current relationships.

CONCLUSION

In summary, in the cognitive therapy of self-injury, it is generally most helpful if clinicians do the following:

- Explain the cognitive model to clients: automatic thoughts, intermediate beliefs, and core beliefs.
- Explain how such thoughts and beliefs support and sustain self-injury.
- Employ Mueser et al.'s five-step model to deal with these dysfunctional, unhelpful cognitions.
- Use collaborative empiricism to evaluate the accuracy of these thoughts. A therapist needs to be careful in eliciting thoughts and evidence *from a client*, rather than providing them.
- Identify common styles of thinking that are unhelpful, are inaccurate, and promote self-harm.

- Over time, identify the core beliefs supporting the intermediate beliefs and automatic thoughts that precede self-injury.
- Transform persistent negative thoughts and core beliefs into more helpful, accurate cognitions that are held with conviction.
- Use homework between sessions to practice the five steps, consolidate progress, and ensure generalization to the natural environment.

CHAPTER 13

Family Therapy

MICHAEL HOLLANDER

The third component of Step 2 in the stepped-care model (See Figure II.1, p. 75) is family therapy. Family therapy is an optional aspect of Step 2, because not all individuals who self-injure want or need family treatment. Some may want to focus their treatment efforts on individual work; others may not have any family members to involve; still others may have family members who refuse to participate.

For those who do want family treatment, such therapy can be a high-risk/high-gain strategy. This is especially true for families in which a child, adolescent, or young adult engages in self-injury. Unless carefully conducted, the treatment can have unintended iatrogenic effects, increasing the likelihood of self-injurious behavior. On the other hand, when crafted and conducted carefully, family therapy can reduce self-injury and increase effective family functioning.

Family therapy for self-injury generally has four overarching goals: (1) educating family members about the functions of self-injury; (2) decreasing any behaviors within the family that trigger self-injury; (3) establishing (or reinstating) age-appropriate roles for parent(s) and child; and (4) decreasing the unbridled expression of emotion, while increasing effective communication about the internal psychological states of family members.

COMMON THEMES IN FAMILIES WITH A PERSON WHO SELF-INJURES

There are very few experiences that are more frightening, confusing, or worrisome to parents than having a child who engages in self-injury. The behavior flies in the face of an important parental function: that of protecting the child's body and well-being. Having a child who self-injures can often lead parents to experience intense levels of guilt. Sometimes this guilt becomes debilitating and can quickly compromise effective parenting skills. Often parental confusion leads to a wholesale sense of uncertainty, followed by helplessness and inaction. Alternatively, some parents' emotional distress leads them to become "certain" about the meaning and function of the behavior in a marginally informed way. Unfortunately, even when parental understanding is accurate, the manner in which parents present their ideas is often very problematic for the adolescent. Such ideas may be paired with quick attempts at problem solving that are much too short on validation. When this occurs, the likelihood that emotional dyregulation will be part and parcel of parent–child interactions is greatly increased. Parents whose understanding is inaccurate and who are pushed by emotional distress may search for confirming evidence to support their view, closing their minds to what their child is saying. This pattern of family transaction often leads to great discord between the adolescent and parents and to increased tension between parenting partners.

Siblings can further complicate the picture. Parents often struggle with how to explain the self-injuring child's difficulties to the other children in the family. Parents are quite right to worry about scaring younger siblings; however, pretending that "all is well" may engender confusion and unspoken fear. Older children, especially adolescents, frequently become judgmental and impatient with their self-injuring sibling. They may condemn their sibling's behavior vociferously, as well as their parents' (mis)management of it. Alternatively, an older sibling may become oversolicitous and protective toward the self-injuring sibling, unwittingly reinforcing the dysfunctional behavior.

Self-injuring adolescents not uncommonly feel lost and estranged from their families. The shame and guilt surrounding the behavior, and their worry about parental reactivity, often lead them to avoid seeking support when they need it most. They can also blame their parents for the self-injury when the parents' efforts to manage the behavior are ineffective or even punitive. For these, and a whole host of other reasons, family therapy often *seems* to be a good idea. Mental health professionals almost reflexively prescribe family therapy in these situations—yet it is almost as common for the treatment to blow up and make matters worse. Why is this such a frequent outcome, and what can be done about it?

PROBLEMS WITH STANDARD FAMILY THERAPY

Of all the psychotherapeutic modalities, family therapy may be the one that requires clients to be most skillful in managing their emotions. Imagine that you are an adolescent sitting with your parents and a therapist, and that the focus of the discussion is your "problematic" behavior. Such situations are bound to evoke powerful feelings in all the participants, especially the adolescent. As a group, youth who self-injure are well known to have poor capacities to manage and modulate their emotions effectively (Walsh, 2006; Klonsky, 2007, 2009; Nock, 2010). In fact, self-injuring is usually the most effective strategy these teens have for managing intense emotional experiences. Consequently, traditional open-ended family therapy is often too emotionally intense for these clients to manage. All too often, they storm out of the room or stay put while emotionally shutting down. Although either of these behaviors may seem ineffective from one perspective, it makes perfect sense from another. Family therapy for these clients is akin to teaching people to swim by throwing them out of a boat in the middle of a deep lake. Some people would quickly give up trying to get to shore and just go under, like our emotionally shut-down clients. Others would flail about for the longest time, exhausting themselves unproductively, like our clients who exhibit intense emotional displays. In either case, learning how to swim spontaneously is not likely to be the outcome. In order for family therapy to be effective, the person who self-injures is required to tolerate intense emotions without any avoidance or escape behavior. By and large, we are asking them to do something they don't have the skill set to do.

Parents come to treatment worried, annoyed, often ashamed, and feeling guilty. Healthy interpersonal development for the child, such as independence and autonomy, has usually been derailed by the self-injury. The situation is an emotional time bomb that requires real clinical acumen. Often the therapy blows up, and all participants become frustrated, hopeless, and despairing. On the other hand, as outlined above, there are some very compelling reasons to prescribe family therapy. The following is a way of conducting family treatment that minimizes unbridled emotional dysregulation and maximizes positive outcomes.

ASSESSMENT AND PSYCHOEDUCATIONAL PHASE

Before proceeding directly to family therapy, the clinician needs to assess the capacities of the family members for emotional experiencing. This early phase is also used to develop clarity about the goals of the family treatment. In addition, the clinician uses this period to help family members understand the functions that self-injury serves in the child's life. Psychoeducation about self-injury will help modulate parental worries and support family members in gaining a more compassionate understanding of the self-injuring child's dilemma. It is critical for the therapist finds the "wisdom" in the self-injuring behavior and to help the family understand the reasons behind it. This is not tantamount to endorsing the behavior, but only to help make sense of it.

I recommend taking the first two to three sessions to complete the assessment phase. During this time, family members can be oriented to the idea that the first several sessions are going to focus on assessing their current capacity to do family work, and on developing a consensus about the issues to be addressed. In addition, the members should be helped to understand that as important as family work is, other interventions may be needed before family treatment can be pursued. At the end of the orientation, family members and the clinician should have a good sense about whether family therapy is indicated at this time, what is going to be discussed in treatment, and what changes the family can expect (Hollander, 2008).

Assessing the Family's Capacity for Validation, Distress Tolerance, and Emotion Regulation

It is often useful to begin the assessment phase with a discussion that focuses on the family's strengths. Doing so helps the family start on a more balanced and hopeful note. It also keys the clinician to areas of resiliency within the family. In addition, it is useful to explore times in the family's history when its members functioned more effectively.

During this phase, the therapist should assess each family member's capacity to validate and to understand the perspectives of others. Any blatantly hostile or judgmental comments should be blocked by the therapist and reframed in more behaviorally specific terms. Such reframing should be neutral, while addressing the speaker's emotional state. Most often, hostility and negative judgments arise from either hurt feelings (sadness) or worry (fear). When these moments arise, the therapist will have the opportunity to get a sense of each family member's capacity to tolerate distress, regulate emotions, and be interpersonally effective (Linehan, 1993a, 1993b). If the family has real trouble with validation, distress tolerance, and emotion regulation, it is likely that some skill building will need to take place before family treatment proper is initiated.

Developing Treatment Goals

An essential aspect of assessment is developing a collaborative set of clearly defined behavioral goals. The clinician should begin to probe for areas of conflict and for each member's theory about why things got off track. The clinician needs to be quite active in this part of the treatment and ever vigilant for signs of emotional dysregulation. In this phase of the assessment, the therapist needs to be skilled in thinking about issues from a dialectical perspective (Linehan, 1993a; Hollander, 2008). The therapist's interventions are aimed at articulating and clarifying the wisdom in each participant's point of view. The therapist has to stay empathically in tune with each family member.

It is often very difficult for us as clinicians to find and maintain compassion and empathy for each family member. Sometimes we are too focused on an adolescent's distress; at other times we may find the adolescent's behavior so reprehensible that we shift toward the parents' perspective. Alternatively, we may experience the parents as excessively angry and rigid toward their child's behavior and lose sight of their emotional pain. Often parents present as so anxious that they come across as excessively needy, helpless, and confused, demanding that we "fix" their child. Whatever the case, it is essential that the clinician find compassion for each participant; without this capacity, the clinician cannot formulate goals that will ultimately enhance *family* functioning, as opposed to working on individual goals. When therapists encounter difficulty generating compassion, or notice that they are losing it, it is useful to get a consultation from a colleague or another team member.

As the assessment phase winds down, the clinician begins to formulate a treatment plan in collaboration with the family. An important part of the treatment plan is deciding who will come to family treatment. The therapist, in conjunction with parents and the self-injuring youth, will have to be part of this process. In my experience, the critical participants are the self-injuring client and the parents. For the most part, siblings can be asked to join on an issue-by-issue basis. It is important to make the goals clear and to obtain a commitment from each participant to the work ahead. All too often, therapists skip this part of the treatment because they assume that everybody is more or less on board. I recommend that eliciting this commitment be a clearly delineated, structured, and formal part of the assessment phase. The commitment should focus on attendance, doing homework, and working toward the shared family goals. Furthermore, it is useful to plan regular reviews about the treatment. If the treatment is going to be ongoing and weekly, a review every 10–12 sessions is a reasonable time frame. The function of the review is to monitor progress toward goals and to introduce new goals if warranted. The key here is to avoid conducting an aimlessly wandering therapy.

The end of the assessment phase marks a crossroads in the treatment. There are several avenues the therapist and family may take. One direction would be for the therapist to recommend that the family spend time developing the emotion regulation and interpersonal skills to do family treatment. For example, the therapist may suggest that the first several months of treatment be primarily focused on helping the family acquire the DBT skill set. Included in this recommendation would be helping family members practice validation and develop a familiarity with the adolescent and parent secondary targets (Miller et al., 2007). If the family as a whole seems to have sufficient capacity to manage family therapy, then treatment can proceed. Finally, there may be families whose level of dysfunction might rule out family treatment. For example, families where there is a history of past or ongoing abuse may not be good candidates for this kind of intervention. It is incumbent upon the therapist to be clear, direct, and transparent when making these recommendations.

FAMILY THERAPY PROPER

After the goals are identified and the decision about who will attend is settled, family therapy proper can begin. If the family therapist is not the individual therapist for the self-injuring youth, a plan for communication between the two needs to be established. In either case, the therapist needs to be comfortable being quite active at managing the treatment hour, so as to minimize affective dysregulation while also letting things play out when this is appropriate. The therapist has to be like a fly fisherman who knows where to cast, when to let the line drift, and when to hold the line taut. It is incumbent on the therapist to find the wisdom in each participant's perspective and to give clear voice to it, while not validating ineffective behavior. An important job of the therapist is to help each participant begin to value the other members' perspective and to develop each participant's capacity to be open and truly curious about others' points of view. The bedrock of such an approach is the capacity for family members to develop genuine curiosity about each other's behavior. This requires that certainty about another person's motivations and intentions be challenged, and that a more open and inquisitive perspective be adopted.

The mortal enemy of such an approach is emotional dysregulation. Intense emotions are likely to compromise participants' abilities to remain curious about each other. Under the sway of unbridled emotions, people's cognitive abilities generally fall apart in one of two ways. First, family members' thinking can become overly rigid, in a way that blocks communication and empathy. Fixed ideas about the motivations behind another's behavior do not lead to dialogue and understanding. Alternatively, people can go in the opposite direction and become paralyzed with uncertainty—acting confused, disorganized, and unable to take a stand or make a decision. Either of these states can lead participants to become attached to an array of myths and misconceptions about the psychological states, behaviors, and motivations of others. Such a process usually culminates multiple misattributions about another family member. These misconceptions are experienced as invalidating and generate more emotional dysregulation. When this occurs, the adolescent is at risk for engaging in more self-injury. Therefore, it is of utmost importance that therapists take an active role in helping the family emotionally manage these moments in treatment. The techniques associated with mentalization-based treatment (Bateman & Fonagy, 2006) can be quite useful in these moments.

Family treatment works best when it has some social ritual and clear structure. Starting with small talk at the beginning of the hour can be a nice way to make the transition into the session. Noticing a new hairdo or outfit, chatting about a sports team, or remarking on the unusual weather are benign ice breakers. The small talk should only last a few minutes before it is time to get into the agenda for the meeting. Setting the agenda is a collaborative process among all participants. The therapist, however, needs at times to take the lead on deciding the order of the agenda. The family therapist has to develop a decision tree or a process to aid in prioritizing issues. Using the target hierarchy from DBT is one helpful rubric to use in ordering priorities (Linehan, 1993a; Miller et al., 2007). For example, if self-injurious behavior has occurred during the past week and it was triggered by family interaction, this would be the highest-priority target in the session. Self-injurious behaviors that were triggered by events outside the family are usually not grist for the mill. A family chain analysis (Linehan, 1993a; Miller et al., 2007; Hollander, 2008) can be conducted to help each participant begin to understand his or her particular contribution to the problem—and, equally important, what all participants might do differently next time to avoid making these contributions. The next highest target would be any behavior, including the therapist's, that might have interfered in moving the treatment forward. Lowest in priority would be all the other issues that are compromising quality of life in family functioning.

Once an agenda has been developed, the therapist should review any homework that was assigned from the last session. Any issues centering around noncompliance with assignments needs to be actively understood.

Chain analyses can be used for this challenge as well. Following the homework review, the discussion should shift to the items on the agenda. At this point, the therapist has to take an active role in managing the time spent on each agenda item and making sure that the family members remain curious, open, and validating of each other's perspective. Conflict between members will inevitably arise. It is the job of the family therapist to help each family member understand what is missing in his or her own perspective, as well as the kernel of wisdom in the other's. The therapist's stance is one of neutrality—not overidentifying with either the self-injuring youth or the parents. Like a traffic cop, the therapist has to manage the flow of emotional expression, stopping unbridled emotional displays, while encouraging the tentative attempts of a member to be understood. It can be very hard work, but work that helps families heal.

As the therapy hour winds down, it is often useful for the therapist to briefly summarize the session. The important topics discussed are reviewed, and skillful behavior on the part of the participants should be highlighted and reinforced. As a general rule, it is also useful to assess each participant's emotional state before the hour is over. This gives the therapist a chance to help emotionally dysregulated members use skills to lower their emotional intensity. After this assessment, homework can be assigned, and the hour concludes with a bit of small talk.

CONCLUSION

In summary, family therapy can be an important component in the treatment of self-injury. It is important for clinicians conducting such therapy to do the following:

- Understand that not all families are capable of using the treatment immediately. Families that are prone to explosive emotion dysregulation may require interventions such as DBT in order to become ready for family treatment.
- Family therapy begins with validation, assessment, and some psychoeducation about the functions of self-injury.
- Family therapy should be structured, with clearly defined and mutually agreed-on behavioral goals. Family treatment should not be aimlessly wandering.
- Each session should work from an agenda. Using a format such as the DBT targets is recommended; in this format, self-harm behavior

is prioritized, followed by threats to the treatment, and concluding with quality-of-life issues for the family.

- Generally, family therapy includes the parent(s) and the self-injuring youth. Siblings may attend on occasion to address specific issues.
- Family therapy can be among the most triggering of psychological treatments. Asking youth to be the focus of extended discussion of their problem behaviors is a lot to ask and can be immensely dysregulating.
- The therapist has to consistently validate all family members, avoid taking sides, and emphasize the wisdom in each member's perspective.
- The therapist must walk a fine line—decreasing the unbridled expression of emotion, while increasing effective communication about the internal psychological states of family members.

CHAPTER 14

Psychopharmacological Treatment

GORDON P. HARPER

The fourth component of Step 2 in the stepped-care model (see Figure II.1, p. 75) is psychopharmacological treatment. Like family therapy, this form of treatment is considered optional, in that not everyone who self-injures requires such intervention. This is especially true for individuals who have self-injured only one or two times, or for those involved in a brief social contagion episode. Unfortunately, studies to date have not focused on the percentage of self-injuring persons who have received psychopharmacological treatment. This chapter discusses those who are most likely to benefit from this type of intervention. It also emphasizes the importance of a detailed assessment, and reviews the agents that have been shown to have the most efficacy.

Pharmacotherapy can help many individuals with self-injurious behavior. Symptoms by themselves do not, however, lead directly to choice of agent or class of agents. Clinical pharmacotherapy, while informed by experience with other clients (both individually and in clinical trials), consists of focused assessment, hypothesis generation, and empirical trial.

THE BIOLOGY OF SELF-INJURY

How Do We Understand What Is Wrong?

All efforts to help individuals with self-injury are directed ultimately at the brain, the source of all thinking and behavior. But as pharmacotherapy, unlike psychosocial interventions, is directed at the mediating neurological structures, it is useful to put self-injury in biological perspective.

All animals, not just humans, protect the self. Self-protective behavior—turning away from harmful stimuli—can be seen in nonhuman primates, in other mammals, and in other vertebrates (birds, reptiles, fish). Even invertebrates protect the self: Worms withdraw from heat or dryness, and cockroaches scuttle away from the light. "Higher" animals like mammals visibly care for the body, through such behaviors as grooming and licking. Harming or mutilating the body represents an overriding of deeply preserved evolutionary behavior—a derangement of developmental biology.

In culturally prescribed body modification, as described in Chapter 5, culture modifies the biological program. But the psychosocial context of such practices differentiates such behavior from what is called "self-destructive." Culturally prescribed mutilation can also strengthen the individual's connection to the group, as in religiously prescribed circumcision or in scarification among some sub-Saharan groups (Favazza, 1996). But pathological self-injury differs from culturally prescribed mutilation, because it occurs without the sanction of the group. Such behavior does not affirm the self. It violates a powerful biological imperative.

The emergence of self-protection in higher mammals is highly contingent. Clinical experience and animal experimentation indicate that self-protection does not emerge "automatically," as in birds or fish, but only when facilitated by the caregiving environment.

Several domains of development are implicated. For example, children normally identify with caregiving adults and grow up to care for themselves. But such identification is distorted in many survivors of abuse or neglect. Similarly, reciprocal caregiving relationships typically develop in humans and other primates. But they can be distorted in humans and in nonhuman primates who have been deprived of expectable nurturance. Stimulus seeking occurs in typical development, but can be prolonged or take malignant form in individuals with cognitive or perceptual deficiencies, in survivors of trauma, and in those who grow up in isolation. Distorted self-care behavior can be seen even in nonhuman mammals—for instance, in the canine "acral lick syndrome" (Rapaport, Ryland, & Kriete, 1992). Self-injury also occurs in individuals with distorted mood, especially depression, or delusional thinking, as in psychosis. Self-care and self-protection can also be blocked by dysfunctional environments—that is, when self-harm is inadvertently reinforced (cf. Mace, Blum, Sierp, Delaney, & Mauk, 2001).

Mediating Mechanisms

Inquiry into biological models of self-injury is motivated both by the wish to understand behavior physiologically and by the wish to develop effective pharmacotherapy. In some disorders, the neurological mechanisms are well worked out. For instance, parkinsonism arises from the death or dysfunction of dopaminergic cells in the nigrostriatal pathway, and supplementation with dopaminergic agents enhances function (Cookson, 2003).* In self-injury, the pathways are less clear; remediation is largely empirical.

A review of the current evidence implicating biological systems is beyond the scope of this chapter, but such reviews are available elsewhere (Villalba & Harrington, 2000; Tiefenbacher, Novak, Lutz, & Meyer, 2005). For current purposes, it suffices to note the following:

1. Several different systems play a role in self-injury: the limbic system (a subcortical brain system regulating mood, affect, and pain); dopaminergic systems leading to and within the cortex; serotonergic systems; and the endocrine system that leads from the hypothalamus to the pituitary to the adrenal glands and other secretory organs (the so-called "HPA axis") (Tiefenbacher et al., 2005).

2. Several different kinds of evidence are relevant: the physiology of typical individuals and of those with major developmental disorders, in whom self-injury is much more common than in the general population; results of inducing lesions, surgical or pharmacological, in animals; and responses to pharmacological trials.

3. Some of the evidence is intriguing. For instance, one study has found that self-injury is directed to body sites that are biologically distinct from nontargeted areas (e.g., to sites with altered skin temperature) (Symons, Sutton, & Bodfish, 2001).

---

*The suffix "-ergic," as in "dopaminergic" or "serotonergic," designates neural pathways in which a neurotransmitter acts. For instance, in a dopaminergic pathway, dopamine is released from one nerve, crosses a short space (the synaptic cleft), and activates the next nerve. Agents that enhance the availability or activity of a transmitter are called "agonists," and those that limit availability or activity are called "antagonists." Thus medicines like fluoxetine (Prozac and others) and sertraline (Zoloft and others) are serotonin agonists. Because they act by blocking the reuptake of serotonin from the synaptic cleft, they are called "selective serotonin reuptake inhibitors," or SSRIs.

4. Biological studies, like clinical observations, make clear that self-injury does not arises from dysfunction in a single pathway or mechanism, but is a heterogeneous class.

5. Correspondingly, many pharmacological agents have been used in treating self-injury: antidepressants, antipsychotics, and mood stabilizers (Shapira, Lessig, Murphy, Driscoll, & Goodman, 2002); anxiolytics and opiate antagonists (Sandman et al., 2000); alpha-agonists (Macy, Beattie, Morgenstern, & Arnsten, 2000); and, in animals, the calcium-channel blocker nifedipine (Blake et al., 2007).

6. Published studies vary in methodology from uncontrolled single-case reports to well-controlled clinical trials, and caution is indicated in interpreting their results. A Cochrane Controlled Trials Register review (Hawton et al., 2009) found "promising results" for problem-solving therapy, provision of a card for emergency contact with services, depot flupenthixol (a first-generation antipsychotic not available in the United States), and long-term psychological therapy for female clients with BPD and recurrent self-harm. The review could not recommend any treatment as well-established.

7. Clinical epidemiology and animal studies suggest that self-injury must be understood both in terms of long-term vulnerability (associated with developmental disorders or arising from such life experiences as neglect or abuse) and in terms of current conditions that act upon such a background.

As an example, consider the role in self-injury of serotonin (also known as 5-hydroxytryptamine), a neurotransmitter that is critical to the maintenance of mood and a feeling of well-being. Drugs that enhance serotonin availability include fluoxetine (Prozac and others), sertraline (Zoloft and others), paroxetine (Paxil and others), fluvoxamine (Luvox and others), citalopram (Celexa), and descitalopram (Lexapro). Serotonin agonists are effective in treating clinical depression. The evidence for such efficacy is well established in adults; controversy attends the use of SSRIs in children and adolescents (see a recent statement at *www.nimh.nih.gov/health/topics/child-and-adolescent-mental-health/antidepressant-medications-for-children-and-adolescents-information-for-parents-and-caregivers.shtml*).

A role for serotonergic pathways in self-care, and the role of serotonin deficiency in self-injury, is suggested by several kinds of evidence. For instance, controlled clinical trials in people with disorders in the obsessive–compulsive spectrum show reduced self-injury, especially hair pulling or other damage to the skin and its appendages. Some individual case reports document striking responses, even life-saving, to SSRIs in clients with severe skin picking (O'Sullivan, Phillips, Keuthen, & Wilhelm, 1999; Velazquez, Ward-Chene, & Loosigian, 2000). As mentioned above, the same effect is seen in dogs with a syndrome in which excessive licking leads to erosion of the skin (Rapaport et al., 1992).

But data have also raised the possibility that some SSRIs may increase problem behavior, especially in the young. Case reports document *emergent* skin-picking behavior (Denys, van Megan, & Westenberg, 2003; Weintrob, 2001) and suicidal ideation when clients begin SSRIs. Such reports indicate how incomplete is our knowledge of the biology of skin picking and other self-injurious behaviors. They also mandate close attention to individual clients whenever a pharmacological trial is initiated—no matter how impressive published results for groups of clients may be.

FOCUSED ASSESSMENT

Pharmacotherapy must be guided by focused assessment. Drugs must not be prescribed as "magic-bullet" therapy just because a client engages in self-injury.

Current Behavior

The behavior to be treated must be characterized. The following questions can guide assessment:

> What does the behavior consist of?
> What is the pattern of the behavior?
> When does it occur?
> Does it occur when the client is frustrated? Anxious? Angry? Sad?
> How long has it been present?
> Does it occur in a predictable sequence?
> Does it occur in response to identifiable triggers or precipitants?
> Are certain caregivers repeatedly present?

Associated Clinical Syndromes

What diagnoses does the individual have? Both lifelong developmental syndromes and acute psychiatric disorders must be considered. A developmental disorder itself may be undertreated. With regard to depression and other acute psychiatric disorders, Haw, Houston, Townsend, and Hawton (2002) found a high prevalence of depression in clients with self-injury, and Tsiouris, Cohen, Patti, and Korosh (2003) showed decreased self-injury with treatment of depression and other disorders. Psychotic disorders must also be considered—including presentations in which frank psychotic symptoms may not be apparent, but the client shows severe mental disorganization.

Current Context

Which elements of the client's current context are relevant to the self-injury? Are caregivers' responses unintentionally reinforcing self-injury? Does caregiver fatigue, therapeutic uncertainty, or unacknowledged anger at the client play a part?

In response to disruptive behavior, an adolescent hospitalized on a psychiatric unit was restricted from contact with peers and participation in unit activities. She inserted small objects under her skin and into body orifices, necessitating trips to emergency medical facilities. Efforts to "keep her safe" included one-on-one staffing; "small-obs restrictions" (limited access to small objects); and trials of antipsychotics, antidepressants, mood stabilizers, and opiate antagonists. The behavior continued. Only when the staff members acknowledged their reaction to her (fear, anger, helplessness, and hopelessness), stopped sending her to another hospital after each self-injury incident, and developed a more hopeful relationship with the client did the behavior decrease. *In an adverse and pathologically reinforcing environment*, pharmacological interventions were of no avail.

Similarly, Mace et al. (2001) have reported greater short-term efficacy in reducing self-injury via behavioral interventions, compared to pharmacological interventions.

Life Context

What is the client's life situation? What are his or her future prospects? Lack or loss of a "future vision" may constitute part of the existential trap in which despair and regression occur. Who, among family members, other caregivers, and in- and outpatient team members, holds that future vision?

Adaptive Perspective

To implement the future vision, the clinician must define the best level of functioning that can be anticipated for the client. Have educational, vocational, and family assessments defined how the client can best be expected to function while self-injury symptoms continue or abate?

Hypothesis Generation

On the basis of focused assessment, the clinician identifies factors that may be contributing to the self-injury. These should be stated in language that points to possible intervention. They should also be stated in terms that specify the degree to which each factor has been recognized or treated. Such factors constitute a formulation or set of hypotheses, put in operational terms. For instance, the clinician might cite such factors as these (see Mace et al., 2001):

- Poor frustration tolerance (long-standing) associated with developmental disorder (possibly undertreated)
- Possible undertreated depression
- Severe cognitive and affective disorganization, without frank psychosis, but possibly responsive to antipsychotic medication
- Mix of competencies and vulnerabilities, presently underevaluated
- Whether the client's clinical team and family are at an early stage of finding a way to talk about the client's strengths and challenges and their adaptive implications
- Unrecognized dysfunctional responses by caregivers, with unintended reinforcement of self-injury

Listing all possible contributing factors explicitly makes it easy to see whether important domains—like the developmental, existential, or social context—have been omitted. From such a list of possible contributing factors, the clinician chooses for intervention those most susceptible to intervention and most likely to make a difference in the target symptom.

EMPIRICAL TRIALS

One of the advantages of stating factors as testable hypotheses is that a clinicin does not have to "commit" him- or herself to a particular formulation ("It's this . . . "). Rather, such a list leads to empirical trials of possibly useful agents.

When depression is a possibility, either because of significant depressive symptoms or because a client may be suffering from despair that is difficult to articulate, a trial of antidepressant medication is indicated. Both newer antidepressants (the SSRIs and others) and first-generation antidepressants (amitriptyline or nortriptyline, imipramine or desipramine) may be considered. Although side effects complicate treatment with first-generation agents more than with SSRIs, side effects of the SSRIs are increasingly recognized, both during treatment and on withdrawal. With all antidepressants, the emergence of activation must be watched for, whether or not clients have a diagnosis of bipolar disorder.

Anxiety in self-injury is sometimes manifest, sometimes only inferred. Treatment with anxiolytic agents—especially benzodiazepines like loraze-pam (Ativan and others) or diazepam (Valium and others)—is sometimes useful, but in some clients such agents exacerbate target symptoms. Clinical observation of such disinhibition on benzodiazepines is consistent with evidence from the treatment of self-injury in monkeys, in which 50% showed decreased self-injury and 50% showed worsened self-injury in response to diazepam (Tiefenbacher et al., 2005).

In clients with delusional self-injury, trials of antipsychotic agents are indicated. In addition, second-generation antipsychotic agents—such as risperidone (Risperdal and others) and clozapine (Clozaril and others)—have an increasingly well-defined role in the treatment of self-injury, especially in clients with developmental disabilities. This role goes beyond the treatment of psychotic disorders. Well-designed placebo-controlled clinical trials have shown that risperidone reduces a number of symptoms, including self-harm behavior and symptoms prioritized by parents, in developmentally disabled children (McCracken et al., 2002; Arnold et al., 2003). Individual case reports have shown clozapine to be effective in clients with BPD, psychosis, and self-injury (Chengappa, Ebeling, Kang, Levine, & Parepally, 1999), and in clients with developmental disorders whose self-injury had not responded to risperidone (Beherec et al., 2011). Treatment with antipsychotic agents may be complicated by weight gain and other metabolic side effects with second-generation agents, and by movement disorders with first-generation agents. The risk of bone marrow suppression with clozapine requires regular monitoring of white blood cell counts throughout treatment.

Mood stabilizers include valproate (Depakote and others), carbamazepine (Tegretol and others), lithium carbonate, and topiramate (Topamax). Although mood stabilizers have not been shown to be effective in treating self-injury in controlled trials, individual case reports have shown some benefit (Cassano et al., 2001). Mood stabilizers may be considered as second-line agents in self-injury, particularly when affective instability is prominent, whether or not a client has a diagnosis of bipolar disorder. Side effects of mood stabilizers are diverse and potentially serious, varying with the choice of agent.

The role of endogenous opioids in pain regulation has led to interest in a possible role for opiate antagonists, especially naltrexone (Revia and others), in self-injury (Sher & Stanley, 2008). The hypothesis is that self-injury serves as a behavioral equivalent of an opiate in tension or pain regulation, and that the "relief" experienced with self-injury could be blocked by blocking the opiate receptor. Both clinical experience and the published literature suggest that this benefit occurs infrequently.

The medications called alpha-agonists include clonidine (Catapres and others) and guanfacine (Tenex and others). Compared to other psychoactive medications, they have benign side effect profiles. Their role in treating attention-deficit/hyperactivity disorder (ADHD), tics, and posttraumatic symptoms has been well established. Some case reports suggest a role in treating self-injury (Macy et al., 2000).

CONCLUSION

Clinical experience converges with a provocative and rapidly expanding literature on the biology and pharmacotherapy of self-injury, reinforcing the idea that self-injury is a heterogeneous phenomenon. Clinical pharmacotherapy must be based on the following:

- Knowledge of the literature
- Focused assessment of the individual client
- Generation of hypotheses regarding possible contributing factors
- Close attention to the context in which self-injury is occurring
- Judicious empirical trials, choosing from among very different classes of medication

Medication trials must be undertaken with simultaneous attention to the several dimensions of the client's context:

- Developmental context
- Context of psychiatric disorders
- Existential/adaptive context
- Social context, considering both family members and other caregivers

TREATMENT: STEP 3

CHAPTER 15

Body Image Work

With body image work, we move to the first component of Step 3 in the stepped-care model (see Figure II.1, p. 75). Clients requiring Step 3 care have generally endured serious mistreatment, including physical and/or sexual abuse. These are *not* the relatively healthy individuals from the general population described in Chapter 4. Because of the mistreatment they have endured – along with biological vulnerabilities—these clients often present with multiple problems beyond nonsuicidal self-injury. These challenges include complex PTSD symptoms, occasional suicidal ideation/behaviors, body alienation, eating disorders, and substance abuse. Body image work is a good place to start with individuals who have such complex problem configurations. Treatment that focuses on body alienation may be more acceptable to individuals who are not yet ready to deal with complex trauma issues, as discussed in Chapter 16.

As noted in Chapter 12, Beck (2011) has suggested that the negative core beliefs of individuals fall into two basic categories: incompetence and unlovability. I believe that a third type of core belief is often centrally important for those who self-injure: negative body image. It may seem intuitively obvious that many self-injuring individuals have compromised relationships with their bodies. Why else would they cut, burn, punch, pierce, pick, excoriate, or otherwise assault their bodies? It seems unlikely that people who hold their bodies in high esteem would subject themselves to such attacks. But understanding the relationship between self-injury and body image problems is complex. Applying this understanding in providing effective treatment is especially important and is the subject of this chapter.

Body image has been a productive area of research since the 1930s (e.g., Schilder, 1935; Secord & Jourard, 1953; Fisher, 1970; Tucker, 1981, 1983, 1985; Cash & Pruzinsky, 1990, 2002; Muehlenkamp, Claes, Smits, Peat, & Vandereycken, 2011). Some authors have emphasized broad psychodynamic formulations (Schilder, 1935; Fisher, 1970). Others have concentrated on narrower, more behavior-specific topics, such as body size estimation (Thompson, Berland, Linton, & Weinsier, 1987), satisfaction with body parts or areas (Secord & Jourard, 1953; Tucker, 1985), or physical self-efficacy (Ryckman, Robbins, Thornton, & Cantrell, 1982). More recently, Cash and Pruzinsky (2002) have argued that body image is a multidimensional construct that is influenced by myriad biological, cognitive, affective, developmental, and contextual factors. A thorough review of the extensive body image literature is beyond the scope of this book; Cash's work is highly recommended (Cash & Pruzinsky, 2002; Cash, 2004).

For present purposes, "body image" is defined as a complex set of thoughts, feelings, and behaviors related to the physical experience, size estimation, appraisal of, and satisfaction with one's own body. Based on the body image literature cited above and my own research regarding the body image difficulties of self-injuring individuals (Walsh, 1987; Walsh & Rosen, 1988; Walsh & Frost, 2005), I have found it useful to consider six dimensions of body self-concept:

- Attractiveness
- Effectiveness
- Health
- Sexual characteristics
- Sexual behavior
- Body integrity

These are defined below.

THE SIX DIMENSIONS OF BODY IMAGE

Attractiveness

"Attractiveness" refers to whether or not an individual feels attractive and receives feedback from others regarding being attractive. This is a very subjective body image dimension. Many individuals who self-injure are objectively attractive people who consider themselves to be unappealing. Some go so far as to refer to themselves quite unjustifiably as "ugly," "disgusting," even "deformed."

Attractiveness is an important feature of one's life. Particularly during adolescence, but also thereafter, attractiveness has been found to be associated with popularity, self-confidence, social competence, and academic achievement (Ashford, McCroy, & Lortie, 2001). Individuals need to feel reasonably attractive to operate comfortably in social environments. For those who feel patently unappealing, the result can be avoidance of social encounters and withdrawal. Those who believe that others recoil at their appearance may choose to avoid "inflicting this pain" on the environment. Other individuals who feel profoundly unattractive may allow others to exploit them, feeling fortunate to receive any attention at all, even if it is exploitive.

Effectiveness

"Effectiveness" is an entirely different dimension of body image. It pertains to coordination, athleticism, and stamina (see Ryckman et al., 1982). Obviously, one can feel very competent athletically while also feeling very unattractive, or vice versa.

For example, I worked with a woman who was an accomplished athlete, but was extremely pejorative about her attractiveness and engaged in chronic self-injury. Although she was objectively quite pleasant-looking, she frequently referred to herself as "a fat, ugly, disgusting-looking pig." However, she felt quite positive about her physical effectiveness. In high school and college, she had been an accomplished athlete. There seemed to be a link for this individual between her athletic achievements and her self-injury. She reported that "when the physical pain of exercise kicked in," she almost always "got off on it." She was an example of an "endorphin-addicted" self-injuring individual who sought the endogenous opioid release associated with sustained physical exertion. Effectiveness was an isolated area of body image satisfaction for this woman. In all other areas, she presented with extremely negative, self-critical thoughts and beliefs about her body.

Health

The body image dimension of "health" involves both subjective and objective aspects. The objective aspect concerns whether or not an individual has any medically diagnosed conditions or illnesses. Persons with a serious or chronic physical illness can have a very compromised sense of body image (Geist, 1979; Hughes, 1982; Cash & Pruzinsky, 2002). Illness can cause considerable physical discomfort; it may also result in intrusive and/or painful medical procedures. Sustained illness may lead to isolation from family and peers and to interruption of (school or work, recreation, etc.). For people with chronic illnesses, such as diabetes, asthma, arthritis, or other problems, the body can be experienced as a major inconvenience or even as "an enemy." For such persons, the body seems to be rarely working in their best interests; instead, it is experienced as an impediment or obstacle to the life they want to live.

Although such illnesses are sometimes present in self-injuring persons, the far more common situation appears to be individuals who feel unhealthy *subjectively*. These are people who have no diagnosed physical conditions or illnesses, but who nonetheless frequently experience their bodies as unwell. We are all familiar with clients who seem to have an unending series of physical complaints that migrate from one body area to another. These are people who are in frequent, almost daily discomfort, reporting a wide variety of problems (headaches, nausea, backache, muscle cramps, intestinal ailments, etc.). Although it is tempting to refer to such people countertransferentially as "hypochondriacs," a more compassionate and insightful attitude is to view them as body-alienated. Frequent complaints of physical discomfort are one way clients communicate their persistent negative attitudes regarding their bodies. Once physical illness has been ruled out by a physician, the clinician can begin to investigate the sources of body alienation in "the chronically ill but physically well" person who self-injures.

Sexual Characteristics

The dimension of "sexual characteristics" refers to comfort–discomfort with the physical changes in the body associated with puberty. Most individuals are comfortable with passing into physical maturity and acquiring adult bodies. Others, particularly trauma survivors or persons with eating disorders, may experience considerable discomfort related to physical maturation. Some trauma survivors may feel that their bodies are "betraying" them as primary and secondary sex characteristics emerge; their adult bodies may remind them all too much of the bodies of their perpetrators. Other trauma survivors may be especially concerned that having physically mature bodies may result in others' approaching them sexually.

Eating-disordered individuals may be horrified in a different way by growth and other changes in their bodies. Females, especially, may view typical physical growth in hips, abdomen, and breasts as evidence of out-of-control weight gain and imminent obesity.

Sexual Behavior

The dimension of "sexual behavior" refers to comfort–discomfort with sexual activity with oneself and/or with others. As individuals move through adolescence, a normative part of development is becoming sexually active. Optimally, this behavior is one that people pursue with a sense of personal safety, self-respect, and reciprocal intimacy with others. Many self-injuring persons, however, report the body image dimension of sexual behavior to be problematic. Discomfort related to sexual behavior can range from inhibited, phobic attitudes about sexuality to behavior that is hypersexual. Some individuals, usually trauma survivors, are entirely sexually avoidant. They may find the prospect of sexual intimacy in the present to be too encumbered by associations with abuse from the past. Until these individuals have dealt with their trauma histories, the prospect of engaging in sexual behavior with others is intolerable.

Other self-injuring persons, who may also be trauma survivors, engage in behavior that is the opposite of avoidance: They may be unconcerned with safe sex practices and have multiple partners within very short periods of time. For these individuals, the briefest of sexual encounters may be the only type of intimacy they can tolerate. Unsafe sexual encounters may also be reinforcing because the sex acts are simultaneously self-demeaning and potentially self-destructive. For those who are "addicted" to self-defeating forms of behavior, sexual risk-taking can be as exhilarating as self-injury itself. Being exploited by others may be congruent with an overall diminished sense of self-esteem.

Body Integrity

Body integrity is a particularly intriguing and complex dimension of body image. An adequate discussion of the concept requires the use of some rather odd language. "Body integrity" refers to whether or not individuals feel as if they "own" or "occupy" their own bodies. To have a sense of body integrity means to feel comfortable within one's body—to feel that it is of one piece and whole. A sense of body integrity requires freedom from prolonged states of dissociation or feelings of disconnectedness from one's body.

For clients who are fortunate enough to have a strong sense of body integrity, queries that involve such language may seem strange. They may respond to questions about body integrity with, "Of course I feel that I 'own' my body. Without it I don't exist!" For a substantial proportion of self-injuring clients, however, a sense of body integrity is not self-evident or automatic at all.

For example, in responding to questions regarding body integrity on the Body Attitudes Scale (BAS; Walsh & Frost, 2005; a copy is provided in Appendix B), many self-injuring clients indicate that they "strongly agree" with such statements as these:

"Sometimes I feel disconnected from my body."
"Sometimes my body feels out of control."
"Sometimes my body feels like an enemy."

"I would prefer to live without a body."

"I often feel at war with my body."

Strong endorsement of such items suggests the opposite of body integrity—that is, "body alienation." Many self-injuring persons seem to be body-alienated in complex ways, and it is important to target body alienation over the course of treatment.

Individuals who present with self-injury *and* eating disorders may be especially prone to body alienation and related dissociative states. As noted by Muehlenkamp et al. (2011) in their empirical study of individuals with both self-injury and eating disorders, "It appears that dissociation, or detachment from the body may be a particularly salient factor to consider in both understanding and treating self-injury within an eating disordered population" (p. 108).

BODY IMAGE AS A FOCUS IN THERAPY

Asking self-injuring clients about the six dimensions of body image is often an extremely useful activity. It can be productive for at least the following reasons:

1. Most clients have not been asked extensive questions about body image, and it therefore represents new, uncharted territory. Particularly for clients who are "therapy veterans," the topic of body image can open up useful new directions in treatment.
2. The presence or absence of negative attitudes regarding the body often serves to differentiate more disturbed from less impaired individuals who self-injure. The presence of negative attitudes may have prognostic implications for the length of treatment and the course of self-injury.
3. The presence of profound body alienation often points to histories of sexual and/or physical abuse trauma, or other major sources of stress, that need to be explored and resolved.
4. Identifying which of the six dimensions are problematic for an individual allows these dimensions to be targeted quite specifically in treatment.

Body Image as Uncharted Territory

As indicated above, a proportion of clients who self-injure are "therapy veterans." That is, they have seen a number of therapists over several years and have become somewhat jaded about the process. They may hold some modest hope that this new treatment will be different, but it is often no more than a glimmer. One reason for their jaded attitude is that too many therapists in hospitals and outpatient clinics have asked the same list of tired questions. One function of exploring body image with clients is to open a fresh topic for discussion. I find that many clients are surprised when first asked about their relationships with their bodies. Introducing an important new theme intrigues these clients and fosters some hope that this treatment will be more effective than past attempts. Creating hope and optimism is basic to starting any new treatment.

Why is body image raised so infrequently by therapists in general? Body image appears to be a neglected theme in therapy because it is rarely part of graduate school education. Clinicians are taught to focus on the general topics of thoughts, feelings, and behaviors (cognitive behaviorism) or fantasies, drives, and conflicts (psychodynamic treatment), but rarely on the specialized topic of the body. The contention here is that body image is a fundamental building block of self-efficacy and self-esteem (Schilder, 1935; Secord & Jourard, 1953; Cash & Pruzinksy, 2002; Walsh & Frost, 2005) and should be given appropriate prominence in the course of treating a self-injuring client.

Body Image as a Prognostic Indicator

Although I do not have extensive empirical data to support this contention, my clinical impression is that the presence of very negative body image attitudes in clients tends to be a negative prognostic indicator. In general, the more profound the body alienation, the more extended the course of self-injury and the more prolonged the treatment response.

Chapter 4 has discussed self-injury in clinical groups versus the general population. I have found anecdotally that self-injuring persons from the general population who are functioning adequately tend *not* to have profoundly negative attitudes toward their bodies. When such clients are asked about their attractiveness, effectiveness, health, sexuality, and body integrity, they usually do not report extensive negative thoughts or beliefs. Whereas self-injuring adolescents and young adults from the general population may report some age-appropriate self-consciousness about body image, they generally do not cite self-loathing or other extreme attitudes. Moreover, when asked questions about body integrity (e.g., about "feeling disconnected from your body" or "experiencing the body as an enemy"), they tend to looked perplexed and deny any such thoughts or beliefs.

In contrast, clinical populations of self-injuring clients tend to present with high rates of negative body image attitudes (Walsh & Rosen, 1988;

Alderman, 1997; Conterio & Lader, 1998; Walsh & Frost, 2005). These attitudes often show evidence of gross distortions, such as the following:

> "I'm ugly, disgusting-looking. I can't even look in a mirror." [attractiveness]
>
> "I have no athletic ability whatsoever. I have no interest in exercise or sports. I'm completely uncoordinated." [effectiveness]
>
> "My body is always breaking down. I'm sick of the headaches, nausea, and menstrual cramps." [health]
>
> "I'd rather have the body I had as a child. To me, these breasts are disgusting, and my stomach and butt are way too fat!" [sexual characteristics]
>
> "I hate it when anyone touches me. I just want everyone to stay away!" [sexual behavior]
>
> "I'd rather not have a body. All it causes me is pain and shame." [body integrity]

Body Alienation and the Link with Trauma/Major Stress

Many authors have found associations between self-injury and sexual abuse trauma (Walsh & Rosen, 1988; Darche, 1990; Shapiro & Dominiak, 1992; Miller, 1994; van der Kolk et al., 1996; Alderman, 1997; Favazza, 1998; Briere & Gil, 1998; Turell & Armsworth, 2000; Rodriguez-Srednicki, 2001; Paul et al., 2002; Muehlenkamp et al., 2011). Self-injury has also been linked to physical abuse (van der Kolk et al., 1991, 1996; Briere & Gil, 1998; Low et al., 2000), as well as other major stressors (to be discussed later)..

When clients report attitudes of profound body alienation in response to questions regarding the six body image dimensions, the possibility of trauma histories must be considered. The question to be addressed is this: How did they become body-alienated? Often the primary factor in this process is a history of abuse.

In trying to discuss trauma histories with clients, I have found that two very different types of problems tend to emerge. Some individuals are unwilling or unable to discuss their abuse histories; the topic is just too painful and retraumatizing to approach. Others present with the opposite problem: They have talked about their trauma histories so often in treatment that they have become desensitized to the content. They discuss physical or sexual abuse as if they were recounting a grocery list.

The topic of body image often provides an alternative avenue to opening up a productive exploration of abuse history. Body image is frequently a less threatening, more indirect route than direct questioning about trauma. An example of how body image discussion may lead to disclosure of trauma is provided below. For this client, previous direct questions about abuse history had not been helpful.

THERAPIST: How has your self-injury been lately?

CLIENT: Pretty low. Twice in the last week.

THERAPIST: That seems like progress. Six months ago it was about once a day, wasn't it?

CLIENT: Yes. It was *every* day.

THERAPIST: Congratulations!

CLIENT: Thank you. (*smiling*)

THERAPIST: Reflecting back on your past self-injury, how do you think you got in the habit of cutting your body?

CLIENT: Well, I've always hated my body.

THERAPIST: That's strong language. Why do you "hate" your own body?

CLIENT: Oh, it is so complicated . . . (*looking away, clearly uneasy*)

THERAPIST: I can tell this topic is making you uncomfortable, but it may be important. Let's go a little further, and if it's too much, you'll stop me, okay?

CLIENT: Okay.

THERAPIST: Why do you hate your body?

CLIENT: I've always hated my body. I've always felt it was dirty, disgusting . . . (*voice trails off*)

THERAPIST: Are there parts of your body you hate more than others?

CLIENT: (*with great intensity*) Oh, yes!

THERAPIST: May I ask what those are?

CLIENT: Anything to do with sex . . . (*evident shame and discomfort*)

THERAPIST: You're being very brave to pursue this. Can we go a bit further in our discussion?

CLIENT: I guess.

THERAPIST: Is there some part of your personal history that has caused you to hate the parts of your body that have to do with sexuality?

CLIENT: Yes . . . (*long sigh*) . . . I guess I need to talk about it. It has to do with my father.

THERAPIST: This is a topic we haven't talked about before, have we?

CLIENT: No. (*starting to cry*)

THERAPIST: Do you think it's time we started to deal with it so that you can put it behind you eventually? [conveying hope]

CLIENT: Probably . . .

THERAPIST: Good. We'll go at a pace that you can handle, but it's important to resolve this so that you can go on with your life. [balancing risk with the need for hope and change]

CLIENT: Yes. I know you're right. (*wiping her eyes*) . . . It's time now.

This type of dialogue emerges in the therapeutic relationship when a climate of trust and safety has been established. Very often the topic of body image provides access to the trauma history. The topic of the body is intensely personal and intimate. Discussing the body grounds the client in the more visceral, physical aspects of his or her experience. Opening the door via body image allows the work of resolving abuse trauma to proceed. This work, known as "exposure treatment," is a major focus of Chapter 16.

On the Specific Link between Sexual Abuse Trauma and Self-Injury

For self-injuring clients with sexual abuse histories, the link between trauma and bodily harm is not an abstract concept, but rather a concrete experience. The psychological wounds of such trauma often lead quite directly to the bodily wounds of self-injury. Over the years, these clients have taught me a great deal about the links between sexual abuse and their recurrent self-harm. Their instruction has occurred not via didactic discussion, but by sharing their anguished life stories in which sexual abuse played a central role. What these clients have revealed over time are the specific links between their trauma history and their recurrent self-injury.

As discussed in Chapter 9, treatment with such clients begins with a thorough behavioral analysis of their self-injury sequence. What these clients disclose in discussing the sequence can be depicted schematically in Figure 15.1. The *upper* section of the figure refers to the self-injury sequence as discussed by the clients. Although my clients have varied considerably in their use of language, the content can be very similar across individuals.

Over the course of treatment, the disclosures of clients shifts from the self-injury sequence to revealing their abuse histories. The sexual abuse sequences they describe are depicted schematically in the *lower* section of Figure 15.1. First I describe the upper sequence, as my clients have presented it, and then explicate the lower section with an emphasis on the links between the two.

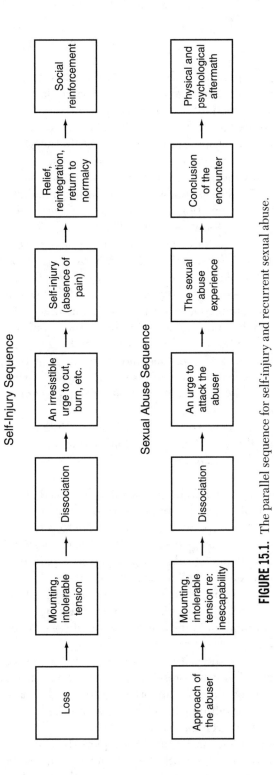

FIGURE 15.1. The parallel sequence for self-injury and recurrent sexual abuse.

217

As the upper portion of the diagram indicates, many clients identify their self-injury as being triggered by some form of loss. For some, the loss involves a blatant rejection in a relationship, a full breakup, or even a death. For others it can be far subtler, consisting of an almost imperceptible slight from a peer, colleague, or family member. Still others experience loss as related to performance problems in such areas as school, work, or athletic competition. Many individuals are reactive to *all* these types of losses.

In Figure 15.1, loss is followed by mounting intolerable affective tension—the escalating emotional discomfort that most self-injuring clients describe as preceding their self-injury. The type of affect varies widely and may include anxiety, sadness, depression, loneliness, anger, shame, or contempt. Regardless of the specific feeling reported, it is experienced as profoundly uncomfortable and requiring immediate relief.

The next step—and it is a key one—is that of dissociation. Many clients report dissociating in response to their escalating affect. They may use very different forms of language to describe the dissociation, such as "I feel like I'm outside my own body," or "It's as if I'm watching myself in a movie," or "I feel disconnected from everyone and everything." Although the specific terminology varies from person to person, the overall experience is generally the same: People report feeling some form of disconnection from their bodies and their immediate experience.

The next step in the sequence is the irresistible urge to cut, burn, or otherwise injure the body. Once individuals with recurrent self-injury reach this point in the sequence, they are unlikely to resist the impulse to self-harm.

Then comes the act of self-injury itself. Of note is that many self-injuring clients report an absence of pain at the time of the act. This anesthesia is probably due to the dissociation experience. There is some sort of profound mind–body disconnection in operation that causes these individuals to feel no pain. Most of them state that they experience pain or discomfort only several hours or even a day after the act.

The next step is the relief from discomfort. The intense affective distress is reduced, and the dissociation experience is terminated. There is a sense of reintegration and a return to "normality"—whatever that may be for the individual.

The final step in the self-injury sequence is the response of others in the environment, if any are present. These reactions vary greatly, ranging from outpourings of effusive support to bitter condemnations of the self-injury. Either way, a self-injuring client may find the responses of others to be gratifying (or reinforcing), as explained below.

The lower sequence in Figure 15.1 depicts the experience of recurrent sexual abuse. It is shown beneath the self-injury sequence because it is postulated here that it serves as the *foundation* for the self-abuse.

The first step in the sequence is the approach of the abuser. In several ways, this action is very much connected to the subsequent experience of loss. Most individuals are abused by someone they know (and trust). The abuser may be a grandparent or parent, the partner of a parent, an older sibling, an uncle or aunt, a babysitter, a teacher, a coach, or a member of the clergy. As soon as the abuse begins, this relationship is forever contaminated—in a word, *lost.*

Another form of loss related to abuse is the destruction of an emerging sense of body integrity. During childhood, a normative developmental task is learning to control one's body and achieve a sense of physical mastery (Ashford et al., 2001). The fragility of achieving this task is easily observed in young children. Whenever they receive a slight scratch or contusion, they invariably become quite upset by their "boo-boo." Their response of alarm and even panic points to how partial a sense of body wholeness and mastery is for young people. Imagine if, instead of a scratch or contusion, the assault on the child's emerging sense of body integrity was genital violation or penetration. It is easy to imagine how disorganizing this would be for children in terms of their relationships with their own bodies.

A third type of loss that clients often report is a retroactive loss of self-esteem. Many young individuals who are sexually abused do not realize at the time that it is wrong or abusive. As many clients have told me, "I thought it was normal to have sex with my abuser until X told me it wasn't." This recognition is shocking to the abused youth and often results in a profound loss of self-esteem and related shame and guilt.

The next step in the sexual abuse sequence is the mounting, intolerable tension. Once children know what is coming, they experience intense affective arousal as the cues preceding the abuse emerge. The emotions commonly involve fear, anger, shame, and guilt—an amalgam of emotions not easily managed by a young child. How do they learn to survive this affect and the related physical discomfort associated with the abuse? The next step in the sequence is dissociation, which is the individual's adaptive response to an impossible, terrifying situation. Dissociation enables the individual simultaneously to escape the emotional distress and the physical pain connected to the abuse. However, one problem with this "solution" is that survivors tend to overlearn this response. In future years, they may dissociate in response to other forms of affective distress that have nothing to do with abusive situations.

The next step is a key one. The individual being abused is inclined to tell others what is occurring, to fight back, and to say "no" to or even attack the abuser. However, abusers are adept at compelling their victims to stay silent and do nothing. Clients have reported such threats as "If you tell anyone, I'll kill you," or "If you say anything, I'll kill your dog." Other abusers are somewhat subtler. They control their victims by using manipulative tactics, such as "It would kill your mother if she knew our special secret," or "If you tell anyone, I'll go to jail, and the family will be broken up."

The effect of these threats—whether subtle or bludgeoning—is that the survivor is compelled to remain silent. A key psychological shift is associated with this silence. Often the survivor comes to *blame the body* for the abuse, or at least to view it as a "collaborator" and thereby permanently contaminated. Some speak of the body with disgust, citing it as the "lure" or "attraction" for the abuser. Others blame the body for physiologically responding to the sexual stimulation, and they feel immense shame. All such self-blame is irrational, but it plagues the sexually abused survivors until they explore it in treatment and resolve it.

The next step in the abusive sequence is the sexual contact and abuse itself. Note that it is positioned directly beneath the self-injury. The two events are often inextricably linked in the minds of self-injuring clients. They disclose such judgments as "I hurt my body because I hate it," or "It is dirty, contaminated, evil, and not really me." They may say, "I can hurt it all I want, because it's not me and I don't care what happens to it." The extent of their body alienation and tendency to dissociate is reflected in such statements.

The conclusion of the sexual abuse encounter signals the end of the particular episode. The abused child returns to whatever "normality" may be for him or her. The final step in the sequence is the physical and psychological aftermath. Note that it parallels the experience of social reinforcement in the self-injury sequence. During the sexually abusive sequence, survivors are forced to endure an aftermath of physical pain and psychological discomfort in silence. This may make the reaction of others to their self-injury all the more reinforcing to receive. After years of enduring abuse in private, at last they can suffer and have someone notice. It does not matter whether the response is nurturing or punitive. Either way, the silence is broken, and a gratifying reaction from others is obtained.

Other Sources of Body Alienation

It should not be assumed that a history of sexual abuse trauma exists whenever clients present with negative attitudes regarding their bodies. There are many other groups of people who may become body-alienated because of trauma or other major stress:

- Individuals with a history of physical (nonsexual) abuse
- Individuals with a history of serious childhood illness
- Gay, lesbian, bisexual, or transgender (GLBT) individuals who are not yet comfortable with their sexuality
- Persons with other idiosyncratic circumstances, such as very unusual physical characteristics

As noted by numerous authors (van der Kolk et al., 1991, 1996; Briere & Gil, 1998; Low et al., 2000), self-injury has also been found to be linked to physical abuse. The factors that produce body alienation in those who have been physically abused can be similar to those that emerge from sexual mistreatment. Survivors of physical attacks may come to blame their bodies for the assaults. Some seem to internalize the loathing that their abusers manifest for them and conclude that they deserve the physical punishment. This internalization can pave the way for subsequent self-assault. Such children often endure parents or other caregivers who rarely hold or physically comfort them. These children may conclude that their "unattractive" or "unappealing" bodies are at fault or to blame.

Sustained or serious childhood illness can also produce body alienation. Those with histories of chronic physical illness, such as asthma, diabetes, arthritis, eczema, psoriasis, or others, can develop very compromised, negative attitudes toward their bodies. If the body frequently causes a child physical pain, limited mobility, social embarrassment, isolation, or other adverse repercussions, it is no wonder that negative attitudes develop.

One example I encountered was a 13-year-old boy with diabetes. Although he occasionally self-injured, he came into treatment primarily because of his serious mismanagement of his diabetic illness. He refused to assess his blood levels consistently; frequently delayed or missed doses of insulin; and ate an unhealthy diet of candy bars, snow cones, and soft drinks. His scores on the BAS were exceptionally negative. In treatment, he said quite directly that he hated his body because it interfered with his desire to play basketball, made him different from his friends, and was a nuisance to manage. This boy was an excellent example of a client who was alienated from his body by the considerable repercussions of his physical illness, rather than by any trauma history.

Another group of self-injuring individuals who have body image problems are GLBT adolescents and young adults. GLBT individuals appear to have higher rates of self-injury than heterosexual youth (Nixon & Heath, 2009). Also, in a sample of disturbed adolescents described in Walsh and Frost (2005), there was a substantially higher proportion of GLBT youth in the self-destructive group. My clinical experience is that the GLBT youth most at risk for body image problems are those who are not "out of the closet." Those who *are* "out" and have a supportive social network appear to do much better. An example of a gay client with considerable negative body image attitudes follows:

James was a 14-year-old struggling with his homosexuality. He frequently cut himself when in a rage or feeling anxious. He generally socialized with girls his age and sometimes stated that he was "dating" one or more of them. Later he would reverse himself and say to his therapist, "Who am I kidding? I'm gay, but I don't want to be." James often presented with anguish about his gayness. He feared his parents' reaction to his coming out. He was convinced, perhaps accurately, that they would kick him out of the house. James frequently ranted, "Why can't I be like everyone else?" Early in treatment, his scores on the BAS were very negative. Only when James came out to his two most trusted female friends did he begin to feel better. They were supportive and did not abandon him, as he had feared.

Some extensive family work enabled James to come out to his family members. They were upset, but James continued to live at home. With this accomplished, his attitudes toward his body and toward life in general improved. His self-injury also markedly declined.

A fourth group of body-alienated self-injuring clients can only be referred to as "idiosyncratic." Their problems with body image emerge from their own unique, or at least unusual, circumstances. Here are some examples of such clients:

- A young woman who had cystic acne on her face and body that caused her considerable social embarrassment. She frequently pierced these pimples with pins or needles.
- An adopted Asian adolescent who was rejecting of her race, in part because she was raised in an all-white suburb. She viewed her race as alien and faceless. She stated that she "hated" her eyes and thought she was ugly. This client pulled out her hair when frustrated.
- An adolescent male who was self-conscious about his short height and slender build. He frequently burned himself after school, particularly when a peer had ridiculed his height or build.
- An overweight 13-year-old female who had been teased for years about her size. She was pervasively self-loathing about her body. After episodes of binge eating, she frequently cut her abdomen.

As these examples suggest, people can become body-alienated for myriad reasons. The task for the therapist is to identify whether body alienation is a problem for a client and, if so, to design treatment strategies to address it.

Targeting Specific Body Image Dimensions for Treatment

Focusing on body image in treatment allows the therapist and client to identify specific dimensions that demand attention. This process can involve asking informally about the six dimensions or using the 36-item BAS provided in Appendix B. The strategy selected depends on individual clients and their receptivity to completing questionnaires. I generally use the more informal approach with adolescents and other clients who are wary or distrustful. However, it is better to use the questionnaire when possible, because it provides more specific, detailed information about all six dimensions. It is also useful to administer the questionnaire recurrently so that change can be tracked.

For argument's sake, let us say that a client completes the BAS during a session and agrees to share it with the therapist. Suppose that the results identify problems with the dimensions of attractiveness, health, and body integrity. These three dimensions can then be explored at length in treatment. One approach will be a cognitive-behavioral one that focuses on identifying the automatic thoughts, intermediate beliefs, and core beliefs supporting the negative attitudes. The goal over the course of treatment is to use cognitive techniques to assist the client in evaluating the accuracy of distorted cognitions, developing more accurate and helpful thoughts, and practicing them both in and out of therapy. Details of the cognitive therapy approach have been recounted in Chapter 12.

Another strategy in working with negative body image attitudes involves building positive body experiences *in vivo*. If the client reports feeling chronically unattractive, he or she may be asked to complete assignments outside therapy designed to enhance feelings of attractiveness. These assignments may involve placing greater emphasis on grooming, obtaining a new haircut or clothes, or going for a complete "makeover." The strategy in negotiating such homework with the client is to make it both fun and adventurous. Chronic negative cognitions about being unattractive or ugly and related behaviors must be challenged with a combination of humor and compassion. The following is an example of such an exchange.

THERAPIST: How are you coming on your attractiveness homework?

CLIENT: Oh, God, not this again!

THERAPIST: 'Fraid so, this again!

CLIENT: Well, I didn't get that haircut . . . (*laughing nervously*)

THERAPIST: I didn't think so. I can be very observant, and this appears to be the same exact haircut as last week.

CLIENT: Well, maybe I'll go this week!

THERAPIST: What's holding you back?

CLIENT: Only 25 years of negative thoughts about being an ugly eyesore! (*laughing*)

THERAPIST: Well, at least you're laughing about what appears to be absurdly inaccurate judgments!

CLIENT: If only I believed it!

THERAPIST: Well, you are getting there, aren't you?

CLIENT: I guess so. I promise next week you'll see a brand new me . . . or at least a new haircut. I really do want to change my hair.

THERAPIST: Great!

Other examples of homework that clients have used to deal *in vivo* with body image dysfunction are provided in Table 15.1. Many of these were suggested by the clients themselves. Although any one of these attempts is likely to produce only modest improvements in body image, the use of several in combination can effect considerable positive change over time.

As with any new skill, the acquisition of these more positive bodily experiences involves extensive, recurrent practice. The therapist needs to monitor follow-through and reinforce the most modest of efforts. Making it fun for the client is important. The strategy is to identify a hierarchy of targets for the appropriate dimensions of body image and to proceed cautiously but emphatically. Readministering the BAS over time usually reveals substantial improvements in the selected body image dimensions.

CONCLUSION

In summary, in providing body image work with self-injurers, it is important for clinicians and others to do the following:

- Understand and work with the six dimensions of body image: attractiveness, effectiveness, health, sexual characteristics, sexual behavior, and body integrity.
- Assess clients in terms of the six dimensions, either informally or by using the BAS.
- Determine whether body alienation is present.
- Ascertain if the client has experienced sexual abuse, physical abuse, serious physical illness, or other forms of trauma/stress linked to body alienation.
- Target specific dimensions of body image for treatment.
- Identify body-related activities that the client can pursue in order to improve body image attitudes and experiences.

TABLE 15.1. Examples of Homework to Improve Body Image

Attractiveness

Going to a skin salon

Charting weight loss associated with a diet

Obtaining electrolysis or derma-abrasion

Consulting a dermatologist

Having orthodontic work done or teeth whitened

Identifying "my top ten most attractive body parts or features"

Effectiveness

Joining a gym

Pursuing a new exercise activity, such as walking, volleyball, racquetball, tennis lessons, dancing

Engaging in a new activity that involves dexterity, such as playing a musical instrument, painting, sculpting, croquet

Health

Charting physical discomfort by body area and linking these areas to an assessment of cognitive, affective, or behavioral antecedents

Initiating a diet or healthier eating

Reducing caffeine or alcohol intake

Asking for a modification of medication regimen

Taking up yoga, tai chi, kayaking

Obtaining a physical and, if the results are good, ignoring future ailments as much as possible

Accepting that physical discomfort is the body's way of expressing feelings and working on modifying those feelings more effectively

Sexual characteristics

Identifying all the positives of having an adult body

Acquiring a variable wardrobe that includes both concealing and revealing clothing

Celebrating an adult body by going to a spa or having a massage

Becoming comfortable with androgyny as a mode of dress and appearance

Acquiring stylish but nonrevealing clothes

Wearing sexually revealing clothing alone in the privacy of one's home

(cont.)

TABLE 15.1. *(cont.)*

Sexual behavior

Accepting that sexual activity is entirely within one's control; one can be sexually active frequently, occasionally, rarely, or not at all

Accepting masturbation

Accepting celibacy

Ensuring safe sex with multiple partners

Working on trauma in order to reclaim one's sexuality

Joining a dating service

Body integrity

Practicing looking into a mirror, extending the time limits

Practicing a body scan meditation with emphasis on wholeness (see Appendix A)

Taking a bubble bath

Walking mindfully, concentrating on the rhythm of breath

Making a snow or sand angel

Relaxing in pleasantly warm water at the beach

Floating on a raft

Having a massage

Doing visual imagery of floating, flying, or rocking

Engaging in any activity that conveys a sense of rhythm, full body coordination, and fluidity, such as washing dishes, raking leaves, shoveling snow, and chopping wood

---

CHAPTER 16

Prolonged Exposure or Cognitive Restructuring for Treating PTSD and Related Self-Injury

This chapter reviews the second component of Step 3 in the stepped-care model (see Figure II.1, p. 75). Step 3 in the model is for individuals who present with multiple self-harm behaviors in combination, including self-injury. Usually persons requiring Step 3 interventions have endured histories of physical and/or sexual abuse or other traumatic/stressful experiences, as described in Chapter 15. Two treatments shown to be effective with these problems are reviewed in this chapter.

A story from the Zen tradition serves as an appropriate introduction to the discussion of trauma treatment:

Never Mind That

A professional dancer, who'd been forced to abandon her career after being pushed in front of a subway train and injuring one of her feet, attended a retreat with Maezumi Roshi (founder of the Zen Center of Los Angeles). Self-conscious about her injured foot, she always kept it covered with a sock.

In her first interview, she asked Maezumi a question about her Zen practice, but he answered, "Never mind that. Tell me about your foot."

"Oh, it's nothing, Roshi," the student answered, trying to turn the conversation back to her practice. "I just had an accident."

Maezumi persisted. Finally she not only told him the story but, weeping, took off her sock to show him. At this Maezumi placed his hand silently on her foot. She looked up to find that he was crying too.

Their exchanges went on like this for some time. Every time she asked the roshi about her practice, he'd ask about her foot instead, and they'd cry together. "You might think you have suffered terrible karma," Maezumi told her, "but this is not the right way to think about it. Practice is about learning to turn disadvantage to great advantage." Finally the day came when the student walked into the interview room and began to tell her teacher about her injury, but it summoned no tears from her.

"Never mind about that," Maezumi told her. "Let's talk about your practice." (Murphy, 2002, p. 74)

This chapter focuses on two forms of treatment for self-injuring clients who have histories of trauma: prolonged exposure treatment (PET; Foa, Hembree, & Rothbaum, 2007), and cognitive restructuring (CR) for PTSD (Mueser et al., 2009). PET is the treatment of choice for PTSD. It has the greatest empirical support to date and has been employed with diverse clientele around the world, including survivors of rape, natural disasters, and war (both civilians and military personnel) (Foa et al., 2007). However, some clients are not able to endure the rigors of PET, which involves substantial, systematic reexperiencing of traumatic events. This is why CR for PTSD is also reviewed in this chapter. It should be noted that CR for PTSD also has strong empirical support as to efficacy (Mueser et al., 2009).

Walser and Hayes (1998) provide a further introduction to this area of work:

The etymology of the word [trauma] gives us a clue about how to approach the issue. "Trauma" comes from the Latin root meaning "wound." Unlike mere pain, wounds involve injury and bodily harm. They produce scars. They take time—perhaps a long time—to heal. (p. 256)

For self-injuring clients, these scars are both internal (psychological) and external (visible on the body).

THE SYMPTOMS OF PTSD

The diagnosis most commonly associated with trauma is, of course, PTSD. Many self-injuring clients diagnosed with PTSD have also received other diagnoses, such as depression, anxiety, panic, and/or BPD. According to Foa et al. (2007) and Mueser et al. (2009), the symptoms of PTSD fall into three basic clusters: (1) intrusion, (2) avoidance, and (3) arousal. Self-injury can often be specifically linked to all three of these clusters.

1. The "intrusion" cluster includes unwanted, recurrent thoughts and images, nightmares, flashbacks, and reactions to reminders of trauma (Foa et al., 2007; Mueser et al., 2009). Self-injuring clients who have survived trauma often report all of these forms of intrusive phenomena. In fact, it is not uncommon for these clients to state that they self-injure in order to *terminate* these experiences. For example, a client may say that if a flashback appears and he or she cuts or burns, "it goes away." This "success" can render self-injury a preferred method for handling intrusive trauma-related experiences.

2. The "avoidance" cluster includes deliberate efforts to avoid thoughts, feelings, behaviors, and environmental cues of trauma. Other symptoms within this cluster are emotional numbing, detachment from others, loss of interest in previous activities, and restricted range of affect (Foa et al., 2007; Mueser et al., 2009). For many individuals, self-injury is the ultimate, preferred avoidance behavior. It can terminate unwanted thoughts (e.g., "I started thinking of my abuser's face"), feelings (e.g., "I feel such shame when I'm naked"), and behaviors (e.g., "I can't possibly wear that close-fitting clothing"). It shifts attention away from the psychological pain of trauma to the intensely preoccupying sequence of self-harm. Some clients say, "For me, self-injury is an escape. Whatever is bothering me is canceled out. Cutting or burning obliterates whatever else is going on at that moment."

3. The "arousal" cluster encompasses diverse problems, including sleep disturbance, interrupted concentration, hypervigilance, and frequent intense states of emotional arousal (Foa et al., 2007; Mueser et al., 2009). Rothbaum et al. (2000) have suggested that the emotional arousal of trauma survivors includes the *primary* emotions of fear, sadness, and anger, and the *secondary* emotions of guilt and shame. Note that these are the very emotions that most self-injuring clients cite as preceding their acts of self-harm. A predominant reason why such clients hurt their bodies is to obtain relief from the arousal states associated with PTSD.

The other arousal problems of recurrent sleep disturbance, poor concentration, and hypervigilance are also commonly reported by self-injuring clients. These states often exacerbate the clients' emotional distress. Sleep disturbance increases emotional vulnerability. Hypervigilance is exhausting in a different way, depleting the attentional abilities of these already overtaxed self-injuring persons.

Thus all three PTSD symptom clusters play a central role in the onset and maintenance of self-injury. For traumatized clients to give up self-injury, they need to achieve mastery over these three symptom clusters via comprehensive treatment.

METHODS OF TREATING TRAUMA

Many forms of therapy have been employed to treat PTSD and its related symptoms. Foa, Keane, and Friedman (2000) have provided a thorough review of these diverse treatment methods. Their book discusses cognitive-behavioral therapy, pharmacotherapy, eye movement desensitization and reprocessing (EMDR), group therapy, psychodynamic treatment, inpatient care, hypnosis, psychosocial rehabilitation, creative therapies, and several others. Foa and colleagues identify cognitive-behavioral treatment as having by far the most empirical support as to treatment effectiveness (Foa et al., 2000, 2007). For this reason, I have chosen to feature two forms of cognitive-behavioral treatment in this chapter.

PROLONGED EXPOSURE TREATMENT

PET consists of systematic methods that help clients deal with the three PTSD symptom clusters. There are five components in PET, as presented by various clinicians and researchers (e.g., Foa & Rothbaum, 1998; Meadows & Foa, 1998; Rothbaum et al., 2000; Foa et al., 2007). These five components are addressed in step-by-step fashion in well-established protocols (e.g., Foa et al., 2007).

Step 1: Information Gathering

The first step in conducting PET is information gathering (Foa et al., 2007). Foa and colleagues recommend using a standardized instrument (e.g., the Standardized Assault Interview) to collect information, when possible.

Meadows and Foa (1998) state that "most clients do not have difficulties during the information-gathering stage" (p. 108). However, I find that some clients have considerable difficulty the first time they disclose information about traumatic experiences. The discussion itself, when the clinician attempts to obtain this information, is often potentially retraumatizing. Thus the information gathering is its own "mini" form of exposure that requires a client to experience multiple trials in order to endure it. In working with self-injuring trauma survivors, the process of acquiring information about childhood abuse is often extremely "hit or miss"; at times it even feels chaotic. Consider this example:

After several months in treatment, a client disclosed an intrusive traumatic dream in which her father was having intercourse with her. The client then became extremely distressed with this content, stated that it was a nightmare, and denied that any similar experience had ever happened in the real world. Three weeks later, the client revisited the content (of her own initiative), and offered that the experience was in fact true and had happened repeatedly. Immediately thereafter, the client retracted the statement, saying that she should not say such awful things about her father. Only a week later did the client remain steadfast, saying that the abuse had happened recurrently, exactly as she had first described it. This remained her position from that point on, and it was supported by an older sibling who had been similarly abused.

The therapist has to allow clients to weave in and out of such content until they have reached firm conclusions as to what has happened and who did what to whom. This process can take weeks and clearly cannot be rushed.

Step 2: Breathing Retraining

The second step in PET is breathing retraining (Foa et al., 2007). Similar versions of this skill have been discussed at length in Chapter 11 of this book and in the Breathing Manual provided in Appendix A. For treating PTSD, Meadows and Foa (1998) recommend a very specific form of breathing practice:

> Breathing retraining is taught by having the client inhale to a count of four, then exhale slowly while saying "Calm" to herself. A 4-second pause is then placed between the breaths, further slowing the breathing process. Initially, the therapist should count and say "Calm" for the client, until a rhythm is established, after which the client may take over. Once the method is learned, clients are instructed to practice breathing for homework, at least twice daily for 10–20 minutes each time. (p. 109)

This technique is designed to help manage anxiety, calm the body physiologically, and teach mastery over unpleasant emotions. I find that this breathing technique is a very useful one, and I recommend it to and practice it with clients. However, it should be noted that early in treatment, not many clients are up to twice-daily practice for 10–20 minutes. They need a great deal of coaching and "shaping" to achieve this level of participation over time.

Another suggestion I would make is to teach a client breathing retraining *before* information gathering is attempted. The breathing techniques can be very useful for clients as they attempt to provide information about their trauma histories. Mindful breathing allows clients to sit with the painful emotions and alarming imagery (or other sensations) for more extended periods of time. This increased capacity enables the treatment to progress with a greater sense of control for the clients.

Step 3: Explanation of Common Reactions to Assault

The third aspect of PET involves explaining and "normalizing" the reactions of clients to discussing their trauma (Foa et al., 2007). The therapist needs to explain the three symptom clusters of PTSD and ask the client which apply. Often there is evidence of all three. As clients begin to deal with trauma-related material, it is common for them to feel as if they are "going crazy." Their intrusive images, flashbacks, and tactile memories may feel like hallucinations. Their terrifying nightmares may make them feel as if they have no control over their own minds and sleep patterns. The intense emotions of rage and shame often feel out of control.

The flood of emotions (or the opposite, emotional numbing) may result in a temporary increase in the frequency or severity of the self-injury behavior. At this point in treatment, clients may feel they are getting worse rather than better. During this challenging phase, a therapist must first ensure that a client is safe. Ascertaining the client's degree of current safety entails conducting a thorough *reassessment* of his or her forms of direct and indirect self-harm (as described in Chapters 3 and 9). Once the therapist is confident that there is no risk of suicide or major self-injury, the task is to reassure the client that this period will pass and progress will resume. Sharing stories about previously successful clients can be reassuring.

Explaining the symptom clusters of PTSD and even predicting relapses of self-injury can be quite helpful to clients during this phase. Clients learn that their distress is normative, that they are not becoming mentally ill, and that their increased self-injury (if any) may be time-limited—especially if they use the replacement skills they have learned.

Step 4: Imaginal Exposure

The fourth step in PET is imaginal exposure, in which the client describes the trauma experiences and memories in great detail while working to achieve emotional relaxation and calm (Foa et al., 2007). The goal is to "expose oneself" (i.e., to experience the trauma memories repeatedly and to master them gradually while defusing their power). Recurrent discussion of the experiences has been found to lower anxiety and to assist clients in differentiating the traumatic experiences from neutral or positive events (Foa & Rothbaum, 1998). Meadows and Foa (1998) recommend providing the following introduction regarding imaginal exposure to clients:

> "Some of the symptoms of PTSD, like nightmares, intrusive thoughts, and flashbacks, are signals that you haven't yet dealt with the memories. So in imaginal exposure, you will deliberately confront the thoughts and memories

without pushing them away. Reliving the assault in your memory lets you process the experience, so that you can file it away in your mind like any other bad memory, rather than have it be so real for you. . . . " (p. 111)

The process of imaginal exposure involves multiple steps:

1. The first is to construct a hierarchy or rank ordering of trauma experiences, ranging from the least to the most upsetting. For constructing the hierarchy, Foa et al. (2007) recommend using a subjective units of distress (SUDs) scale (see Chapter 11) ranging from 0, indicating no distress at all, to 100, reflecting the maximum distress imaginable. An example of a hierarchy that I constructed with a client is provided in Figure 16.1. Some of the content may seem beyond belief, but I assure the reader that it comes from an actual, credible individual. Note that the items on the client's hierarchy are from her past (about 20 years before). This hierarchy is by no means complete, but it is meant to be representative.

It took several weeks to construct this hierarchy with the client. She was able to work on this task only after considerable trust had been established. It was important to explain the purpose of the imaginal exposure to her and to assure her that it would help her with her nightmares, flashbacks, deep sadness, rage, self-blame, and self-injury.

2. Once the hierarchy has been constructed, the treatment proceeds by selecting an item in the *middle* of the hierarchy. Items from the middle are usually chosen first, because the content is reasonably challenging without being too overwhelming.

3. The client is then asked to describe the specific item in the hierarchy in complete detail. The therapist needs to be attuned to aspects of the

Experience	SUDs rating
Seeing my brother at the breakfast table	20
Passing my father in the kitchen when others are present	40
Answering the phone and hearing my father's voice	50
Having my brother grope me over my clothes	60
Having my brother molest me in the barn	70
Having sex with my father in the barn	80
Having sex with my father upstairs while others were in the house	90
Having sex with my father while my mother was "asleep" in the same bed	100

FIGURE 16.1. Imaginal exposure hierarchy of trauma experiences.

experience that the client may want to skip over or avoid altogether. The client needs to be gently brought back to these aspects, so that they can be explored and defused.

4. Any specific incident may have to be discussed multiple times in order to markedly reduce (and, ideally, eliminate) the three symptom clusters.

5. Meadows and Foa (1998) suggest that clients should be asked about their SUDs level every 5 minutes or so during imaginal exposure. As the distress mounts, breathing is employed to manage and reduce the SUDs. I find that when clients report anything above 50–60 SUDs, breathing exercises are indicated. Clients find it supportive when the therapist practices the breathing along with them. As one person said, "It makes therapy feel like a joint enterprise."

6. It is generally a good idea to employ the breathing until the SUDs level drops to 30 or below. If the client reports being stuck at a high level of distress, it may be necessary to take a break. However, doing so runs the risk of further reinforcing the pattern of avoidance. It is best to "hang in there" until the effectiveness of the breathing emerges and the repetition of the discussion results in habituation.

7. Foa and colleagues also recommend having the client talk in the *present tense* during imaginal exposure (Foa & Rothbaum, 1998; Meadows & Foa, 1998). I tend not to follow this recommendation because of adverse reactions from clients. When clients begin talking about their trauma histories, I take great pains to emphasize that *discussing* the experiences is very different from *living* them. I frequently reassure clients that they are safe and in no danger in the present. I find that having clients use the present tense to describe their traumas tends to blur this distinction. Clients seem more likely to feel retraumatized and unsafe. I am in no way claiming that my approach is superior to Foa's; on the contrary, hers is the one with empirical support. Nonetheless, I have had to modify my approach in response to recurrent feedback from clients.

8. Another suggestion from Foa and colleagues is to ask clients to close their eyes during the imaginal exposure (Meadows & Foa, 1998). The intent of this suggestion is to encourage clients to retrieve memories vividly without outside distractions. I have found that many trauma-surviving clients who self-injure do not feel safe closing their eyes in the presence of others. I therefore offer this suggestion without emphasizing it, and am struck by the very high percentage of such clients who choose to keep their eyes open.

9. The process of imaginal exposure moves through the hierarchy until all items have been dealt with and mastered. The pace of this work varies

greatly from client to client. Sometimes a single item can take weeks; other times several items from the hierarchy can be handled in a single session.

10. In doing imaginal exposure, I find it helpful to use replacement skills in addition to breathing. Thus clients working on an item from the hierarchy may opt to listen to soothing music, have a cup of herbal tea, or do walking meditation in the office. It is important to emphasize that the replacement skills are used to reduce the SUDs level in the sessions, rather than to escape the discomfort of the traumatic memory or related experiences.

11. It must be stated that some clients resist overly structured approaches to treatment. This can be particularly true for late adolescent and young adult clients. For those who complain that working with a hierarchy is too formulaic, I am quite willing to proceed informally. Hierarchies can be constructed and worked on without ever writing them down with clients. The risk of using an informal approach is that it can fail to be sufficiently thorough. As a result, key trauma experiences may not be addressed. However, with persistence and acumen, the clinician can avoid this risk as a detailed hierarchy emerges in his or her mind but remains "offline" for the client.

Step 5: In Vivo *Exposure*

The fifth and final step in PET is *in vivo* exposure. This technique is essentially the same process as imaginal exposure, but it brings the treatment into the real world (Foa et al., 2007). I find that many clients need to do imaginal exposure work regarding their trauma memories before they can attempt major changes in their daily living environments. *In vivo* exposure focuses on activities in a client's present life that have been negatively affected by associations with trauma. These are activities that trigger the symptom clusters of intrusion, avoidance, and arousal. As with imaginal exposure, a therapist and client begin by constructing a hierarchy. Clients then progressively expose themselves to these situations *in vivo* in order to achieve mastery. An example of an *in vivo* exposure hierarchy is provided in Figure 16.2. This hierarchy was developed with the same client whose imaginal hierarchy was presented in Figure 16.1. Note that all of the experiences identified were problematic for the client in the present.

As indicated by the SUDs ratings, the items in this hierarchy triggered varying degrees of emotional arousal and avoidance behaviors. For example, if the client saw a photo in the paper of a man who resembled her father, she felt noticeably uncomfortable but could continue reading. However, if she saw a man on the street who resembled her father, or a policeman, she

Experience	SUDs rating
Seeing a photo of a man in the newspaper who resembles my father	20
Walking past a police officer on the street	30
Walking past a man on the street who resembles my father	40
Entering an elevator alone with a strange man	50
Seeing a photograph of my father	50
Having my brother call on the phone	60
Seeing my mother or father at our family home	80
Having my husband approach me sexually "at the wrong time"	90

FIGURE 16.2. *In vivo* exposure hierarchy of trauma experiences.

would immediately experience intense fear. Generally she would cross the street or enter a building in order to distance herself from the approaching man. In a similar vein, if this woman were waiting for an elevator and an unaccompanied man approached, she would not enter the elevator, but wait for another. Obviously, these avoidance behaviors caused the client considerable inconvenience, and she experienced an untoward amount of fear.

The *in vivo* exposure treatment for this client progressed through several steps. First, she brought photos of persons who resembled her father to my office. We practiced looking at these photos until she felt little or no discomfort. She then did the same practice at home. Next, she began to practice *in vivo* exposure on the way to my office. She would intentionally walk by men on the street in situations that would normally be distressing for her. When such men approached, she used her breathing *in vivo* and forced herself not to alter course. She then would discuss the results (including her SUDs levels) in the sessions immediately thereafter. Over time, this client took great satisfaction in her progress. These avoidance behaviors (and related fear) had plagued her for many years, and she was glad to be rid of them.

After this, the client progressed to looking at photos of her father. She did this first in my office and subsequently at home. With practice, she was able to reduce her SUDs to close to 0. Then she took on the challenge of managing her emotions more effectively when her brother called on the phone, and, ultimately, when she visited her mother and father at the old family home. The sexual issues with her husband were more complicated and required couple treatment later on.

One other issue that deserves comment is that the therapist needs to assess for circumstances in the real world that are *legitimately* dangerous.

Although my client might have practiced walking by men in the city during daylight hours, her homework would never have included this activity at night. Some clients have very poor judgment in distinguishing the truly dangerous from the irrationally frightening. They may need considerable help in learning to make this distinction and to protect themselves.

An Example of Trauma Treatment Using Replacement Skills and PET

When Penny began therapy at age 22, she had one of the more severe cases of self-injury I had treated. She had cut her arms and legs hundreds of times, and her extremities had extensive scarring. She had also burned herself occasionally, pulled out her hair, and episodically engaged in bulimia. Penny was an intelligent young woman who was attending college. However, she was already in her eighth semester and was nowhere near graduation, due to a pattern of missed classes, exams, and papers. She was a very capable individual who was nonetheless self-defeating, self-loathing, and self-destructive.

Early in treatment, Penny was very distrustful. She rarely made eye contact and refused to let me see the wounds on her arms. Her responses to questions were often defensive, such as "Why do you want to know that?" or "What business is that of yours?" or "How could that possibly be of interest to you?" Although these questions sound abrupt and off-putting, they were often delivered with a wry, sarcastic sense of humor. Because of her intelligence and wit, I sensed that there was considerable reason to be hopeful.

After several months of gradually conducting a behavioral analysis, I began to get a clearer picture of Penny's self-harm. Penny cut herself in response to three main situations: (1) academic deadlines and pressure, (2) conflicts with peers, and (3) some not-yet-articulated discomfort with body image. Early in treatment, the topic of her relationship with her body was clearly too much for her, so we concentrated on academics and peer issues. We worked on identifying a number of replacement skills. She particularly liked mindful breathing, expressive artwork that included drawing and clay sculpting, and walking meditation. We also practiced breaking down her academic assignments into very small steps so that they were not so overwhelming.

As Penny began to use these replacement skills consistently, her academic performance improved. She used the skills to avoid panic as she was writing a paper or preparing for an exam. She also employed her breathing skills in social situations when she felt herself starting to "tighten up." The result was that over the first 6 months of treatment, her self-injury declined from multiple times per week to a few times per month.

Although all this work was fine and good, therapy had yet to address the heart of the matter: her relationship with her body. She manifested her dislike for her physical self in several ways beyond her self-injury. She said quite explicitly that she "hated" her body; she frequently mocked her appearance with statements such as "Being ugly is not a social asset," "I wish Quasimodo were still alive; I might get a date once in a while," and "I only purchase stainless steel mirrors." She also scored very low on the BAS (see Appendix B).

When the timing seemed right, I asked her how she had come to hate her body so much and why she assaulted it so frequently. These questions opened the floodgates. For many minutes, Penny just wept and could not speak. I listened as calmly as I could and assured her it was good that she could "finally let it out." She then began to tell her tale of abuse and exploitation—which took months to complete.

Penny's story recounted 10 years of abuse. She had been abused from the ages of 6 to 16, first by her father and then by her older brother. The father's abuse involved full intercourse/rape; the brother's, genital touching. Once her history of abuse was on the table, we began full exposure work. First we started with imaginal exposure, followed by *in vivo* exposure. Excerpts from the hierarchies we used in her treatment have been provided above in this chapter.

In doing imaginal exposure with Penny, I found that it was not possible to include every situation of abuse she had endured. Because of the duration and frequency of the abuse, the sheer number of experiences was in the thousands. During the 10-year period, it was not unusual for the client to be raped by her father two to four times per week. Therefore, the hierarchy could not identify every experience but concentrated on *categories* of abuse, such as "being groped by my brother over my clothes," "having sex with my father in the barn," or "having sex with my father upstairs when others were present in the house." (Note that "having sex" was her terminology, not mine.)

Not surprisingly, the retrieval of this material produced incredibly powerful emotions in Penny. She expressed rage, sadness, emptiness, and an overgeneralized fear for many weeks. Over time, she also added great shame and a sense of guilt to the mix. She asked herself endless questions about how the abuse could have gone on for 10 years without discovery or respite. In particular, she attacked herself with questions about "complicity" and "passive acceptance." This portion of treatment involved my helping her to challenge her irrational, self-blaming cognitions. The facts were that her father had long-term alcoholism and a vicious temper. He had beaten his wife frequently over the years and had been known to kill family cats when in a rage. He had also threatened Penny that if she ever told anyone, "the police will come and take you away"—which explained why Penny was so avoidant of police later in life. Many times I actively sided with Penny during this phase in treatment, emphasizing that she had been in a totally powerless situation and bore absolutely no blame.

The most challenging period in Penny's therapy was not the exposure work regarding the sexual abuse. It occurred when Penny realized that her mother had known about the abuse and had done nothing to intervene and protect her. The most flagrant example of this situation was the incident when Penny had been forced to have sex with her father while her mother was "asleep" in the same bed. Retrieving this memory was the cruelest blow for Penny, and it produced a marked short-term deterioration. Although Penny had not self-injured for over 6 months, when she began talking about her mother's role, the self-harm came back with a flourish. She cut herself repeatedly and even burned herself—something she had not done in years. She also became briefly suicidal, stating that she was "thinking of taking pills to end it all." As she worded it at the time, "I always knew my father and brother were bastards, but it's just too much to accept that my mother was too!" During this period, hospitalization was considered but not utilized. We increased the number of sessions and added frequent phone and e-mail contact.

Penny was able to meet this challenge. She eventually directly confronted all three family members regarding their abuse. Penny started with her father and chose to have the conversation in my office with me present. This allowed her to feel safe and not worry about violent retaliation. (I also made sure there were colleagues close by.) Later she also met with her mother and brother privately.

Penny moved beyond her self-injury and trauma. In fact, she turned great misfortune into a vocation: She eventually became a social worker doing protective interventions with abused children.

AN ALTERNATIVE APPROACH: CR FOR PTSD

Although PET is the PTSD treatment with the most empirical support, unfortunately there are many self-injuring clients who are not able to endure the rigors of exposure. That is, they are not able to tolerate the repeated direct exposure to traumatic memories required by the treatment. These clients become alarmingly self-destructive (involving suicide attempts or atypical self-injury) or decompensate into psychotic states. Fortunately, an empirically supported treatment that does not involve exposure is now available: CR for PTSD (Mueser et al., 2009). This treatment does not ask individuals to relive or reexperience the traumatic events that occurred in their lives. Rather, the treatment focuses on the thoughts and beliefs derived from the trauma. The treatment is conducted in highly structured therapy sessions over about 12–16 weeks. Research has shown the treatment to be highly effective, with many individuals reporting that their PTSD symptoms no longer interfere with daily living (Mueser et al., 2009). Clients have also reported improved quality of life.

CR for PTSD is an individual therapy model. In order to determine who meets criteria for the treatment, individuals are asked to complete three assessment questionnaires. These include the Stressful Events Screening Questionnaire, the PTSD Checklist (PCL), and the Beck Depression Inventory (BDI). Progress is monitored thereafter every 3 weeks with the PCL and BDI (Mueser et al., 2009).

Components of the Treatment

The CR for PTSD program includes breathing retraining, learning about common reactions to trauma, and developing skills for managing upsetting thoughts and feelings. These are techniques that, when practiced, reduce PTSD symptoms as well as other symptoms (such as anxiety, distress, irritability, and high levels of body tension). Many individuals even find that their symptoms of depression decrease as a result of this treatment (Mueser et al., 2009). Here is a brief description of the three main components of CR for PTSD:

Breathing Retraining

Breathing retraining is taught and practiced in the first session and assigned as homework over the first 3 weeks of treatment. As in PET, it is taught early in the treatment to provide clients some immediate relief from anxiety and other forms or arousal associated with PTSD. This breathing technique is very similar to that used by Foa and colleagues in PET, as described above. (For details of this and other components of the treatment, see Mueser et al.'s [2009] extremely detailed text.)

Psychoeducation

The second phase of treatment involves psychoeducation. Individuals are taught the common reactions to having experienced traumatic events (i.e., intrusion, avoidance, and arousal). Individuals learn that PTSD symptoms are learned responses that can be unlearned. The CR for PTSD program teaches individuals ways to change these learned responses. During this phase of treatment, clients also learn about common reactions to trauma, such as substance abuse and relationship difficulties.

Cognitive Restructuring

CR is the heart of this treatment. It involves learning how to identify and challenge thoughts and beliefs that contribute to distress. First, individuals learn ways to increase their awareness of distressing thoughts. Mueser et al.'s (2009) five steps are employed over and over again in this phase of treatment (see Chapter 12 for a description and an example of using the five steps). Clients also learn to identify patterns in their thinking that contribute to negative feelings, and ways to challenge and change their thinking to decrease distress. The majority of the treatment sessions focus on these aspects of CR.

Homework is also an important part of this treatment. Individuals receive homework sheets from the Mueser et al. (2009) text as part of each therapy session, to foster better retention of the material and to generalize it to the real world. Homework assignments are negotiated collaboratively and explained fully before each session ends.

Examples of Clients' Success with CR for PTSD

Seven colleagues and I at The Bridge were trained in this treatment intensively during 2010–2011. We employed CR for PTSD to treat individuals who had previously been unable to endure PET. To date, the treatment has been very helpful in assisting clients to achieve considerable relief from their PTSD and related self-injury. Several examples of successful clients follow:

- A 35-year-old woman had been raped by her older brother from the ages of 4 to 10. She was plagued with self-injury, flashbacks, dissociation, and social isolation. These symptoms largely remitted after the treatment.
- A 25-year-old woman had been molested by her mother's boyfriend at age 13. She suffered from depression, anxiety, self-injury, an eating disorder, and recurrent PTSD images and nightmares. All of her symptoms were much relieved by the treatment, with the exception of the eating disorder, which is still being intensively treated.
- A 20-year-old female had not only been raped by her mother's boyfriend, but as a young teen had been sold by him in the sex trade. Her symptoms included flashbacks, dissociation, extreme social withdrawal, self-injury, and recurrent suicidality. All these symptoms were much improved at posttreatment. Flashbacks and dissociation were all but eliminated.
- A 42-year-old male had been incarcerated for 10 years previously attempted homicide; he had tried to murder his mother's abusive husband (his stepfather). His PTSD symptoms included flashbacks, incapacitating shame, social isolation, and substance abuse. The treatment allowed him to view his criminal assault in a much more balanced perspective and to move forward. Of note was that he had committed no other aggression for two decades, yet had been judging himself to be a chronic offender.

CONCLUSION

In summary, in providing treatment for PTSD in self-injuring clients, clinicians and others need to do the following:

- Know the symptom clusters of PTSD (intrusion, arousal, and avoidance).
- Understand how self-injury may be directly linked to, and in fact may be used to *manage*, these three clusters.

- Employ either PET or CR for PTSD, both of which are preferred, evidence-based treatments.
    - PET has the most empirical support for its efficacy with PTSD. It focuses on (1) gathering information, (2) teaching breathing retraining, (3) explaining common reactions to trauma, (4) conducting imaginal exposure, and (5) providing *in vivo* exposure.
    - CR for PTSD is an empirically supported, non-exposure-based treatment that is recommended for those who are unable to endure detailed retrieval of traumatic memories. After formal assessment of PTSD symptoms, it focuses on (1) teaching breathing retraining, (2) providing psychoeducation about the common reactions to trauma, and (3) using the five-step CR process to deal with dysfunctional thoughts and beliefs derived from the trauma.

TREATMENT: STEP 4

CHAPTER 17

Treating Persons
with Multiple Self-Harm Behaviors

When people require Step 4 interventions (see Figure II.1, p. 75), they are facing complex, serious challenges. In the first edition of this book (Walsh, 2006), I referred to such individuals as presenting with "poly-self-destructive" behavior, meaning that they perform multiple direct and indirect self-harm behaviors in combination (see Chapter 3). For example, individuals may present with such direct forms of self-harm as recurrent suicide attempts, atypical/severe self-injury (e.g., self-harm involving multiple sutures, reopening of sutured wounds, genital self-injury, foreign-body ingestion), and common, low-lethality self-injury. In terms of indirect self-harm, they may abuse substances, have an eating disorder, present with diverse risk-taking behaviors, and be recurrently noncompliant with psychotropic medication regimens. These individuals are literally "walking inventories of self-harm behaviors" and are extremely difficult to treat. Such individuals generally require Step 4 interventions, which are discussed in this chapter and the next.

THE NEED FOR A HIERARCHY OF RISK

A common mistake for treaters to make in working with such individuals is to develop treatment goals such as "Client will remain free of self-harm behaviors for 1 month." I have seen such goals formulated in treatment plans over and over again when I have provided consultations to state hospitals, private inpatient psychiatric units, group homes, and residential schools. There are several problems with these types of goals. First, they are too global and nonspecific. Second, they are unrealistic, in that they ask clients who present with *many* self-harm behaviors to forgo them all at once. Third, such goals treat all self-harm behaviors as if they have the same importance, which they do not. High-lethality behaviors are much more important than low-lethality acts and should be addressed differently.

I therefore recommend constructing a "hierarchy of risk" for clients who present with poly-self-destructive behavior. The basic principle for developing a hierarchy of risk is to prioritize the highest-lethality behaviors, then move to the next most risky, and so on. An example of a hierarchy of risk for a very challenging client is provided in Figure 17.1. This client was a 28-year-old female residing in a state hospital when I provided a consultation on managing her self-harm. She had a history of suicide attempts, which needed to be given top priority. If she could make progress on eliminating those behaviors, it would be a considerable accomplishment. And it was unrealistic to think that she could address all of her self-harm behaviors simultaneously.

The topic of her anorexia nervosa was given second highest priority, for two reasons. First, it is a serious and potentially life-threatening eating disorder. In addition, Thomas Joiner (2005) has provided evidence that those with this diagnosis *die by suicide* at higher rates than persons with any other psychiatric diagnosis.

Over the course of 9 months, this client was able to make considerable progress as her self-harm targets became more specific, well-defined, and

---

1. Suicide attempts (history of neck constriction, overdose)
2. Anorexia nervosa (current body weight stable, but episodic fasting, purging)
3. Atypical, extreme forms of self-injury (foreign-body ingestion, reopening of sutured wounds)
4. Hard drug use (past use of intravenous drugs, crack cocaine; currently institutionally sober)
5. Moderate to extreme physical risk-taking behaviors (jumping from moving cars on two occasions)
6. Common, low-lethality self-injury (cutting, abrading, self-hitting)

FIGURE 17.1. A hierarchy of risk for an individual with multiple self-harm behaviors.

realistic. In discussion with her treatment team, she recognized that her suicide attempts, anorexia nervosa, and atypical self-injury behaviors (wound opening, foreign-body ingestion) would prevent her from being discharged to a community setting. With her team, she worked first on her suicidality, then on the eating disorder, and so forth. During this 9-month period, it was *not* a priority that she give up her common, low-lethality self-injury, because it was so far down her hierarchy of risk. This removed considerable pressure on the client to be "perfect" (i.e., to present with no self-harm behaviors at all). With a great deal of intensive DBT (see below) in combination with the hierarchy-of-risk approach, this client was able to move to a community-based residential treatment program within a year.

The practice of using a hierarchy of risk has broad utility. Consider these two case examples addressing very different problems:

Emily was a 19-year-old high school senior in special education classes. She presented with cutting, hair pulling, and frequent smoking of marijuana. Asked by her therapist which of these behaviors she was willing to address, she said the hair pulling. She explained that she found the bald spots on her head socially embarrassing, whereas the cutting and "weed smoking" were only problems in the eyes of others. The therapist employed a cognitive-behavioral approach to address the hair pulling for 5 weeks (see Keuthen et al., 2001), and this was successful. After this "victory," she decided to work on cutting after all.

Samantha was a 40-year-old woman who had been picking her skin for over 20 years. When she entered treatment, she had over 30 lesions on her body in diverse areas. Using a hierarchy of risk, the therapist asked her to identify which body area she would like to address first. Samantha selected her face because it was the most socially noticeable. She then targeted not picking her face, with no expectation she would cease picking other body areas. She also practiced replacement skills diligently (see Chapter 11). Within 6 weeks, her face was wound-free. Buoyed by this success, Samantha next targeted her arms, followed by her legs. The last body area to be addressed was a wound under her hairline. Sam was "pick-free," as she called it, within a year's time.

USING BROAD-BASED TREATMENTS TO ASSIST PERSONS WITH MULTIPLE SELF-HARM BEHAVIORS

Working with persons who have multiple self-harm behaviors requires aggressive, broad-based treatments in order to make progress. Two such treatments are DBT (Linehan, 1993a; Miller et al., 2007; Dimeff, Koerner, & Linehan, 2007), which has been mentioned in earlier chapters and is described further in Chapter 18, and illness management and recovery

(IMR; Mueser et al., 2006). The way in which we employ these two major evidence-based practice models at my agency, The Bridge, is simply conceived: If a client suffers from pervasive emotion dysregulation and unstable interpersonal relationships, we recommend DBT. In contrast, if a client suffers from symptoms of serious mental illness (especially psychosis) with frequent decompensations and relapses, we recommend IMR. Both of these treatments are briefly discussed below.

Dialectical Behavior Therapy

DBT is an empirically validated cognitive-behavioral treatment, informed by the mindfulness practices of Zen Buddhism. It is a multimodal treatment with four major components: (1) weekly highly structured individual therapy (using a hierarchy of behavioral targets and diary cards); (2) weekly group skills training that focuses on four major skill areas: mindfulness, distress tolerance, emotion regulation, and interpersonal effectiveness; (3) as-needed coaching between sessions to assist clients with skill acquisition and generalization; and (4) a weekly consultation meeting for the treatment team, designed to enhance learning of DBT and to provide peer support and supervision. These modes of treatment are designed to teach self-destructive and self-defeating clients to employ healthier emotion regulation and interpersonal skills, and thereby to achieve a new, improved life—a "life worth living" (Linehan, 1993a). Via the consultation team, the treatment is also designed to "treat the treaters"; this phenomenon may be unique to DBT.

As suggested by this list of core components, DBT is a complex, intensive, and comprehensive treatment that is not meant for everybody. As noted by Miller et al. (2007) in writing about DBT with suicidal adolescents,

> [DBT] is not intended for the prototypical teen exhibiting fairly benign mood lability. . . . Nor is DBT intended for an adolescent with a single episode of major depression who makes a first suicide attempt following an acute stressor. . . . We believe that DBT is most appropriate for those suicidal teens who exhibit a more chronic form of emotion dysregulation with numerous coexisting problems. . . . (p. 1)

Put another way, DBT is especially well suited to clients at steps 3 or 4 in the stepped-care model for treating self-harm (see Figure II.1, p. 75). At my agency, The Bridge, we employ DBT according to protocol with clients who have very complex self-harm behaviors. We use DBT with a very diverse clientele, including emotionally disturbed adolescents (see Chapter 18), transition-age youth with major mental health challenges, developmentally delayed adults, women with acquired brain injury and physical disabilities, and adults with serious and persistent mental illness who have spent years in state hospitals.

DBT is often an exceptionally good match for people who present with multiple self-harm behaviors, related profound emotion dysregulation, and chronically unstable interpersonal relationships. Some outcome data pointing to the success of this approach are provided in the discussion of residential DBT for suicidal and self-injuring adolescents in Chapter 18.

Illness Management and Recovery

The counterpart to DBT with poly-self-destructive individuals is IMR (Mueser et al., 2006). This treatment is designed for persons with serious mental illness (especially psychosis) who are prone to decompensation and relapse. It is quite useful in reducing self-harm behaviors in this population, because its very structured, manualized approach is helpful to cognitively disorganized individuals. Moreover, IMR is based on a recovery model that emphasizes personal choice and self-determination (Mueser et al., 2006).

Three types of treatment strategies are utilized in IMR: (1) motivational strategies, designed to assist clients in achieving short- and long-term goals; (2) educational strategies, which provide basic information about the nature of mental illness and strategies for preventing relapses; and (3) cognitive-behavioral strategies. The cognitive-behavioral strategies focus on changing behavior through the use of positive and negative reinforcers; behavior shaping toward goal achievement; modeling of skills and new behaviors; frequent use of practice, role plays, and homework; and CR (as described in Chapters 12 and 16).

IMR is a manualized treatment with 10 modules. In general, we find that completing all 10 modules with seriously impaired clients can take a year or more. Brief summaries of the modules are provided below.

1. *Recovery strategies.* In this module, clients focus on instilling hope; identifying and utilizing strategies toward recovery; identifying important personal goals; and developing specific plans for achieving these goals.
2. *Practical facts about mental illness.* This module provides a message of optimism about the future; assures clients that having a mental illness is not their fault; helps clients identify symptoms and warning signs; and provides examples of people with mental illness who have had meaningful and productive lives.
3. *Stress–vulnerability model.* This module explains how stress and

biological vulnerability play a role in causing symptoms; conveys that treatment can help clients reduce their symptoms and achieve their goals; helps clients become familiar with treatment options; and helps them with decision making.

4. *Building social support.* This module provides information about the benefits of social support; conveys confidence that clients can strengthen their social connections; and helps clients identify and practice strategies for connecting and becoming closer to more people.

5. *Using medication effectively.* This module provides accurate information about medications for mental illness, including advantages and disadvantages; provides an opportunity for clients to talk openly about their beliefs about and experiences with taking various medications; helps clients to weigh the advantages and disadvantages of taking medications; and, for clients who choose to do so, helps them develop strategies for taking medications regularly.

6. *Reducing relapses.* This module helps clients to identify triggers and early warning signs of impending relapse; helps clients to develop relapse prevention plans; and encourages clients to include family members and other supportive people in developing and implementing such plans.

7. *Coping with stress.* This module conveys a sense of confidence that clients can reduce stress and improve their ability to cope with stress effectively; helps clients identify the life events and "daily hassles" that can cause them stress; helps clients to identify and practice strategies for preventing some sources of stress and managing others; and encourages clients to include family members and other supports in their plans for coping.

8. *Coping with problems and symptoms.* This module conveys confidence that clients can deal with their problems and symptoms effectively; helps clients identify problems and symptoms they experience; and introduces a step-by-step method of solving problems and achieving goals.

9. *Getting your needs met in the mental health system.* This module conveys confidence in clients' making their own decisions; provides information about mental health services and benefits that will help clients make decisions; encourages clients to discuss the services they are receiving or would like to receive; and provides strategies for effective self-advocacy.

10. *Drug and alcohol use.* This module provides clients with information about the effects of alcohol and substances on mental illness; discusses how reducing or stopping use of substances can help

them to achieve their recovery goals; encourages discussion of the pros and cons of using substances; and helps clients who desire to stop using substances to develop a three-step plan for achieving this goal.

A free copy of the IMR manual is available online (*http://store. samhsa.gov/product/Illness-Management-and-Recovery-Evidence-Based-Practices-EBP-KIT/SMA09-4463*). As should be evident from the description of the 10 modules, IMR places heavy emphasis on clients' personal choice, identification of their own recovery goals, and empowerment. This philosophy especially resonates with clients who have lived in state hospitals, where their lives have been highly regimented with little personal choice or freedom. Clients often experience IMR as exceptionally liberating, in contrast to many of the therapeutic interventions they have previously received.

This chapter concludes with a case example in which IMR played a central role in a person's recovery from institutionalization and self-harm.

Zoe was a 31-year-old female who had been institutionalized since age 15. She carried a diagnosis of schizoaffective disorder. Her long tenure in the state hospital was due to suicide attempts by overdose, frequent episodes of foreign-body ingestion and head banging, chronic low-lethality self-injury, and sexual risk-taking behaviors. As an inpatient, Zoe had participated in DBT but discontinued it after 6 months, saying that it was too regimented for her. Also during her inpatient stay, she was offered CR for PTSD (see Chapter 16), which helped her considerably with her symptoms derived from incestuous abuse during childhood.

Finally, at age 31, Zoe was referred to a community-based group home that employed IMR as its core treatment model. Zoe became "hooked" right away, because IMR starts with clients' defining their own recovery goals. Zoe used IMR conscientiously to identify her triggers, warning signs, and relapse behaviors. She employed her coping skills quite well, but needed massive levels of staff support to avoid returning to the state hospital. Despite occasional brief stays at a local inpatient setting, Zoe has now been out of that hospital for 2½ years. She states, "I couldn't have done it without IMR."

CONCLUSION

- This chapter recommends using a hierarchy of risk with individuals who present with multiple self-harm behaviors. A hierarchy of risk targets one self-harm behavior at a time, starting with the most lethal or physically damaging.
- People with poly-self-destructive behavior require complex, multimodal treatment to recover. Two such treatments are DBT and IMR.

Both treatments are evidence-based, highly structured, and manual-ized.

o DBT is especially well suited to individuals with pervasive emo-tion dysregulation and chronically unstable interpersonal relation-ships.

o IMR is an excellent match for individuals with psychosis or other serious mental illness. It is a treatment that emphasizes personal empowerment and self-determination.

CHAPTER 18

Residential Treatment Targeting Self-Injury and Suicidal Behavior in Adolescents

with LEONARD A. DOERFLER and ARIANA PERRY

This chapter presents the final component of Step 4 in the stepped care model (see Figure II.1, p. 75). In a stepped-care model, some clients do not respond to the first three steps of service. These are individuals for whom outpatient skills training, various forms of cognitive-behavioral treatment (including PTSD treatments), brief hospitalizations, and outreach/home-based services have not proved effective. This chapter focuses on the residential treatment of self-injury and related problems in adolescents. Clearly, this is a form of treatment that is used only when less intensive forms of treatment have failed.

The term "residential" refers here to community-based group homes, residential treatment centers, and special education boarding schools. This chapter does not discuss treatment of self-injury in forensic or correctional facilities, which is reviewed in Chapter 24.

Residential treatment of self-harm behaviors is among the most under-researched topics in the field of self-injury. As I was preparing my first study of residential treatment of self-injury (Walsh & Doerfler, 2009), I was able to locate only a few empirical investigations of inpatient treatment, and none whatsoever regarding group home or residential school settings.

The absence of empirical research from group homes/residential schools is regrettable, because the number of children and adolescents being served in such settings has increased substantially since the 1980s (since the 1980s Connor, Doerfler, Toscano, Volungis, & Steingard, 2004). Moreover, "Analyses suggest that the growth in residential treatment has been accompanied by decreased access to inpatient treatment and that residential treatment centers increasingly serve as an alternative to inpatient psychiatric care" (Connor et al., 2004, p. 498). Some of the influences behind this increase have been the emergence of managed care and related efforts to reduce expensive inpatient treatment. The view of managed care professionals is that residential treatment is a cost-effective alternative to inpatient care. Whether it is an effective treatment alternative has yet to be established.

THE LITERATURE ON RESIDENTIAL TREATMENT OF SELF-INJURY

Many of the earliest citations in the clinical literature regarding self-injury came from inpatient settings (e.g., Offer & Barglow, 1960; Podvoll, 1969; Pao, 1969). Generally, these reports described the forms of the behavior and speculated as to motivations and psychodynamics. They did not discuss treatment at length. The 1970s and 1980s brought preliminary efforts to use empirical methods to study self-injury, primarily in hospital or group home settings. For example, Ross and McKay (1979) studied the prevalence, clinical correlates, and relationship dynamics of self-injury in a large residential school for girls. They reported that in a sample of 136, an astonishing 86% of the girls had self-injured, representing one of the more dramatic social contagion episodes on record. Rosen and I studied adolescents from both inpatient and group home settings and reported associations among histories of abuse, body alienation, and self-injury (Walsh & Rosen, 1988). Although we and Favazza (1987) discussed the treatment of self-injury, we did not provide empirical assessment of treatment efficacy.

Only recently have researchers turned to the evaluation of treatment effectiveness related to self-injury. Muehlenkamp (2006) reviewed the empirically supported treatments of self-injury and concluded that two variants of cognitive-behavioral treatment have been evaluated most extensively: problem-solving therapy (PST; D'Zurilla & Goldfried, 1971; D'Zurilla & Nezu, 2001) and DBT (Linehan, 1993a, 1993b; Miller et al., 2007). Only a few inpatient applications of PST or DBT have been empirically evaluated; to date, none exist for group home or residential school applications.

As noted by Muehlenkamp (2006), in a meta-analysis of 20 studies involving PST conducted by Hawton and colleagues (1998), the majority either failed to produce reductions in self-injury or failed to produce reductions that were superior to those for controls. Therefore, Muehlenkamp (2006, p. 170) concluded that "overall, the research regarding the effectiveness of PST is inconclusive."

The findings regarding the residential treatment effectiveness of DBT appear somewhat more promising. DBT was originally presented as an outpatient treatment for suicidal women with BPD. In the first randomized clinical trial (RCT), which has been described in Chapter 11, DBT was found to significantly reduce psychiatric hospitalizations, parasuicide attempts, medical severity of parasuicide, and treatment dropout in comparison with a TAU control condition (Linehan et al., 1991). (Note: In this and other DBT studies, the operational definition for "parasuicide" resembled but was not identical to the definition of self-injury used in this volume. Parasuicide included the common forms of self-injury, but also such behaviors as nonfatal overdose.) Since this first evaluation of DBT, a number of additional RCTs have been conducted (see Miller et al., 2007), but none have involved inpatient or community residential settings.

I have located three non-RCT studies that evaluated the effectiveness of DBT in treating self-injury on an inpatient basis. Barley et al. (1993) described an effort that transformed a psychodynamic inpatient unit into a inpatient DBT program. Drawing on a sample of 130 patients, they reported a significant decline in parasuicide, in comparison to the previous treatment regimen. They also compared the new DBT service to another inpatient unit (without randomization) and found significantly lower rates of parasuicide on the DBT service.

Katz, Cox, Gunasekara, and Miller (2004) described a 2-week inpatient program for adolescents. They modified Miller et al. (2007) 16-week outpatient DBT protocol and provided individual DBT twice per week, plus daily skills training groups, diary cards, and behavioral and solution analyses. Using standardized measures, Katz et al. compared 26 adolescents receiving DBT with 27 patients receiving TAU; they examined depression, suicidal ideation, hopelessness, parasuicidal behavior, hospitalizations, and other variables. Results were that the DBT group had significantly fewer behavioral incidents on the ward than the TAU group. At a 1-year follow-up, both the DBT and TAU patients demonstrated significantly reduced parasuicidal behavior, depression, and suicidal ideation. Thus the results were equivocal as to any unique DBT effects.

Bohus, Haaf, et al. (2000) applied standard DBT in a 3-month inpatient program for adult women. Treatment of a sample of 24 yielded significant reductions in self-injury at 1 month postdischarge. This study did not employ a control group. Bohus et al. (2004) then performed a follow-up study comparing inpatients receiving DBT with a waiting-list/TAU group. Subjects were again evaluated at 1 month postdischarge and showed significantly less self-injury than the controls (31% vs. 62%). However, 31% still represents a substantial portion who were self-injuring.

From these findings in inpatient settings, Miller et al. (2007) concluded that "there are no data suggesting that inpatient treatments are effective at reducing suicidal behavior and [nonsuicidal self-injurious behavior]" (p. 33). This conclusion seems to be more conservative than warranted. Granted, there are no RCTs in support of the effectiveness of inpatient DBT in treating nonsuicidal self-injury, but some encouraging findings at least point in the right direction. This brings us to a discussion of the community-based residential treatment of self-injury in adolescents.

COMMUNITY-BASED RESIDENTIAL TREATMENT OF SELF-INJURY

As noted above, to date there are no empirical studies regarding the treatment of self-injury in group homes or residential schools. This is unfortunate, in that such settings can provide treatment that is both intensive and extensive. Clients are in care many hours per day over extended periods of time. Such a treatment duration offers considerable opportunities for teaching and practicing new skills that may assist clients in learning to give up self-injury and other self-harm behaviors. Of course, the intensity of residential settings can also have associated risks. Having multiple people live together who present with emotion dysregulation and dysfunctional behaviors can sometimes exacerbate these difficulties. One example is the social contagion of self-injury, which is discussed at length in Chapter 20.

Connor et al. (2004) have argued that "residential treatment needs to progress beyond the one size fits all approach and develop more specific and empirically proven treatments for the specific needs of [distinct] populations" (p. 497). Toward this end, The Bridge of Central Massachusetts, a nonprofit human service agency for which I serve as Executive Director, decided in 1999 to implement evidence-based practices in its group homes and supported housing programs tailored to meet the needs of diverse clientele. Among the groups we serve are suicidal and self-injuring adolescents. In reviewing the literature on the treatment of self-destructive people, we concluded that DBT was the most promising, empirically validated approach for the adolescents we serve. After being intensively trained in DBT, we took on the project of transforming a generic, "TAU" group home for teens into a comprehensive DBT program. The components of this program are briefly described, after which some outcome data are provided.

DBT FOR ADOLESCENTS AT THE BRIDGE

In May 2001, The Bridge opened Grove Street, a 10-bed program that serves male and female youth between the ages of 13 and 19 years. The program is located in a three-story, single-family-style home in a middle-class neighborhood. The adolescents served by Grove Street have had significant difficulties managing their emotions and have displayed impulsive and self-destructive behaviors. They are often depressed, anxious, and aggressive, and have had problems with substance abuse, eating disorders, and attention deficits. Most have had multiple, extended psychiatric hospitalizations. For an adolescent to be admitted to this residence, the severity of the disturbance must be expected to worsen without intensive clinical intervention; there must be a documented assessment that the adolescent or his or her family would be placed at risk if the adolescent were to live at home; and less restrictive settings must have previously been attempted and deemed unsuccessful.

The Grove Street program offers the forms of DBT treatment summarized in Table 18.1. The table indicates how the provision of DBT at Grove Street differs from Linehan's (1993a) original outpatient DBT formulation. A full-time, intensively trained, master's-level therapist provides the individual DBT and skills training in the program.

As the table indicates, a number of modifications have been made to standard outpatient DBT. These changes were made to accommodate the emotional and behavioral challenges and developmental capabilities of the adolescent clientele. For example, adolescents with short attention spans tolerate 1-hour group meetings much better than 2½-hour sessions. Also, teaching skills via activity-based learning is generally more effective than more formal, didactic instruction. A behavior management point-and-level system based on DBT targets is employed, in order to provide more trials for skills practice and generalization. All residential staff members are trained in the DBT principles of validation. Their counseling focuses on conveying acceptance, while also fostering the learning of new skills that reduce problem behaviors and enhance quality of life. The residence also offers family therapy, as well as skills training with parents and children participating conjointly. The emphasis is on generalization of DBT skills to the home environment during treatment and postdischarge. Youth and families are coached to use their DBT skills at home on weekends during the youth's routine passes.

Despite these modifications, the program strives to provide DBT according to protocol. As in standard DBT, individual therapy in the residence focuses on the standard DBT targets and uses chain analyses and

TABLE 18.1. Provision of Standard Outpatient DBT versus Grove Street DBT

Treatment modality	Standard outpatient DBT	Grove Street
Individual therapy	Provided by outpatient clinician	Provided by clinician on site
Group skills training	Led by clinician and co-leader; one 2½-hour group session per week	Led by clinician and several residential counselors; two 1-hour group sessions per week
Diary cards	Client self-monitors	Residential staff members prompt and monitor daily
Coaching in crisis	Clinician (by phone)	Clinician or residential counselors on site
Structuring the environment	Informal, as needed	Program structure based on DBT targets
Family therapy and skills training	Not included except by Miller et al. (2007)	Family therapy on site at least monthly; family members learn DBT skills
Consultation team	All clinicians on team weekly	DBT clinician and residence staff members weekly
Pharmacotherapy; case management	Outpatient as needed	Provided on site

diary cards tailored to the needs of each youth. Also, the DBT skills training covers all the skills in the manual within a 6-month time period, consistent with Linehan's time frame for outpatient treatment.

OUTCOME DATA FOR THE GROVE STREET PROGRAM (2001–2010)

Client Characteristics

Since the original publication on Grove Street outcomes (Walsh & Doerfler, 2009), my colleagues and I have updated the data set and analyses. These data are from 9 years of program operation (2001–2010). During this period, the program has served 66 adolescents. Of these, 47 have been females and 19 males. The age range has been from 13 to 19 years, with a mean of 16.59. Length of stay for the clients has ranged from 1 month to 26 months, with a mean of 10.03 months.

The funder for the program, the Massachusetts Department of Mental Health, refers all clients, and the program has no right of refusal. All clients who come to the program have received multiple DSM-IV-TR diagnoses, with the following distribution for the 66 clients: major depressive disorder, 65.15%; bipolar (I or II) disorder, 59.09%; oppositional defiant disorder, 34.85%; PTSD, 45.45%; substance abuse disorder, 16.67%; ADHD, 43.94%; anxiety disorders, 16.67%; eating disorders, 16.67%. Note that many clients have received five or more diagnoses, perhaps suggesting that previous caregivers had struggled to understand these clients' dysfunction. Grove Street does not provide its own diagnoses for clients. (Note: No clients have been diagnosed with BPD because technically this diagnosis cannot be employed until age 18.)

Because Grove Street is a single DBT-oriented adolescent residence with no sustained waiting list, there has been no opportunity to assign subjects randomly to different treatment conditions, and subsequently to compare them. We did devise an alternative strategy that permits some statistical comparisons. We noticed early in the process of operating the program that clients who had participated in (and in most cases completed) two full courses of DBT seemed to do better. A "course" consisted of 6 months of treatment during which all the skills in the DBT manual (Linehan, 1993b) were covered. Our interpretation was that the first round of DBT allowed the clients to learn the skills in a preliminary way, and the second round enabled them to consolidate this learning and to apply the skills in their day-to-day lives more consistently and effectively. The second round also offered more opportunity to generalize the use of the skills to the home environment after discharge.

We therefore decided to compare two groups: clients who had participated in more than one round of DBT (defined here as 7 months or more of residential care) versus those who had received one round or less (6 months or less). The first group is referred to as the "more-DBT group." Their lengths of stay in the program ranged from 7 to 24 months, with an average of 12.73 months. The comparison group is referred to as the "less-DBT group." Their lengths of stay ranged from 2 to 6 months, with a mean of 4.23 months. Therefore, the two groups differed *substantially* in the amount of DBT they received. Our hypothesis was that clients who completed more-DBT would do better on all outcome variables.

The more-DBT group comprised 45 individuals, or 68% of the total served. This group included 28 females (62%) and 17 (38%) males; the racial composition was 39 white, 3 Hispanic, and 3 black. The less-DBT group consisted of 21 youth; there were 19 females (90%) and 2 (10%) males, and the racial composition was 14 white, 6 Hispanic, and 1 black. Therefore, the two groups were different as to gender, but quite similar as to race.

Differences between the DBT Groups

We then performed analyses to compare the clients who received more DBT versus less DBT, using 2 × 3 analyses of variance. We compared the two treatment groups across three time periods: (1) 6 months prior to enrolling at Grove Street, (2) the first 6 months at Grove Street, and (3) 6 months after discharge. We also looked at three clinically relevant variables: (1) psychiatric hospitalizations, (2) incidents of self-injury, and (3) suicide attempts. We selected these problems because they played a central role in the placement of these youth in residential care.

The findings were that the adolescents showed significant improvement (both statistically and clinically) over the time periods examined. The between-group "treatment" effect was found for some variables, but not for others.

Number of Psychiatric Hospitalizations

The findings regarding psychiatric hospitalizations included a significant effect for time (i.e., a significant decrease in hospitalizations over the three time periods). There was also a significant group effect (the less-DBT group had more hospitalizations at all three time periods than the more-DBT group). The interpretation of the findings is that both groups showed equal improvement over the course of treatment, but that the less-DBT group started off worse and continued to be worse during both treatment and follow-up. Figure 18.1 presents the data for psychiatric hospitalizations.

Rates of Self-Injury

The findings for self-injury were that there was no significant effect for more versus less DBT, but there was a significant effect for time (a significant decrease in the number of self-injury episodes). Both groups, regardless of length of treatment, showed similar decreases in self-injury episodes. Quite remarkably, self-injury dropped to almost zero during the 6-month follow-up period for both treatment groups. Such success is rare in outcome studies focusing on self-injury. See Figure 18.2 for these outcome results.

Number of Suicide Attempts

As shown in Figure 18.3, the pattern for suicide attempts was the same as for self-injury episodes. There was a significant effect for time (a significant decrease in the number of suicide attempts), but no significant effect for more versus less DBT. This indicated that both DBT groups showed similar

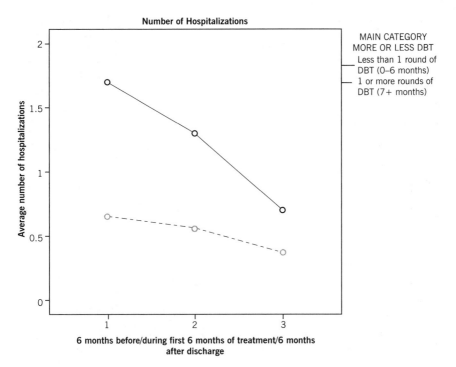

FIGURE 18.1. Number of psychiatric hospitalizations for the groups receiving more versus less DBT.

decreases in suicide attempts over the course of treatment. Moreover, at the 6-month follow-up, the number of suicide attempts was virtually zero. Suicide attempts (and corresponding risk) decreased dramatically after discharge from Grove Street (even for the less-DBT group).

Residency after Discharge

We also performed analyses comparing the more- and less-DBT groups and level of placement at pre- and postdischarge. Findings are depicted in Table 18.2. There were no significant differences between the groups in type of placement level *prior* to entering the Grove Street program. This was important to establish, because it suggested that the two groups were not substantially different at point of intake. That is, they came from similar types of placements, suggesting similar levels of dysfunction.

However, there was a statistically significant difference between the groups in terms of placement level during the first 6 months *after* leaving

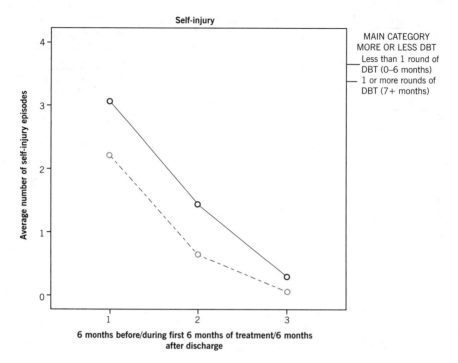

FIGURE 18.2. Episodes of self-injury for the groups receiving more versus less DBT.

Grove Street. As shown in Table 18.3, the adolescents who received one or more rounds of DBT were significantly more likely to be living in their family homes (67% vs. 43%) or in an adult group residential setting (27% vs. 10%). In contrast, adolescents who received one round or less of DBT were more likely to be admitted to a hospital setting (33% vs. 2%) or to be living in a locked residential setting (14% vs. 4%). In addition to quality-of-life considerations, the more-DBT clients were clearly living in less expensive treatment settings—or, better yet, at home with their families.

Summary of the Results

Although the results were not entirely consistent with our hypotheses, it was gratifying to note that both the more- and less-DBT groups showed significant decreases over time in both self-injury and suicidal behavior. Both types of self-harm behaviors were all but extinguished at 6 months postdischarge. These were very encouraging findings.

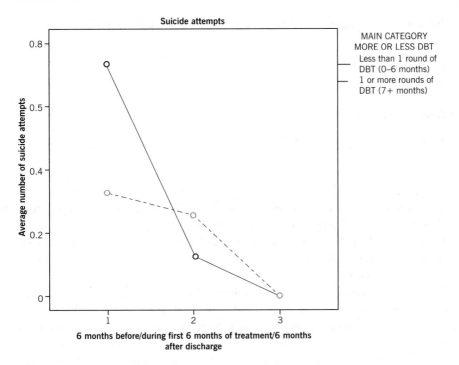

FIGURE 18.3. Suicide attempts for the groups receiving more versus less DBT.

TABLE 18.2. Placement Level during 6 Months before Entering Grove Street

	Less than one round of DBT	One or more rounds of DBT
Hospital	$n = 4$ (19%)	$n = 7$ (16%)
Locked residential	$n = 10$ (48%)	$n = 14$ (31%)
Group residential	$n = 5$ (24%)	$n = 10$ (22%)
Family home	$n = 2$ (10%)	$n = 14$ (31%)

TABLE 18.3. Placement Level during 6 Months after Leaving Grove Street

	Less than 1 Round of DBT	1 or More Rounds of DBT
Hospital	$n = 7$ (33%)	$n = 1$ (2%)
Locked Residential	$n = 3$ (14%)	$n = 2$ (4%)
Group Residential	$n = 2$ (10%)	$n = 12$ (27%)
Family Home	$n = 9$ (43%)	$n = 30$ (67%)

Findings consistent with our hypotheses were that, over time, the more-DBT group showed significantly fewer psychiatric hospitalizations than the less-DBT group. The more-DBT group also was significantly more likely to reside at home or in a less restrictive treatment setting at 6 months postdischarge than the less-DBT group. Both of these findings suggest the predicted "dosage" effect.

There were of course multiple limitations to the data presented here. The sample was very small ($N = 66$) and was drawn from a single treatment setting in Massachusetts. Two groups were compared as to treatment effects, but there was no random assignment. The two groups were not comparable as to gender distribution. Moreover, there was some evidence that the less-DBT clients were more dysfunctional, in that they had higher rates of hospitalization than the more-DBT group at all three time periods. Better outcomes for the more-DBT group could have been due to preexisting differences in levels of disturbance and dysfunctional behavior in the two groups. It is possible that the less-DBT clients experienced poorer outcomes not because they received less-DBT, but because they were substantially more impaired.

Other influences that could have played a role in the positive outcomes for the more-DBT group include maturation effects, regression to the mean, or other historical/ contextual influences that are unknown. Another concern is that treatment was evaluated only at 6 months postdischarge. Ideally, additional assessments would have been performed at 1 and 2 years postdischarge.

On the positive side, the data and results reported here do represent a step forward. This study appears to be one of the first regarding the treatment of self-injury and related problems in a community residential setting. The findings are encouraging because residential DBT appeared to work quite well for a large proportion of clients in terms of reduced rates of hospitalizations, self-injury, and suicidal behavior, as well as higher rates of successful return to family living. This contribution is important, in that large numbers of self-injuring youth are treated in such settings, and empirical

3366

evaluation is warranted. Future studies in such residential settings should include larger/more diverse samples, employ randomized assignment and control groups, and perform more sophisticated statistical analyses.

SOCIAL CONTAGION OF SELF-INJURY IN RESIDENTIAL PROGRAMS

A final topic for this chapter is the phenomenon of social contagion of self-injury. As just reviewed, one advantage of residential treatment settings is that intensive treatment can be provided over extended periods of time. However, congregate living can also lead to an exacerbation of problems. One such dilemma that has been frequently reported in the literature is the social contagion of self-injury. This topic is discussed at length in Chapter 20.

I speculate in Chapter 20 that the following dimensions may influence social contagion of self-injury:

- Desire for acknowledgment (e.g., "Pay attention to me")
- Desire to punish (e.g., "See what you've made me do")
- Desire to produce withdrawal (e.g., "Perhaps now you'll leave me alone")
- Desire to coerce others (e.g., "If you don't do X, I'll cut myself")
- Competition for caregiver resources (particularly in residential settings, where staff resources can be scarce)
- Anticipation of aversive consequences (e.g., "If I assault someone else, I'll go to jail; if I cut myself, the penalties are modest")
- Direct modeling influences (i.e., behavior is influenced by modeling alone without apparent contingencies)
- Disinhibition (i.e., behavior is produced by witnessing self-injury in others)
- Peer competition (i.e., behavior is produced by the wish to be the "best" at self-injury)

Note that the first six items and the final item in this list can be conceptualized as consistent with Nock and Prinstein's (2004) functional approach. That is to say, these influences for self-injury contagion involve negative social reinforcement (e.g., producing the withdrawal of others or avoiding aversive consequences) or positive social reinforcement (e.g., receiving attention, coercing others). However, the role of modeling effects such as direct imitation or disinhibition may not fall within their framework.

Nonetheless, the important topic pertaining to self-injury contagion in residential settings is how to prevent it when possible, and how to manage it when it does occur. In Chapter 21, I discuss a protocol for responding to self-injury in school settings, as well as basic principles for managing and preventing contagion in such settings. The same basic principles can be useful in preventing or managing self-injury contagion in residential program or inpatient settings. These principles are now adapted to a residential context:

1. Encourage clients who self-injure to stop talking about the behavior with fellow residents. Explain that such talk is triggering, is conducive to contagion, and may thereby "hurt your friends."

2. Instead, these clients should talk to trusted adults (such as residential counselors, therapists, or parents) *in private* about their self-injury.

3. Consistent with this approach, self-injuring clients in the residential milieu are expected to cover up wounds, scars, and bandages, as these visual cues can also be triggering.

4. Group treatment methodologies should concentrate on skills training and avoid or prohibit discussions of self-injury.

5. Individual therapy should be the modality where self-injury is worked on in depth.

6. Clients who defy these respectful requests may receive negative consequences in the residential program if their behavior is deemed conducive to contagion (e.g., such clients may be dropped to safety level, lose privileges, and be required to perform a DBT repair).

An Empirical Study of Self-Injury Contagion at Grove Street

In the Grove Street DBT program, we have striven to be consistent with the six principles listed above. Toward this end, the program has very clear rules about client communication regarding self-injury. Within the program, it is a major rule violation for clients to discuss self-injury or exhibit their wounds or scars in the midst of peers. In addition, skills training groups have strict rules about not discussing details of self-injury or other self-harm behaviors. Instead, self-injury is discussed at length in individual DBT, with an emphasis on data collection via diary cards and on behavioral chain analyses. Problem solving and skills practice in individual therapy prioritize learning healthy mindfulness, emotion regulation, distress tolerance, and interpersonal effectiveness skills to replace self-injury. Data have already been presented indicating that the program has been quite successful in reducing rates of self-injury and suicide attempts.

In order to measure whether self-injury contagion was occurring in the Grove Street program, we conducted an empirical study replicating an ealier design (Walsh & Rosen, 1985). For a 2½-year period, we collected daily data on the occurrence or nonoccurrence of self-injury. We then analyzed the distribution of self-injury occurrences to determine whether the behavior had occurred in statistically significant clusters or bursts. The result was that no significant clustering was found; rather, the distribution of self-injurious acts appeared to be entirely random. Given our previous problems with self-injury contagion in group settings (Walsh & Rosen, 1985; Rosen & Walsh, 1989), we tentatively concluded that the strategies identified above to prevent social contagion of self-injury have been effective.

CONCLUSION

- Some clients who self-injure and present with other dysfunctional behaviors fail to respond to such interventions as outpatient treatment, short-term hospitalizations, or outreach/home-based services.
- Such clients may respond to residential treatment that offers highly specialized, intensive, targeted services.
- One such treatment described in this chapter is a residential program for adolescents that provides DBT according to protocol.
- Some outcome data for this program suggest that DBT has been effective in reducing psychiatric hospitalizations, self-injury, and suicide attempts in the youth served.
- Some of the positive outcomes were affected by amount of DBT, suggesting a "dosage effect." The clients who received more DBT (7 months or more) was more likely to live at home or in less restrictive settings after discharge than those who received less DBT (6 months or less).
- Residential settings are underresearched as to treatment effectiveness. The outcome study of the residential program reported here is one of the first ever published.
- Strategies to prevent social contagion of self-injury in residential programs have been reviewed, with some data to suggest the effectiveness of such strategies.

PART III

Specialized Topics

INTRODUCTION

Part I of this book has reviewed definitions and contexts of self-injury; Part II has discussed the assessment and treatment of self-injury according to a stepped-care model. This concluding section of the book looks at specialized topics related to self-injury. The first of these chapters (Chapter 19) focuses on self-care for clinicians and other professionals. Self-injury tends to provoke intense reactions in caregivers, in part because it often involves recurrent bodily harm. Stressed reactions in treaters are understandable and should not be judged negatively. Rather, caregivers need strategies to cope with self-injury so that they can maintain a compassionate and therapeutic frame in working with clients.

The other topics covered in this concluding section provide good examples for why caregivers might react powerfully to encountering self-injury. The topic of social contagion of self-injury—especially among youth—is discussed in Chapter 20, along with some specific strategies to prevent the phenomenon. An evidence-based protocol for responding to self-injury in school settings is reviewed in Chapter 21.

The book concludes with detailed discussions of some very alarming self-harm behaviors. These include a scholarly yet practical discussion of the "choking game" by Amy M. Brausch in Chapter 22. Kenneth L. Appelbaum provides a trenchant discussion in Chapter 24 of self-injury in correctional settings, where self-harm behaviors can be especially severe. Also falling into the "severe and alarming" category are the discussions of foreign-body ingestion (Chapter 23) and major self-injury (Chapter 25), which bring the volume to a close.

CHAPTER 19

Managing Reactions to Self-Injury
A Guide for Therapists and Other Caregivers

Favazza (1998, p. 265) has written that the treatment literature on self-injury "is basically one of countertransference." Although I hope that this statement is somewhat of an exaggeration, there is little doubt that self-injury can produce extreme reactions in caregivers. Many authors have discussed the negative responses of treatment professionals to self-injuring clients, including Linehan (1993a), Alderman (1997), Conterio and Lader (1998), Hyman (1999), Farber (2000), and Shaw (2002). As an example of such a reaction, Alderman (1997) has vividly described her experience of working with her first self-injuring client:

> Although I had been studying in the area of self-injury for some time, seeing the fresh jagged wounds on [the client's] arms had a major impact on me. I felt as if *I* had been wounded. I imagined the great amount of pain this girl must have felt in order to cut herself, and I felt quite sad. I wanted her to talk to me about the pain, to tell me about what she was going through when she hurt herself. I wanted her to promise me she would never injure herself again. I wanted to make her stop. And, as commonly experienced in any therapeutic relationship, what I wanted and what the client wanted were two different things. She continued to injure herself. I continued to want her

to stop. Eventually, I became discouraged and frustrated because she wouldn't do what I wanted. (p. 192)

Alderman's remarks are an appropriate introduction to this topic. This chapter reviews the considerable range of negative reactions of caregivers to self-injury; it also offers some suggestions for how to manage these responses. Although this chapter is written primarily for professionals, the concepts presented may also be relevant for family members and significant others.

Consistent with the theoretical framework of this book (see Chapter 6), the reactions of caregivers to self-injury can be conceptualized as biopsychosocial phenomena. Therapists, nurses, physicians, residential counselors, case managers, educators, and other professionals respond to self-injury physically, psychologically, and interpersonally. Of greatest concern are the responses that threaten to harm clients and derail the treatment. As noted by Linehan 1993a, "Therapy-interfering behaviors on the part of the therapist include any that are iatrogenic, as well as any that unnecessarily cause the patient distress or make progress difficult" (p. 138).

Some of the negative reactions that I have encountered in professionals working with self-injuring clients include the following:

- *Biological responses.* Therapists may report increased heart and respiration rate, nausea, light-headedness, physical arousal and agitation, episodic insomnia, or other psychosomatic symptoms in response to self-injury.
- *Psychological responses.* These consist of three elements:
  o *Cognitive.* Therapists may present with confusion, disorientation, indecisiveness; pejorative judgments regarding self-injuring clients; pessimism regarding the treatment; self-doubt regarding professional competence; exaggerated "savior" fantasies.
  o *Affective.* Therapists may experience anxiety, fear, shock, disgust, panic; or anger, frustration, bitterness, rage; or sadness, discouragement, hopelessness, helplessness.
  o *Behavioral.* Therapists may present with excessively sympathetic, emotionally charged, or agitated responses; employ pejorative language (both technical and slang) to refer to clients; attempt to coerce, control, and extinguish the behavior via the use of demanding safety contracts; withdraw, avoid, transfer, or terminate treatment of clients; or abandon typical professional boundaries by becoming overly involved with clients or preoccupied with their self-injury.

- *Social/environmental responses.* Professionals sometimes punish clients for their self-injuring behavior by withdrawing privileges, suspending them from school or treatment settings, or the like. They may also intervene inappropriately in clients' lives outside of treatment, such as imposing unnecessary psychiatric hospitalizations, violating confidentiality by contacting adult clients' significant others or employers without permission, or warning other clients to "avoid" the self-injuring clients.

And these biopsychosocial phenomena represent only a partial list.

Why does self-injury produce such intense reactions in professionals trained to help those in distress? Therapists and other caregivers are human beings who have the same adverse reactions as anyone else to self-inflicted bodily harm. Self-injury violates the expectation that all people naturally seek to avoid pain and seek pleasure. Most forms of self-injury cause immediate tissue damage that is shocking to see. Blood, wounds, scabs, scars, and sutures are violations of the usual human bodily form. Blood and related bodily fluids present some risk to others of acquiring serious and even fatal diseases.

Encountering the wounds of self-injury often produces a visceral, automatic recoiling in others. To withdraw from or avoid those who have intentionally damaged their own bodies may be "wired into" the human organism. The impulse to escape may be especially intense when the behavior is at the level of major self-injury or self-mutilation. When people disfigure their eyes, faces, breasts, or genitals, or cause themselves extensive physical damage that requires medical attention, almost any human being is likely to be shocked and want to withdraw (at least temporarily).

How then should caregivers learn to manage and overcome such understandably negative responses? They need to "unlearn" typical reactivity in each of the biopsychosocial realms in order to manage their own distress and to fulfill their roles as caregivers. Clients have every right to expect that professionals will respond compassionately and therapeutically to their self-destructive behavior. In order to become effective caregivers in response to self-injury, professionals need to acquire and employ at least the following set of skills.

PHYSICAL SELF-SOOTHING

Professionals need to be able to calm themselves when they find themselves reacting physiologically to self-injury. A basic way to achieve this calming state is to practice and employ the breathing skills (and other self-soothing techniques) presented in Chapter 11. Breathing skills are well documented to be useful in slowing respiration and heart rate, and thus in fostering a sense of physical calmness (Foa & Rothbaum, 1998; Williams et al., 2007). It is very difficult for a therapist to feel anxious or agitated when his or her body is in a state of relaxation. In other words, professionals treating self-injuring clients need to use the very same replacement skills in managing their emotions as their clients are learning over the course of treatment.

COGNITIVE RESTRUCTURING

The main way in which professionals can manage their negative reactions to self-injury is through cognitive self-monitoring and CR. Intense biological, affective, behavioral, and social/environmental reactions begin with thought processes. If the professional interprets routine, low-lethality self-injury as a "suicidal crisis," he or she is likely to overreact to the situation. Therapists who require of themselves that their clients "get better" rapidly will inevitably find themselves frustrated when the self-injury persists for months. Professionals who question their own competence because clients recurrently self-injure need to modify unrealistic expectations. Clinicians who think they should be able to control the behavior of adolescents and adults and "make them get better" are only setting themselves up for needless conflicts and power struggles. A dispassionate, patient attitude is crucial in conducting therapy with those who self-injure.

Many authors have written about the challenges of dealing with negative judgments of and behavior toward self-injuring clients (Alderman, 1997; Favazza, 1998; Farber, 2000; Linehan, 1993a). Unfortunately, it is not unusual to hear professionals use pejorative language when referring to self-injuring clients or their behavior. I have often heard caregivers use the following terms:

- "Manipulative"
- "Attention-seeking"
- "Just a suicide gesture"
- "Just behavioral" (i.e., indicating that the client is not truly upset, just using the behavior strategically)
- "Gamey" or "game-playing"
- A "bad borderline" (i.e., insulting the client with an unflattering psychiatric diagnosis)
- "Faking"
- "Contrived"

- "Exploitive"
- "Beating the system"
- "Con man/woman"

When caregivers employ such terminology in referring to their clients, they are well on the way to having lost a helpful perspective. Professionals who make such statements are usually suffering from serious "compassion fatigue." Peer supervision or a regularly scheduled staff consultation team (Linehan, 1993a) can be helpful in reducing the frustration of such therapists and getting them back on track. Therapists should assume that they will occasionally have adverse reactions to self-injuring clients. That is to say, counterproductive thoughts and feelings are all but unavoidable. It is no disgrace to experience such negative responses unless they go unacknowledged and unaddressed. The rule of thumb is that clinicians should deal with negative reactions when they are still *at cognitive and affective levels,* before they emerge *behaviorally* in the therapeutic relationship itself.

If a therapist is experiencing distress in response to self-injury in clients, I would also suggest that he or she employ Mueser et al.'s (2009) five steps, as described in Chapter 12. This process enables professionals to identify the following:

1. The *situation* that has triggered the distress—for instance, "My client keeps self-injuring, and it appears to be getting worse."
2. The *feelings* generated by this situation, such as fear and a sense of failure and hopelessness.
3. The *thoughts* underlying these feelings, such as "It's my fault she's not getting better. I shouldn't work with people who self-injure."
4. The *evidence for and against* these thoughts. Sample of evidence for: "Her rate of self-injury has remained steady for 4 months; she is not getting better." Sample of evidence against: "I've worked successfully with other self-injuring clients, and treatment has taken time with these others as well. She is progressing in other areas."
5. *Developing new, more accurate, and more helpful thoughts,* such as "I'm using an evidence-based treatment with this client and working hard. It usually takes time, and all I can do is influence her, not control her."

REGULATING AFFECTIVE RESPONSES

In my opinion, therapists experience three main categories of negative emotions in relation to self-injury in clients:

1. Anxiety, fear, and related avoidant emotions
2. Frustration, anger, and related aggressive emotions
3. Sadness, discouragement, and related hopeless/helpless emotions

The task of the therapist is to recognize the occurrence of such emotions and to "turn them" into therapeutic responses. For example, anxiety and fear can be transformed into positive attentiveness. Avoidant feelings, such as anxiety and fear, suggest that the clinician is on alert for danger. Therapists can use such "alarm responses" productively by becoming finely attuned in assessing and monitoring the self-injury. Hypervigilance can be a strength when it is used to understand all the details and nuances of the self-injurious behavior.

Anger can also be a useful response if it is transformed into a commitment to assist the client and strategically "fight" the problem. The primary utility of aggressive feelings is the energy they provide the therapist in committing to help the client acquire and employ useful replacement behaviors. A certain amount of fierceness can also be useful in compassionately challenging the self-denigrating cognitions and self-loathing emotions of clients. This is particularly true for abuse survivors, who frequently suffer from irrational self-blame and need the therapist to model appropriate indignation directed at the abusers.

Sadness and discouragement on the part of therapists have no place in the treatment of self-injury. Clients quickly discern any pessimistic attitudes in the minds of their treaters. The negativism of a therapist instantaneously becomes the hopelessness of a client. The way to transform discouragement into proactivity is to return to the wealth of techniques available in the psychotherapeutic repertoire. The spectrum of therapeutic interventions, including psychopharmacology, cognitive therapy, replacement skills training, body image work, and exposure treatment, offers the therapist an extensive range of options. It is very rare that all these methods can be exhausted without some measure of therapeutic success.

MANAGING NEGATIVE BEHAVIORS

Alderman (1997, p. 196) has presented an extensive list of counterproductive therapist behaviors that may emerge in relation to self-injury:

- Being late for, or forgetting, sessions
- Being inattentive during sessions
- Refusing to discuss self-injury in sessions
- Being argumentative with clients

- Making judgmental statements to clients
- Using self-injury contracts coercively
- Threatening a client with hospitalization
- Raising fees inappropriately

I hope that such behaviors are rare among treaters of self-injuring clients. I also believe that if caregivers become aware of their pejorative judgments (such as those listed in the section on CR above) early enough, their behavior with clients will never deteriorate to such an extent. In order for therapists to manage their behavior appropriately in sessions, the following basic "rules to live by" are helpful to keep in mind:

- Self-injury is generally not about suicide and should not be treated as a suicidal crisis. If therapists remind themselves that self-injury is an alarming behavior but not a life-threatening crisis, they are more likely to remain calm, strategic, and helpful.
- The best interpersonal approach in responding initially to self-injury is to employ a low-key, dispassionate demeanor in combination with respectful curiosity (see Chapter 7).
- Clients are slow to give up self-injury because they rely on it for affect regulation. Therapists should understand why their clients employ self-injury and should be patient in their expectations for change.
- To give up self-injury, clients need to learn replacement skills that are at least as effective as self-injury.
- The emphasis in treatment should be on learning new skills rather than on giving up self-injury. Addition is easier than subtraction.

INTERVENING APPROPRIATELY IN CLIENTS' ENVIRONMENTS

Interventions in the living environments of self-injuring clients should generally be positive and nonintrusive. Clients should not be punished for self-injuring. Self-injury is the problem for which they seek or require treatment. The behavior should not be viewed as a form of noncompliance, defiance, or provocation. Coercive interventions in a client's living environment should generally be few and far between. If self-injury is properly viewed as non-suicidal, then immediate protective interventions in the environment are usually not necessary. Arranging outpatient intervention is generally the more appropriate course. Whenever possible, interventions in clients' living environments should involve their consent. Thus, if a therapist wants to speak with a spouse, partner, or close friend, explicit written permission from the client should be obtained. However, there are some exceptions to this rule, including the following:

• *Self-injury in minors.* When children or adolescent minors self-injure, their parents or guardians should be notified immediately. A detailed protocol for dealing with self-injury in minors in school settings is presented in Chapter 21.

• *Circumstances when the behavior has passed beyond common, low-lethality self-injury into atypical/severe self-injury.* When clients self-injure their eyes, faces, breasts (in females), or genitals, or if they inflict damage requiring medical intervention, they sacrifice their right to direct their own treatment (at least temporarily). In such cases, protective interventions such as psychiatric evaluation and/or hospitalization should be pursued for the clients' own safety.

• *Circumstances when the self-injury is worsening and may shift to suicidal behavior.* These circumstances are even more alarming than the ones just described. In some situations, persons who engage in frequent self-injury discover that the behavior is "no longer working." Such clients may attempt to gain relief by increasing the level of physical damage or by shifting to hurting other areas of the body. If these methods still fail to provide relief, the individuals can become actively suicidal—at which point protective interventions are required.

CONCLUSION

By and large, therapists are able to treat self-injuring clients with equal measures of compassion, optimism, and technical skill. The entire professional identity of caregivers is based on their desire to help and relieve distress. Self-injury can tax the best intentions of clinicians, but with proper self-monitoring and the use of skills, professionals can avoid the pitfalls. Becoming actively aware of the risks of negative thoughts, feelings, and behaviors can serve to inoculate professionals against acting counterproductively in the treatment. Clients deserve care that is fresh, positive, and technically proficient.

In summary, it is helpful in providing treatment to self-injuring clients if professionals and other caregivers do the following:

• Remain aware of the inevitable risk of negative responses to self-injury.
• Carefully monitor their cognitive, affective, and behavioral responses to self-injury.

- Remain alert to pejorative language regarding self-injuring clients as a tipoff to negative reactivity.
- Manage and diffuse pejorative judgments and negative emotions regarding self-injury before they are acted on in the treatment.
- Practice the same skills that clients learn, in order to deal effectively with negative responses to self-injury.

CHAPTER 20

Social Contagion and Self-Injury

The topic of the social contagion of self-injury has a long history that has been reviewed in Ross and McKay (1979), Walsh and Rosen (1988), Favazza (1996), Taiminen, Kallio-Soukainen, Nokso-Koivisto, Kaljonen, and Helenius (1998), Farber (2000), Nock (2008), and Walsh and Doerfler (2009). Rosen and I have defined "self-injury contagion" in two ways: (1) when acts of self-injury occur in two or more persons within the same group within a 24-hour period (Rosen & Walsh, 1989); and (2) when acts of self-injury occur within a group in statistically significant clusters or bursts (Walsh & Rosen, 1985). These two definitions have different emphases and are not incompatible.

Social contagion episodes have generally been reported in children, adolescents, or young adults living in institutional or treatment settings, such as orphanages (Holdin-Davis, 1914), inpatient units (Offer & Barglow, 1960; Crabtree & Grossman, 1974; Kroll, 1978; Taiminen et al., 1998), prisons (Virkkunen, 1976), juvenile detention facilities (Ross & McKay, 1979), group homes (Walsh & Rosen, 1985; Walsh & Doerfler, 2009), or special education schools (Rosen & Walsh, 1989). Self-injury contagion has yet to be studied extensively in normative settings, such as public schools, universities, and the community at large. Only a few informal reports exist regarding contagion in these locales (e.g., Walsh & Rosen, 1988; Farber, 2000).

Although the phenomenon has been reported anecdotally for almost 100 years, Rosen and I were the first to provide some empirical evidence of self-injury contagion (Walsh & Rosen, 1985). We studied a group of 25 adolescents in a community-based treatment program over a 1-year period. We found that self-injury occurred in statistically significant clusters or bursts, whereas other problems (e.g., aggression, substance abuse, suicidal talk, and psychiatric hospitalizations) did not.

Taiminen et al. (1998) replicated our findings in Finland. They studied a group of 51 adolescent psychiatric inpatients over a 1-year period. They also found that self-injury occurred in statistically significant clusters. Of particular interest in their report was that two subjects self-injured for the first time while on the psychiatric unit. Taiminen and colleagues concluded that a majority of self-injury events in closed adolescent units may be triggered by contagion, and that *self-injury can spread to adolescents previously naive to self-injury.* Thus treatment programs can be hotbeds of contagion where iatrogenic effects emerge. Clients who go to such settings to receive help may instead acquire new problematic behaviors such as self-injury. Such risks make the need to understand, manage, and prevent contagion all the more important.

MOTIVATIONS REGARDING SELF-INJURY AND CONTAGION

When individuals are asked why they self-injure, they usually cite intrapersonal (internal psychological) reasons as being most important. This internal explanation would seem to be contrary to an interpersonal or contagion explanation for self-injury. For example, Osuch, Noll, and Putnam (1999) studied a sample of 75 adult inpatients who self-injured. They collected self-report data and employed a factor analysis to explore the motivations for self-injuring. Six factors emerged, in this order: (1) affect modulation, (2) desolation (desire to escape feelings of isolation or emptiness), (3) self-punishment and similar motivations, (4) influencing others, (5) magical control of others, and (6) self-stimulation. The first three and the last involve intrapersonal dimensions, whereas the fourth and fifth factors concern more interpersonal arenas. For this sample, then, the interpersonal factors appear to have been less important.

In a similar vein, Nock and Prinstein (2004) found intrapersonal motivations to be more powerful than interpersonal in predicting self-injury. They proposed and evaluated four primary functions of self-injurious behavior: (1) automatic–negative reinforcement (e.g., removal of unpleasant affect), (2) automatic–positive reinforcement (e.g., to feel something better, even if it were a different form of pain), (3) social–negative reinforcement (e.g., to avoid punishment from others), and (4) social–positive reinforcement (e.g., to gain attention from others or communicate unhappiness).

Nock and Prinstein's (2004) sample consisted of 108 adolescents admitted to an inpatient psychiatric unit. The group yielded a sample of 89 individuals who had self-injured at least once. The authors performed a factor analysis on patient self-report data and found that the "items related to the automatic–reinforcement functions were endorsed much more frequently than items related to the social–reinforcement functions" (p. 889). More than half of these self-injuring adolescents reported engaging in the behavior "to stop bad feelings." Items on the automatic reinforcement subscales were endorsed by 24–53% of the participants, whereas items on the social reinforcement subscales were endorsed by only 6–24%. They concluded that the participants "reported engaging [in self-injury] in order to regulate emotions much more frequently than to influence the behavior of others" (p. 889).

Rodham et al. (2004) reported similar results in their study of adolescents who performed deliberate self-harm. Their sample included 220 self-cutting youth (ages 15 and 16) from school settings in England. The most frequently selected reasons for cutting (from a list of eight options) were intrapersonal in nature. These included such items as "I wanted to get relief from a terrible state of mind" and "I wanted to punish myself." Interpersonal items such as "I wanted to find out if someone really loved me," "I wanted to get some attention," or "I wanted to frighten someone" were cited much less frequently (Rodham et al., 2004, p. 82). The authors concluded that youth who self-cut were more likely to cite depression, escalating affective pressure, or a need to take their minds off problems than interpersonal items such as reacting to arguments with others or seeking attention (Rodham et al., 2004).

These findings would appear to suggest that interpersonal issues are generally of lesser importance in supporting self-injury. However, Nock (2008) has conducted some more recent work that sheds some additional light on the role of social reinforcement in supporting self-injury. As he notes, "nonsuicidal self-injury is maintained by social reinforcement in at least a substantial minority of instances" (Nock, 2008, p. 159). He has elaborated a three-component theoretical model regarding social reinforcement of self-injury: (1) Self-injury may be a signal of distress, a culmination of a behavioral series such as speaking, yelling, crying, scratching, and cutting; (2) self-injury may be a signal of strength (e.g., "My self-injury demonstrates that I am dangerous—look what I am capable of"); or (3) self-injury may reflect a desire to affiliate with a valued social group (e.g., the commonly voiced statement "There's a special bond among cutters").

Nonetheless, Nock is still talking about a "substantial minority" of people who self-injure; this phrase seems to contradict much of the current anecdotal information emanating from U.S. public schools and universities, where self-injury is now rampant. A number of explanations can be proposed to explain the discrepancy between the empirical reports cited above and the anecdotal information emerging from community settings regarding self-injury contagion.

One explanation is that for the studies cited above, contagion elements may not have been operative in the samples employed. The samples may have consisted of people who were not intensely engaged with each other, and therefore interpersonal factors may not have been salient. (Proximity alone in inpatient units or schools does not necessarily produce engagement.)

Another explanation for why self-injuring participants in these studies emphasized intrapersonal motivations over interpersonal aspects may be related to the limitations of self-report data. Individuals may be loath to admit two types of motivations for self-injuring. First of all, most human beings are unlikely to concede that they deliberately *imitate* the behavior of others. This is especially true for behavior that is viewed as negative or pathological. Imitation is generally viewed as a weak, low-status behavior. From an early age, children are socialized to avoid being "copycats."

In addition, people are unlikely to admit that their self-injury is *strategic* or *instrumental*. They are disinclined to acknowledge that their acts are intended to "manipulate" others. Such behavior is likely to be condemned as devious and exploitive. A much more acceptable reason to self-injure is a desire to reduce psychological pain. Affect regulation is a preferable rationale to being viewed as a "copycat" or a "schemer." Citing pain generates compassion; citing imitation or manipulation generates disdain or resentment.

INTERPERSONAL DIMENSIONS SUPPORTING CONTAGION

Interpersonal aspects play a central role in contagion episodes. These interpersonal factors include at least four categories of behavior: (1) limited communication skills; (2) attempts to change the behavior of others; (3) response to caregivers, family members, or significant others; and (4) additional peer group influences.

Limited Communication Skills

Desire for Acknowledgment

One reason why multiple people self-injure within a group may be that they lack effective communication skills. Many individuals say that they self-injure in order to let others know that they are angry, sad, anxious, or depressed. When asked why they do not use words to communicate this discomfort, they are dismissive of verbal communication, saying that it is not powerful enough to convey the intensity of their message. They believe that for others to really understand their distress, the communication must be concrete, visible, and dramatic. They fear that otherwise their distress will be viewed as insignificant and will be ignored or not taken seriously. Or, as Nock (2008) has indicated, some individuals live in environments where their significant others fail to respond to less dramatic forms of communication, such as talking, yelling, and crying. These people may be inadvertently shaped into self-injuring because more subtle forms of communication are ineffective.

Desire to Punish

Sometimes self-injury is intended as an attack or an accusation. It can be a dramatic expression of "Look what you've done to me!" The feelings that tend to accompany this form of self-injury are rage and vengefulness. The assumption of this type of motivation is that the others in the immediate environment will react to the self-harm with fear or guilt. If the response of others is dismissive or even neutral, the communication will have failed.

Attempts to Change the Behavior of Others

Desire to Produce Withdrawal

In many cases, self-injury within a group is intended to do more than communicate; it is designed to change the behavior of others. In some instances, the goal is to shock and offend in order to provoke withdrawal. For example, a peer group consisting of five boys in a high school shared an interest in Gothic clothing, alternative music, and violent video games. On the periphery of this group were other males and some females who wanted to be included, in part because of access to marijuana. The original five members began burning each other with cigarettes. This scared off the hangers-on, which was exactly what the core group intended.

Desire to Coerce

Self-injury can be an effective means to coerce others to behave as desired. The term "coercion" is used here in the sense presented by Patterson (1975), meaning "to control others by inflicting pain." When parents or significant others become aware of self-injury in a loved one, they often experience intensely painful reactions, such as fear and panic. Parents may become hysterical when they first learn that their child is cutting or burning. They may feel desperate to do whatever it takes to stop the behavior. Small groups of youth may choose to exploit this reactivity. This is not to say that they do this in an entirely conscious or deliberate way. Rather, it is a primitive type of coercive communication—an ultimatum taking the form of "Give me what I want, *or else!*"

Response to Caregivers, Family Members, or Significant Others

Competition for Caregiver Resources

A third category of influences that inadvertently reinforces self-injury contagion involves behavior directed specifically at caregivers. In treatment settings, caregivers include direct-care staff members, therapists, and administrators; in schools, they include teachers, coaches, counselors, and administrators; and in families, they include parents or any significant other adults.

Self-injury is sometimes inadvertently reinforced in such settings by the competition for scarce resources among caregivers. Both professionals and family members have to attend to many competing demands. Self-injury can be a very effective means of gaining extra attention within a milieu, because it is hard to ignore and it places caregivers in a difficult position. To attend to the behavior in a solicitous, supportive fashion runs the risk of reinforcing it. To ignore it is ethically questionable and has been found to escalate the severity of self-injury acts in some instances (Offer & Barglow, 1960; Lester, 1972).

Self-injuring persons are generally aware of the dilemma facing caregivers. Some choose or feel compelled to exploit the situation by relying on self-injury to dominate a milieu. Non-self-injuring individuals may observe that self-injury results in a person's receiving medical assessment, therapy appointments, skills training practice, extra medication, and the like; the temptation becomes considerable to follow suit and obtain the benefits offered by self-injury. When a contagion episode erupts, the rate of self-injury may skyrocket as individuals perceive the availability of caregivers to be declining. They become motivated to have the most recent or most severe self-injury in order to have the solicitous attention shifted to them.

Anticipation of Aversive Consequences

In some settings, such as treatment programs, clients learn to differentiate desirable from aversive consequences. They recognize that violence or substance abuse may get them suspended or even expelled from a program. In contrast, they realize that self-injury tends to result in less radical and punitive consequences. Self-injury may therefore be differentially rein-forced. If clients feel a need to express intense emotion, they may learn to inhibit violence because of legal consequences or physical restraint within the program. Self-injury can be a more advantageous and strategic act. The emotions get expressed, but the consequences are modest and may even be inadvertently positive, as discussed above.

Additional Peer Group Influences

Direct Modeling Influences

Bandura (1977) established long ago that some behavior is markedly influ-enced by direct modeling influences. Human beings often imitate the behavior of others even when no external contingencies apply. An example would be a youth imitating the self-injury of a peer even when no emotional relief or social reinforcement is expected or forthcoming.

Berman and Walley (2003) conducted an interesting experiment to test the contagion hypothesis regarding self-inflicted aggressive behavior. They examined the influence of a self-aggressive model on self-aggressive behavior in others under controlled laboratory conditions. A sample of 94 adults was given the opportunity to self-administer shock while competing with a fictitious opponent in a reaction time task. Participants observed the opponent self-administer either increasingly intense shock (a self-aggressive model) or constant low shocks (a non-self-aggressive model). Results sug-gested that social information influenced the expression of self-aggressive behavior: Berman and Walley found that participants attended to the oppo-nent's shock choices in both model conditions and chose shocks consistent with those of the observed model.

One reason why people self-injure within a group may thus be the influence of direct modeling effects. Several youth have said to me, "I saw my friend do it, so I said, 'What the heck, I might as well try it.'" These adolescents seemed unmindful of contingencies when they performed the self-harm.

Disinhibition

A second group effect that plays a role in producing contagion is disinhi-bition. In these circumstances, the self-injuring behavior of one person reduces or eliminates the inhibitions of another regarding self-injury. Some-times this sequence happens quite explicitly, as when one person says to another, "Come on, try it, you may like it." Or it can happen via more distant observation; for instance, one individual stated, "I saw the scars on her arms and figured if she could do it, so could I. It's not like she's particularly tough or anything."

Peer Competition

In some groups of self-injuring youth, a competition develops. Individuals may try to outdo each other in terms of the type of weapon employed, extent of physical damage, level of disfigurement, number of wounds, or body area(s) assaulted. In such cases, the typical human instinct for self-protection is turned upside down, and extreme behaviors rule. The most common examples may be youth who "play chicken" by burning each other with cigarettes. The "winner" is the one who tolerates the most pain and refuses to "give up." The victor achieves a certain brief status by being deemed the toughest or most courageous.

THE ROLE OF PEER HIERARCHIES

Another way to understand contagion is to identify peer hierarchies that influence the behavior. Matthews (1968), Ross and McKay (1979), and Rosen and I (Walsh & Rosen, 1988) have all noted that "high-status instigators" may play a role in the spread of self-injury through a group. One way to assess whether peer influences of this type are operational within a group is to create a sociogram, such as the one provided in Figure 20.1. As discussed in Rosen and Walsh (1989), each box in the figure represents a student who self-injured over a 10-month period while enrolled in a special education school. For this study, an "episode of contagion" was defined as any occasion when two or more individuals self-injured within a 24-hour period. Such episodes are represented in the sociogram as a line connecting two students. As shown in Figure 20.1, students 8 and 9 shared the most contagion episodes: six during the 10-month period.

Although some co-occurrences of self-injury could have been coincidental, we believe that if they happened recurrently, interpersonal factors were in play. This conclusion was supported by comments from the students themselves when we interviewed them. For example, students 4 and 7 stated that students 8 and 9 were individuals they looked up to and liked to "hang out with." They reported enjoying the "action" that students 8 and 9 created in the milieu, saying, "It's never boring when they're around. They drive the staff crazy!" Students 4 and 7 also said they liked the attention they received

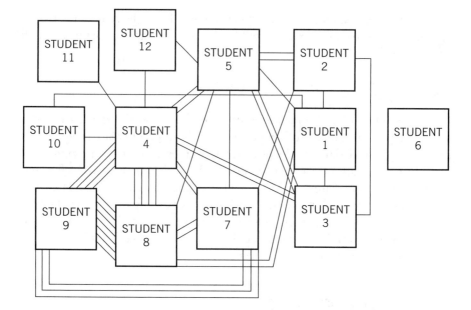

FIGURE 20.1. Schematic representation of self-injury contagion over a 10-month period.

from 8 and 9 when they self-injured. During these periods, students 4 and 7 felt more accepted and more important in the overall peer group.

Constructing a sociogram of a peer group and debriefing self-injuring individuals make it possible to determine the highest-status and most influential members of the group. This determination enables caregivers to target those individuals for intervention, in order to manage and reduce contagion. Taiminen et al. (1998) employed the same sociogram technique in their study of adolescent inpatients.

Ross and McKay (1979) used a similar strategy in attempting to diffuse what was perhaps the most extensive contagion phenomenon in history. Their study of a Canadian training school for girls revealed that 86% of those incarcerated (117 of 136) had carved their bodies at least once. Ross and McKay reported that the administrators at the school tried various methods to diffuse the contagion, such as manipulation of contingencies. Dispensing more attractive awards or more severe punishments did not work; in fact, the contagion only got worse. Only when the school staff decided to "co-opt" the high-status leaders in the peer group did their interventions lead to success. Once the peer leaders were on board, the contagion episodes markedly declined.

DESIRE FOR GROUP COHESIVENESS

Another major reason why momentum toward self-injury develops within a group may be a desire for cohesion. Many self-injuring individuals state that there is a special bond between people who cut, burn, or otherwise harm themselves. The source of the cohesiveness appears to be both inclusive and exclusive. Those who share the problem of self-injury have taken a step most people are unwilling to take. Once that "club" has been joined, the members feel they share a unique experience that is intensive, risky, and intimate. They may choose to share details of how it feels to lacerate the skin, or what they do with the blood, or how they clean the wounds. These are conversations that foster a rather exclusive intimacy; those who have not self-injured cannot participate. Persons who are part of a self-injury contagion episode often believe that they understand each other's pain at a visceral level. They may state that "no one understands a cutter like another cutter," or that no one else can provide such empathic forms of support.

When a contagion episode is unfolding, a sense of escalating excitement often develops. People within the group may feel a sense of intimacy and exhilaration that they are unable to achieve through other means. Contagion episodes can be intensely invigorating until the inevitable "crash" happens. Self-injury contagion cannot really provide sustained and stable intimacy within a group.

A CASE EXAMPLE OF SELF-INJURY CONTAGION

The following case example demonstrates many of the interpersonal dynamics discussed above.

Several years ago, I worked with a woman who was the captain of her college lacrosse team. At the same time, I shared on-call duties with a colleague who was the therapist for another member of the team. I came to know about the second client's situation as a result, because I was this client's "backup" therapist when my colleague was unavailable. Through both these clients, I learned about a sustained contagion phenomenon that involved five women on the lacrosse team. These women tended to have very stormy relationships—ranging from those involving sexual intimacy, to close personal friendships, to vehement disagreements and relationship breakups.

Among the major measures of psychological distress in this group were the frequency and intensity of their self-injury. All five had self-injured at some point in their college careers. My client had done so hundreds of times. She was by far the "leader" in terms of self-destructive behavior within the group. The rate of self-injury for the others in the group ranged from 2 or 3 times to 50 (for my colleague's client).

Early in the treatment of my client, whom I call Ms. O, a contagion episode developed for this group. The cluster of self-injury began after the lacrosse team lost a game. At the start of the season, expectations had been high for this team, because its record the previous year had been good and it included many returning athletes. Nonetheless, the team lost three of its first four games. Particularly vexing was the third loss, which occurred despite a noticeably weaker opponent.

On the evening after the loss, Ms. O cut herself eight times on her forearm and several more times on her calf. Immediately after this action, she walked down the hall of her dorm and entered the room of one of her teammates (modeling influence). The teammate gasped as she saw the blood running down her friend's extremities and said, "What have you done?!" Ms. O replied, "I'm sick of this shit! The team sucks, our record sucks, and most of all, I suck!" (This statement belied the fact that Ms. O was clearly the best player on the team.) She then burst into tears and, as she told me later, "made a fool of myself crying for several minutes" (limited communication skills). The woman to whom Ms. O had vented was Ms. Z, the group member with the second most experience in self-injury. After beginning treatment with my colleague, she had not self-injured for several months. However, that evening she cut herself about four times on her forearm. As she later explained to my colleague, "Seeing all that blood and hearing the crying was just too much for me. I couldn't contain myself any longer" (disinhibition).

Ms. Z then let Ms. O and another team member know that she had hurt herself. Ms. O felt guilty, believing that Ms. Z would not have relapsed but for her, so she cut herself several times again the next afternoon (limited communication skills; competition; desire for cohesion?). Ms. X, the other individual Ms. Z had informed, quickly told two other team members within their group "that Ms. O is cutting herself like crazy." Ms. X and the other two members of the group then rallied around Ms. O, expressing their concern in effusive ways. They brought Ms. O flowers and took her to lunch. With this level of support, Ms. O appeared to stabilize. She began spending inordinate amounts of time with the teammates who had supported her so intensively (cohesiveness achieved).

Before long, Ms. Z began to feel ignored. She felt "closed out" by this tight new group and wondered whether she had done something wrong. In response to this feeling of isolation, Ms. Z cut herself several more times and made sure that Ms. X and the other two team members were aware of the incident (limited communication skills; competition for scarce resources). The attention of the group then shifted back to Ms. Z. One member of the team gave her a massage because she "seemed so stressed out." Another made a dinner for her so she "could stop all this cutting."

Eventually Ms. X and the two members of the team who had the least experience with self-injury (i.e., two or three times) decided to scratch their arms while together (disinhibition; limited communication skills; competition for scarce resources; desire for cohesion). They reported feeling overwhelmed by all the support provided to Ms. O and Ms. Z. Their behavior seemed to pay off as the attention of the group shifted briefly to meeting their needs—even though they tended to be lower-status members of the group (cohesiveness achieved).

The episode concluded as it had begun, with another incident from Ms. O. In response to all the uproar, she cut herself more deeply, resulting in 11 sutures on her left arm (disinhibition; competition). The extent of the damage caused by this act of self-injury seemed to shock the group members and cause them to step back from the round of self-injurious acts. No further self-injury ensued for several weeks.

Oddly, the performance of the lacrosse team improved after this contagion episode. As one of the women stated, "The cutting wasn't a good thing, but it did bring us together. We were so close afterward that we played better as a team."

OTHER UNUSUAL ISSUES RELATED TO CONTAGION

Pseudocontagion Episodes

It should also be noted that "pseudocontagion" episodes sometimes occur (although rarely). In these circumstances, a burst of self-injury in a group may pertain less to interpersonal issues than to intrapersonal dilemmas experienced in parallel fashion. For example, a peer group may learn of the imminent departure of a favorite teacher or staff member. If the group is not cohesive, each member of the group may experience emotional pain independently in relation to the loss. In such groups, little communication is exchanged about their common experience of loss. In a pseudo contagion episode, individuals start self-injuring at the same time due to the experience of a common trigger. The episode may look like an interactive contagion phenomenon, but it is not. Rather, it is a series of relatively independent events happening at the same time in parallel fashion.

Electronic Communication Contagion Episodes

Relatively recent phenomena are contagion episodes that involve people who have never met face to face. These have become possible because of electronic communications media, such as message boards, chat rooms, texting, YouTube, and websites. I have treated multiple clients in psychotherapy who frequently participate in chat rooms or Facebook exchanges devoted to self-injury. Others frequently view videos of people cutting themselves on YouTube (see Lewis et al., 2011). Most or all of the mechanisms described above related to contagion can influence behavior in electronic milieus. Members may use disclosures regarding self-injury to communicate intense feelings (e.g., "I can't believe you ignored my messages for two days! I ended up cutting myself"), coerce others ("Without your help, I would cut myself"), model for others ("I always use an X-ACTO knife; it's so precise"), compete with others ("That's nothing, I just cut myself 12 times . . . "), and disinhibit others ("Knowing that you cut yourself today means that I may have to"). Pecking orders also emerge in these milieus, whereby those who self-injure with the greatest "conviction" have the highest status. Some self-injuring individuals go so far as to create their own self-injury websites. Most claim to have developed these websites to provide support and help others, but the content on the sites is often more triggering than therapeutic.

Perhaps the chief anomaly of these electronic versions of contagion episodes is that episodes emerge among people who have never met face to face. Members seem to take it on faith that the disclosures of self-injury are accurate and truthful. There is no way to know whether the self-injuries described have really happened (even with photographic "evidence") or are the creations of those with vivid self-injurious imaginations. This lack of validation was previously impossible in face-to-face groups.

CONCLUSION

- The ultimate goal in trying to understand the complex factors related to social contagion of self-injury is to learn how to manage and prevent it.
- Social contagion is often the result of underdeveloped social communication skills and peer modeling. It occurs primarily in adolescents and young adults.
- Understanding a contagion episode generally involves looking carefully at unintended positive and negative social reinforcers.
- Recently, the Internet has played a key role in the social contagion of self-injury. In assessing self-injury, professionals need to look not only at personal relationships with others who self-injure, but also at Internet influences (e.g., websites, chat rooms, and YouTube videos devoted to self-injury).

The next chapter presents a protocol used in public schools to respond to self-injury. One of the goals of this protocol is to prevent self-injury contagion in school settings.

CHAPTER 21

A Protocol for Managing Self-Injury in School Settings

Since the first edition of this book was published in 2006, the protocol for schools described in this chapter was incorporated into the Signs of Self-Injury Prevention Program developed by Screening for Mental Health and The Bridge (Jacobs, Walsh, & Pigeon, 2009). This program has two components: (1) a manual and educational DVD for school staff (which includes the protocol described below), and (2) an educational DVD and discussion guide designed for high school students. The DVD for students includes three chapters with youthful actors depicting dilemmas regarding self-injury in peers. The DVD has two take-home messages for youth: (1) If you become aware of self-injury in a peer, let him or her know you care, and tell a responsible adult (such a school counselor); and (2) avoid discussing the details of self-injury with peers, as this tends to trigger the behavior in others (i.e., an anti-social contagion message).

My colleagues and I recently evaluated the Signs of Self-Injury Prevention Program (Muehlenkamp, Walsh, & McDade, 2009). The study employed a sample of 274 adolescents from Massachusetts (mean age = 16.07 years, 51.5% female, 73% European American). We found that the program did not produce iatrogenic effects (i.e., there was no evidence that the program triggered self-injury). We also found that the program increased accurate knowledge about self-injury and improved help-seeking attitudes and intentions among students (Muehlenkamp, Walsh, & McDade, 2009). In addition, school staff members reported that the program was user-friendly and well received by school personnel.

This program has since been employed throughout the United States and in Germany and Japan. As a result, the school protocol presented below can be said to have been widely distributed and employed. Information regarding this program can be accessed online (*www.mentalhealthscreening.org/ programs/youth-prevention-programs/sosi*).

SCOPE OF THE PROBLEM

Since the beginning of the 21st century, many middle schools and high schools in the United States and other countries have experienced an explosion of self-injury among their students. On average, there is an estimated prevalence rate of 15–20% for adolescents in school and community samples in the United States and Canada (Heath et al., 2009). This phenomenon often produces confusion and alarm in school staff members who are not used to dealing with high rates of self-harm. Such reactions are entirely understandable; schools, after all, are institutions of learning, not mental health clinics.

In order for school personnel to respond effectively to self-injury, they need a systematic approach, such as the protocol presented here. In order for this protocol to work effectively, staffers must first receive several hours of training. This training should include at least the following:

1. Staff members begin by learning about the full range of self-destructive behaviors, including direct and indirect self-harm (as presented in Chapter 3). Personnel in schools who are responsible for the first line of assessment need to understand and ask about the entire spectrum of self-destructive behavior. This involves going beyond the presenting problem (e.g., self-injury, substance abuse, eating disorder) and asking about all forms of direct and indirect self-harm (see Chapter 3, Figure 3.2). This enables the staff to discern whether a student has one or more self-destructive behaviors, and, if so, to determine whether he or she is in a crisis requiring immediate intervention. In many schools, the role of providing a preliminary assessment is assumed by a social worker or psychologist, but in some cases the point person can be a guidance counselor, a nurse, or even a vice principal or principal.

2. Next, staff members should be trained in differentiating self-injury from suicidal behavior (as presented in Chapters 1 and 2). They need to learn which behaviors should be considered suicidal (e.g., the use of a gun, overdose, hanging, jumping from a height, and ingestion of poison) and which

should be considered self-injurious (e.g., most forms of self-inflicted cutting, burning, abrading, hitting, biting, and excoriation). Staff members need to be cognizant that the former behaviors may result in death, but that the latter are unlikely to. Whenever school professionals are unclear about the distinction between self-injury and a suicide attempt, they should always rely on mental health professionals to make the determination.

3. Staff members also need to understand that certain types of self-injury require immediate assessment by a psychiatric emergency service—namely, those that involve significant tissue damage requiring medical treatment (such as suturing) or those that involve face, eyes, breasts, and genitals. (See Chapter 9.)

4. Staff members should be aware that body modification (e.g., tattoos and body piercings obtained from professionals) is not the same thing as self-injury. (See Chapter 5.)

5. Staff members should learn that the best way to respond to common self-injury is with a low-key, dispassionate demeanor and respectful curiosity (as described in Chapter 7). The behavior should not be responded to hysterically, but it should also not be dismissed, minimized, or "normalized."

6. Staff members should understand that the problem of self-injury is complex, and that biological, environmental, and psychological factors combine to produce the behavior. These various factors must be addressed to eliminate the behavior (as discussed in Chapter 6). Treatment usually takes time, and school staff should not expect rapid extinction of the behavior. Requiring that students return to school only after their self-injury is eliminated is completely unrealistic.

Once these various training topics have been addressed with the staff, a school is in a position to implement a protocol to deal with self-injury. The advantage of having a written protocol is that staff members will know how to respond to self-injury systematically and strategically. An established protocol is comforting to staff, students, and parents alike.

The protocol presented below has been used effectively in many school settings. However, it does not represent a "boilerplate" solution that can be implemented in every school. Each school needs to decide on the components of its own protocol. These should be tailored to meet the unique needs of each educational culture and environment. The protocol that follows describes steps in assessing and responding to self-destructive behavior, including self-injury. It describes staff members' responsibilities and expected interactions with students and their families.

PROTOCOL FOR DEALING WITH SELF-DESTRUCTIVE BEHAVIORS

1. Any school staff member should contact the designated point person (e.g., a school social worker, guidance counselor, psychologist, or nurse) *immediately* when a student presents with any of the following behaviors:

   a. Any suicidal talk, threats, "joking," notes, poetry, other writings, artwork, cell phone texts, Internet postings, or other communications that have suicidal themes.

   b. Any instances of self-injury, such as wrist, arm, or body cutting; scratching, burning, or hitting; picking of wounds; crude self-inflicted tattoos; disfiguring hair pulling and removal; or excessive accident proneness.

   Note: Self-injuries of this type are generally not suicidal in intent and are generally not likely to result in death. However, they do indicate serious psychological distress, and they require professional assessment and treatment as soon as possible.

   c. Eating-disordered behavior, such as self-induced vomiting, sustained fasting, marked ongoing weight loss or gain, or use of diet pills or laxatives.

   d. Disclosures regarding risk-taking behaviors, such as the following:

   • *Physical risks* (e.g., walking in high-speed traffic, walking on an elevated railroad bridge, straddling the edge of a high roof)

   • *Situational risks* (e.g., getting into a car with strangers, walking in a dangerous area of a city alone late at night)

   • *Sexual risks* (e.g., having many sexual partners, having unprotected sex with strangers)

   e. Substance use behavior that exceeds "normal" adolescent experimentation, suggestive of abuse or addiction (e.g., students' getting high before school or drinking alcohol or smoking marijuana multiple times per week).

   f. Discontinuance of prescribed medications without the prescribing doctor's permission.

   g. Other behaviors that suggest serious emotional distress or dyscontrol, such as uncontrollable crying, explosive anger, frequent fights, extreme reactions to minor events, serious isolation, or extremely poor hygiene.

2. Once the school social worker, psychologist, or nurse receives information about any of the behaviors listed above, he or she will contact the student discreetly and will confidentially investigate the report.

If requested, the social worker, psychologist, or nurse may keep the identity of the referring school staff person confidential.

There are three possible outcomes based on the information obtained from interviewing the student, peers, and school staff:

a. *If the incident is deemed minor and/or already resolved*, there will be no action beyond the interview with the student. The student will be encouraged to contact the social worker, psychologist, or nurse in the future, should he or she again become distressed.

   Note: The school staff person who contacted the social worker, psychologist, or nurse will be advised of this outcome as soon as is feasible within the confines of confidentiality. This feedback loop is important, so that the referring staff member knows that his or her report resulted in an intervention.

b. *If the incident is deemed important and requires additional intervention*, the child's parent or guardian will be called by the social worker, psychologist, or nurse immediately and briefed on the situation. Whenever possible, the student will be advised in advance that the social worker, psychologist, or nurse is calling the parent or guardian. The purpose of the call will be explained as ensuring that the student has adequate support, protection, and assistance. The social worker or nurse will emphasize that the call has no disciplinary or punitive purposes. Also, whenever possible, the call to the parent or guardian will be made *with the student present*, so that he or she is aware of the specifics of the communication.

c. When a student presents with any of the self-destructive behaviors listed above, the parent or guardian will be asked to pursue a number of possible options to assist the student:
   • Initiating outpatient counseling for the child and/or family.
   • Seeking psychotropic medication for serious cognitive or emotional disturbance (e.g., depression, OCD or other anxiety disorder, thought disorder).
   • Agreeing to the child's receiving enhanced academic and/or counseling supports within the school setting itself.
   • Providing releases of information to the school, so that the social worker or nurse may communicate with any outside professionals who are assisting the student.

d. Once the social worker, psychologist, or nurse has made a recommendation for professional help, he or she will recontact the parent or guardian within 1 week to ascertain whether or not the referral has been pursued. The social worker or nurse will emphasize the importance of this referral and the need for action, if none has been taken. Repeatedly failing to take action in support of the mental health needs of a child may be grounds for filing a neglect or abuse report on the parent or guardian, as mandated by the state's child protection agency.

Note: Again, the school staff person who contacted the social worker, psychologist, or nurse will be advised of this outcome as soon as is feasible within the confines of confidentiality. This feedback loop is important, so that the referring staff member knows that his or her report resulted in an intervention.

e. *If the incident is deemed to be an emergency or crisis involving imminent risk,* the social worker, psychologist, or nurse will arrange for an immediate screening at the local psychiatric emergency service and/or police intervention. Examples include a student's disclosing a specific plan to overdose, shoot him- or herself, hang him- or herself, or jump from a dangerous height on that day. In such circumstances, parents or guardians will be informed of the situation as soon as the crisis is handled and stabilized.

Note: Once more, the school staff person who contacted the social worker, psychologist, or nurse will be advised of this outcome as soon as is feasible within the confines of confidentiality. This feedback loop is important, so that the referring staff member knows that his or her report resulted in an intervention.

IMPLEMENTING AND USING THE PROTOCOL WITH SELF-INJURY

The protocol presented above employs formal language designed to produce consistent responses in school staff to a variety of self-harm behaviors. In order to explain how the protocol works in the real world, it is useful to provide a case example:

Amy is a 14-year-old freshman in high school. One day her friend, Beth, tearfully discloses to the school social worker, James, that Amy has been cutting herself. Beth tells James that she feels guilty saying anything about Amy's cutting, because she promised her friend that she wouldn't tell. However, Beth is afraid that her friend may die from her "suicide attempts," and so she "just can't keep it a secret any more." The social worker reassures Beth that she has done the right thing. He tells Beth that cutting usually won't result in death, but that it is an indication of serious distress. He tells Beth that he will take over from here and see that Amy gets some help. He also assures Beth that he will try not to reveal his source of information, in order to protect her friendship with Amy.

Within an hour, James catches Amy between classes and asks to speak with her. He jokes, "Don't worry! You're not in trouble!" Amy looks relieved to hear she hasn't "done anything wrong." In his office, James tells Amy gently that he has learned that she has been cutting herself. Amy dissolves in tears and asks, "Who told you that?" James says that this is less important than learning more about her self-harm. He then begins to assess the nature of her cutting. He learns that she has been cutting her left forearm and left leg "for about 3 months." He asks to see the cuts on her arm, and is relieved to see that the tissue damage is modest and that the number of cuts is under 10. Amy states that the cuts on her leg "are about the same as on my arm, but not so many." James's preliminary assessment is that Amy's self-injury is of the common, low-lethality type and not a psychiatric emergency.

James then continues his informal assessment and learns from Amy that she has not hurt herself in other ways, has no suicidal plans or history, and is not a risk taker. She reports that she occasionally smokes marijuana or drinks a beer on weekends, but that her substance use is not frequent. Amy denies having an eating disorder and is not taking any psychotropic medication.

From this information, James concludes that Amy is in no immediate risk, but that she does require help on an outpatient basis for her self-injury. His next step is to call Amy's mother with Amy present in the office. He explains that he is going to call her mother in order to get Amy some help with her cutting behavior.

On the phone with the mother, James follows the school protocol. In speaking with the mother, he first explains that he is not calling because of any disciplinary problem. However, he's learned that Amy has been cutting her arm and leg with a razor for about 3 months. The mother expresses shock at this information and exclaims, "Why would my daughter want to kill herself?" James attempts to reassure the mother that self-injury usually doesn't have much to do with suicide, but is indicative of serious emotional distress. He explains that cutting has unfortunately become a relatively common problem among teens. He then asks the mother whether she would be willing to pursue outpatient counseling for her daughter to help with the problem. He also suggests that an assessment regarding medication might be indicated. Amy's mother responds affirmatively, saying that she will follow up on both suggestions immediately. James then provides the names and numbers of three local counselors, all of whom have an affiliation with a psychiatrist. He asks that the mother call him back when the appointments have been scheduled. The mother agrees, and the phone call ends.

Amy seems relieved that her "big secret is out" and that her "mother isn't mad." James sends Amy back to class and says he'll check on her tomorrow to see how she is doing. As a postscript, the mother calls the next day to say that a therapy appointment has been scheduled in 3 days and that the therapist will arrange for a psychiatric consultation regarding medication. James promises to stay in touch with the mother to monitor Amy's progress.

Of course, not all situations proceed as smoothly as this example. The reactions of family members are highly variable. Some parents or guardians are dismissive and insist that a child is "just doing it for attention" or that the behavior is "part of some fad." These individuals need to be counseled to be more sympathetic and responsive. Other parents or caregivers may present with extreme reactions, such as becoming enraged at the child for his or her "misbehavior" or for "embarrassing the family in the community." Such reactions are usually indicative of other family problems that may need to be addressed via outpatient family work. Usually, it is best for the school staff to suggest gently but firmly that such a family obtain some "short-term counseling" in order to learn how to deal more effectively with the "challenging adolescent." Defining the problem as residing in the adolescent may be necessary at first, to move a family past defensiveness and distrust of mental health professionals.

Some self-injuring youth have few or no family resources. They may be living in a short-term foster home, in a respite program, or with a minimally involved distant relative. In such cases, the school may need to take the initiative in obtaining mental health services for the child. Many schools have a mental health clinician on site who has been assigned by a local mental health clinic. Such services may be billable through third-party insurance. These resources can be an important source of support for students without family members who will arrange follow-up care.

MANAGING AND PREVENTING CONTAGION

Another common problem that schools face is dealing with epidemics or contagion episodes of self-injury, as described in Chapter 20. In these situations, multiple students who know each other self-injure within short periods of time. Such students often appear to be communicating frequently about self-injury, in effect, triggering the behavior in each other. In some situations, the contagion is immediate and direct: Youth self-injure in each other's presence. Peers may share the same tools or implements, or may even take turns injuring each other.

As noted in Chapter 20, youth may trigger self-injury in each other because (1) the behavior produces feelings of cohesiveness (e.g., as one teen said, "There is a special bond among people who cut themselves"); (2) the behavior has powerful communication aspects (e.g., "My friend must really be upset to cut herself so many times"); (3) the behavior may be viewed as outrageous and provocative (e.g., "It really freaks out my parents when we do this"); and (4) the behavior may also be inadvertently reinforced by adults (e.g., "Finally, my parents believe I'm in a lot of pain").

School professionals should consider three main interventions in order to minimize the risk of contagion: (1) reduce communication about self-injury among members of the peer group; (2) reduce the public exhibition of scars or wounds in the school milieu; and (3) treat the behavior via individual counseling methods and *not* group therapy, with a few exceptions.

Reducing Communication about Self-Injury

When students talk to each other about self-injury, this generally has a very triggering effect. Youth may compete with each other to produce more cuts or burns or to use grislier methods of self-harm. Students may also take turns assuming the role of caregiver and victim. As one adolescent exclaimed to me, "My group of friends is so crazy! Someone is always cutting! There is always someone who needs help!"

A strategy that sometimes works to reduce contagion is for the school staff to explain to individual students that talking (or texting or posting) about self-injury has a negative effect on peers by making self-harm much more likely. Many students injure themselves without remorse, but feel guilty about behaving in a way that may hurt their friends. Appealing to them to reduce or cease communications about self-injury can work with those who have a social conscience. As one adolescent said to me, "It's my business if I cut myself in the privacy of my own home, but I don't want to be responsible for others doing this stuff." Of course, some youth do not mind triggering the behavior in others and may even take delight in "playing uproar." When such youth deliberately and repeatedly trigger self-injury in others, disciplinary action may be needed to reduce the climate of contagion. On rare occasions, students may have to be suspended for refusing to behave in nontriggering ways within the school milieu. Such students may need to agree in writing to reduce their contagion-generating behaviors in order to return to school.

Managing Students Who Exhibit Their Scars or Wounds

A related problem occurs when students openly show their scars or wounds while at school. Such individuals may wear short-sleeved shirts, short pants, or short skirts that place their scars in open view within the school community. Viewing these scars or wounds can be very triggering for vulnerable students. My recommendation when a student exhibits scars or wounds is first to meet with the student alone. A direct request is made to the student that he or she cover the scars with clothing (or jewelry, a bandana, or some other means) when at school. Merely covering the wounds with a large bandage is not acceptable, because it is all too obvious that wounds are underneath. Many students will agree to covering their scars, once an explanation regarding social contagion is provided.

For students who are not responsive, the next step is to involve parents. A staff person explains to family members that visible wounds or scars are triggering to others in the school community. Parents are asked to assist in monitoring the student's choice of clothing. Most families are responsive to this request, and the problem rapidly declines.

A few students and families are not helpful, however, and a more limit-setting approach becomes necessary in these cases. Families may be asked to provide extra sets of clothing to be stored at school, so that these can be used when the students' attire on a given day is ill advised. In some cases, students may need to be sent home and directed to return only when they have changed into less scar-disclosing attire.

Using Individualized Methods, Not Groups, in Treating Self-Injury

A number of years ago, I was asked to consult at a middle school that was experiencing an epidemic of self-injury. I learned that eight females in the seventh grade, all of whom knew each other, had been cutting for several months. The social worker who worked with the girls was convinced that they were influencing each other to cut. She attempted to deal with the situation by establishing what she called a "cutters' group." She told me she knew she "had a problem" when she was approached by another girl who asked, "How bad do I have to cut myself to get into the cutters' group?"

The school social worker's assessment was correct: She did have a problem. Despite her best intentions, she had inadvertently contributed to a contagion episode. My recommendation to this staff person was that she disband the "cutters' group" and refer the girls out for individual therapy. She proceeded to follow this suggestion, using the protocol described above. A year later, she reported that none of the eight girls was still cutting.

This anecdote has a basic message: It is often exceedingly dangerous to treat self-injury in groups, because open discussion of self-injury's antecedents, behavior, and consequences runs the risk of being exceptionally triggering. A much more strategic course is to refer clients to individual therapy, where they can focus on their specific needs for replacement skills, cognitive therapy, and resolution of trauma.

A notable exception to this rule is to use groups for replacement skills training. Such groups should be governed by strict rules that prohibit discussion of the details of self-injury. Members are told, "It's very important that you discuss self-injury in great detail, but you should do this in individual therapy, *not* in group therapy." The focus in these groups is on learning, practicing, and generalizing the use of skills in the real world. Replacement skills, as presented in Chapter 11, can be taught quite efficiently to groups of

self-injuring youth as long as the focus remains consistently on skill acquisition. Maintaining this focus can often be quite challenging for therapists,
because members find talking about self-injury so alluring. Quick redirec-
tion to the skills training topic of the day is important for the success of the
group. A brief excerpt from a group session illustrates this process:

GROUP LEADER: Hello, everyone. Let's begin by reporting on last
week's homework, which was mindful breathing. Who brought
their Mindful Breathing Tracking Card?

MEMBER 1: I did. I had a good week in terms of using my breathing.

GROUP LEADER: Great! What happened?

MEMBER 1: Well, I practiced four times, which is good for me. And I
even used it once when I felt like cutting.

GROUP LEADER: Great! It's good to be able to use breathing skills when
you're distressed. Did it help?

MEMBER 1: Yes, I was able to calm myself down and not cut.

MEMBER 2: (*breaking in*) Breathing doesn't usually work for me when I
get an urge to cut. When I get really pissed, I go into my bedroom
and just . . .

GROUP LEADER: (*quickly raising his hand in a "stop" gesture and inter-
jecting gently but firmly*) Remember, we don't get into details about
self-harm behaviors in group, but it is important for you to explore
that in individual therapy.

MEMBER 2: Oh, yeah, I forgot.

GROUP LEADER: (*turning to look at Member 1*) Okay, what were you
saying about using your breathing?

Running skills training groups with multiple self-injuring adolescents
generally requires co-leaders. The primary leader can be responsible for
the skills training topic of the day, and the secondary leader can focus on
preventing triggering behavior as well as other tasks (such as scanning the
group for anyone who looks distressed). Skills training can be effectively
taught in groups, but the leaders need to be focused on their mission and
alert to detours that may produce contagion. Examples of skills groups that
have been run effectively in schools include those focusing on self-soothing
skills, violence prevention, dating skills, and grief groups (for students who
have lost a parent through death). All of these groups have assisted self-
injuring youth in learning new skills that enable them to reduce the frequency of self-harm.

CONCLUSION

This chapter has focused on managing self-injury in school settings.

- The components of a thorough staff training sequence have been reviewed.
- A protocol for responding to self-destructive behavior in students has also been discussed.
- Finally, specific suggestions have been offered to prevent and manage social contagion in school populations.

For more extensive discussions of social contagion, see Chapter 18 and especially Chapter 20.

CHAPTER 22

Asphyxial Risk-Taking (the "Choking Game")

AMY M. BRAUSCH

Adolescents have been engaging in various risk-taking behaviors for decades. One type of risk-taking behavior that seems to have reemerged within the past 5 years is the "choking game." Although the colloquial term for this activity implies a benign and enjoyable experience, the behavior can have severe consequences and can even result in death. Recent publications, particularly from the medical community, have called for researchers and practitioners to use a different label when describing this activity. The preferred term is "self-asphyxial risk-taking behavior" (SAB). Adolescents typically engage in this activity in groups. They use various means to cut off the supply of oxygen to the brain on themselves or each other, with the desired effect of dizziness, a "head rush," and a simulated experiencing of "getting high." The dangers of this activity extend beyond the act of losing consciousness. Many adolescents who participate in SAB experience hypoxic seizures; some have suffered brain damage; and the behavior can result in accidental death.

Adolescents have used a wide variety of techniques for achieving the desired effect. One technique involves self-induced hyperventilation, followed by applied pressure to the neck or chest until the individual loses consciousness. Other techniques involve adolescents' using a "sleeper hold" on one another, again with the goal of briefly losing consciousness. Adolescents have also been observed using various apparatus (ropes, dog leashes, belts, etc.) as ligatures around the neck and then loosening them to prevent serious injury. One particularly alarming trend in this behavior is adolescents' posting videos and photos of the activity on social networking sites, such as Facebook and YouTube. A recent study conducted a search on You-Tube for videos of adolescents participating in SAB (Linkletter, Gordon, & Dooley, 2010). Researchers identified 65 videos, and all of them featured two or more individuals. Of all the videos, more than half included individuals estimated to be between the ages of 12 and 18; 72% of all participants were European American; and 90% of all participants were male. Although all participants who lost consciousness regained it, over half of the observed individuals experienced hypoxic seizures.

Data collected by the CDC (2008) provide some insight into who might be most at risk for death from SAB. Among all reported deaths resulting from SAB between the years 1995 and 2007, the majority were in youth between the ages of 11 and 16. Boys were much more likely to die from SAB than girls, and almost all of the youth who died were alone at the time of death. Although at least one study (see below) reported higher rates of prevalence for SAB in rural areas, the CDC (2008) noted that it has received reports of SAB deaths from all over the United States.

PREVALENCE

The CDC (2008) reported that between 1995 and 2007, SAB resulted in 82 deaths among children and adolescents. The majority of these deaths were reported from 2005 to 2007, and 86% were male. A handful of published studies have tried to estimate prevalence rates for the behavior. A survey of youth in Ontario and Texas reported that about 7% of middle and high school students had participated in the behavior, and 68% affirmed that they were familiar with the activity (Macnab, Deevska, Gagnon, Cannon, & Andrew, 2009). The 2008 Oregon Healthy Teens survey revealed that 5.7% of eighth graders throughout the state had participated in SAB (Ramowski, Nystrom, Chaumeton, Rosenberg, & Gilchrist, 2010). Although males and females engaged in the behavior at equal rates, participation was more prevalent among youth who lived in rural areas. Other factors that seemed to increase the likelihood of SAB were (1) self-reported use of alcohol or other substances, and (2) reporting at least one mental health risk factor (Ramowski et al., 2010). Finally, a study that analyzed data collected about health and risk behaviors from a rural area in the Midwest found a 16% rate of participation in SAB among high school students (Brausch, Decker, & Hadley, 2011).

IDEAS ABOUT THE FUNCTIONS OF SAB

As clinicians and researchers continue to investigate the precipitating events and emotional states of individuals who engage in self-injury, the exploration of the underlying causes and motivations for SAB are just beginning. Very little information has been published about the behavior outside the medical community, and those sources tend to focus on its physiological consequences and/or warning signs that an adolescent may be engaging in it. As mentioned above, the Oregon Healthy Teens survey established some preliminary links between SAB and concurrent risk behaviors, such as substance use and at least one mental health factor (which the survey authors defined as suicide ideation, gambling, having an unmet mental health need, and/or self-rated mental health as "fair" or "poor") (Ramowski et al., 2010).

A recent study explored the potential overlap between SAB and self-injury in a large sample of high school students (Brausch et al., 2011). Students were divided into four groups: those who had engaged in both SAB and self-injury, those who engaged in self-injury only, those who engaged only in SAB, and students who reported neither activity. Statistical analyses showed significant differences among the four groups on measures of suicide ideation and behaviors, substance use, and disordered eating behaviors. Specifically, adolescents who had engaged in both types of risk behaviors reported the highest levels of suicide ideation in all four groups. This group also reported the highest levels of unhealthy eating and exercise behaviors, as well as the most substance use. Results of this study thus indicate that adolescents who have been involved in both SAB and self-injury may also report other concurrent risk behaviors, including suicidal ideation and attempts.

A recent follow-up study attempted to gather more specific information about SAB and its possible functions (Brausch, 2011). The questionnaire developed for the study was modeled on existing self-injury assessments that focus on both occurrence and functionality of the behaviors. The questionnaire was completed by 215 college students at a public Midwestern university. Eighteen students responded that either they had choked themselves or someone had choked them as part of the "choking game" at least once. Everyone who reported choking themselves noted being in a group at the time. Slightly more than half indicated that they had passed out as a result. Frequencies of SAB ranged from 1 to 20 times, with the modal response falling between 2 and 4 times. Ages when the behavior occurred ranged from as young as 10 for the first time to 20 for the most recent time. Most students reported engaging in the behavior between the ages of 11 and 15. Of the students who noted that other people had choked them or pressed on their chest as part of the "choking game," the majority reported losing consciousness as a result. Frequencies ranged from 1 to 10 times, with most students reporting 1–4 instances of the behavior. The age range was slightly older for this behavior, with the majority of students reporting it between 13 and 17 years. Regardless of self- or other-administration of the asphyxial risk-taking, the majority of participants reported believing that the behavior was dangerous and noted that they did not videotape or take pictures of the activity. Various reasons were endorsed for engaging in SAB, but a few responses were given most often. Students marked "to see what it felt like" as the most common reason for trying the behavior, and "to have fun," "to feel a rush or get high," and "to feel more part of a group" as the other most common reasons. Results from this preliminary investigation of the possible functions of SAB suggest that many adolescents participate at first out of curiosity, as part of a group situation, or for sensation seeking. Research in this field is just beginning, and much more information is needed before we can draw any definitive conclusions about the motivations, intent, and functions of SAB.

WARNING SIGNS

Although awareness of SAB is not as widespread as awareness of other self-harming behaviors, the CDC (2008) has identified several warning signs of SAB; parents, school personnel, peers, and health care providers can be on the lookout for these. One warning sign that an adolescent may be engaging in SAB is overhearing discussions of the activity by any of its many aliases. The behavior has been labeled as the "choking game" in popular media outlets within the past few years, but it is also known by many other names among adolescents. These include "pass-out game," "space monkey," "suffocation roulette," "fainting game," "blackout," "flat-liner," and "space cowboy." Participation in SAB may also manifest itself in observable physical features, such as bloodshot eyes, pinpoint bleeding under the skin on the face, and red marks around the neck. Other warning signs include an adolescent's complaining of frequent, severe headaches and seeming disoriented after spending time alone. Some parents report noticing that their adolescent children are significantly increasing the amount of time they spend alone; they may also note a change in behavior, such as increased or uncharacteristic irritability or hostility. Parents may notice a child wearing high-necked shirts frequently (even when these are not appropriate for the weather), or may find items such as dog leashes, cords, or jump ropes in their child's room. Some parents have noticed wear marks on the furniture in their child's room as the result of tying ropes or other items to things like bedposts multiple times. Lastly, they may come across photos or videos of their child and/or child's friends engaged in SAB stored on the child's cell phone or posted on Facebook (CDC, 2008).

EDUCATION, PREVENTION, AND INTERVENTION

Although the consequences of other risk-taking behaviors have been integrated into school curricula (e.g., Drug Abuse Resistance Education [D.A.R.E.] for substance abuse prevention), very little if any mention is typically made of SAB in schools, medical offices, or mental health agencies. The increasing reports of accidental deaths from SAB in newspapers and other popular media in recent years may have helped to increase awareness. However, it can be assumed that most parents are not aware of this behavior, and research has found that many adolescents do not consider the activity dangerous (Macnab et al., 2009). Many parents who have shared their personal accounts of losing a child to SAB note that they had never heard of the "choking game"; even those who had usually state that they never would have thought their child would try it. Obviously, greater education about and awareness of the behavior and its dangerous consequences are needed.

Parental involvement and monitoring may play a large role in preventing SAB. Many parents who are involved in their children's lives take an active role in limiting access to potentially dangerous materials and media. For example, experts strongly recommend that parents use parental blocking tools on home computers to protect their children and adolescents from online pornography and predators. One recommendation for prevention of SAB is for parents to utilize these monitoring tools to censor sites such as YouTube, so that adolescents are unable to access videos of the "choking game." It is also recommended that parents have monitoring policies and agreements in place with their children regarding cell phones and Facebook accounts. Moreover, it is important to educate parents and teachers about the many aliases for the "choking game" (see above), so that adults can recognize when adolescents are making references to the activity in texting, e-mailing, or social networking.

Another convenient way for parents to help prevent SAB in their children is to work on establishing and maintaining open communication about many sensitive and relevant topics for their children's age group. Parents are frequently encouraged to engage their children in conversations about many developmental issues (sexual behavior, drug and alcohol use, bullying, etc.). Experts also recommend that parents watch television with their children and engage them in discussions about what they are viewing, the message a particular program is portraying, and how the message fits with the family's value system. Frequent and honest communication between parents and children that focuses on problem solving, critical thinking, and making healthy choices may help adolescents more easily recognize dangers and act accordingly. Because of the limited data available at the time, the CDC (2008) statement about the "choking game" *did not* recommend that parents directly discuss the activity with their children, because practices for prevention of the activity had not been studied. Instead, the CDC encouraged parents to be aware of the activity, its aliases, and its warning signs, and to discuss it with their children if they suspect that the children may be involved in it. These recommendations may change as more information about prevalence, risk factors, and prevention is obtained and disseminated. However, an adolescent who has talked with a parent about the potential dangers of other dangerous activities may then choose not to participate in SAB if he or she encounters it among peers. Adolescents who report feeling more supported by parents and greater family cohesiveness show decreased involvement in risk-taking behaviors overall (Garnefski & Diekstra, 1996).

On a broader level, at least one organization has been founded with the sole mission of providing education, increasing awareness, and prevention of SAB. The most active organization is a nonprofit called GASP, which stands for Games Adolescents Shouldn't Play (*www.gaspinfo.com*). This group was founded and is run by volunteers who have been directly affected by the consequences of SAB. GASP directs its educational efforts to three main audiences: school personnel, parents, and medical professionals. The organization has developed educational tools that are available for download on its website or by request mail. These tools include brochures, a slideshow presentation to be used in school settings, and a short video aimed at teens that highlights the dangers of the activity. One major goal of the organization is to integrate information about SAB into the D.A.R.E. curriculum, which has an established presence in schools across the United States. Other goals include implementing an SAB prevention program in all 50 states and all Canadian provinces and territories, as well as designing an official GASP-certified trainer program.

Education efforts should also encourage adolescents to disclose the behavior (whether it is their own or another adolescent's) to a trusted adult, so that education and intervention can occur on an individual basis. Similarly, if an adolescent discloses the behavior to a parent, the parent may consider talking with parents of other children or adolescents who may also be involved. Once parents or teachers are made aware of a youth's participation in SAB, the youth can be monitored more closely and referred for appropriate services and intervention.

Information on specific interventions for SAB is quite limited. However, an important first step is careful and detailed assessment of the behavior, its frequency, history, and functions. Previous studies have found at least some overlap between SAB and substance use, suicidal ideation, disordered eating symptoms, and other impulsive behaviors (e.g., Brausch et al., 2011). It is recommended that intervention approaches and techniques be selected on the basis of the youth's motivation for engagement in SAB and any other concurrent risk-taking behaviors. For example, an adolescent who cites "getting high" as a primary motivation for engaging in SAB may also have experimented with other substances and would be likely to benefit from a substance abuse treatment framework. Adolescents who endorse motivations for belongingness in a group may have underlying self-esteem issues or problematic peer relationships; these would lend themselves to using problem-solving techniques, social skills training, assertiveness training, and/or self-confidence building. Moreover, according to Walsh's "poly-self-destructive youth" theory, a subgroup of adolescents who engage in one risk-taking behavior are more likely to experiment with additional risk-taking behaviors (Walsh & Frost, 2005). The "choking game" may be just another sensation-seeking experience for adolescents who thrive on adrenaline rushes and strongly believe that they are invincible. Treatment for these adolescents may rely on techniques from motivational interviewing to help these youth recognize potential consequences of risky behavior and the impact of those consequences on their goals for the future. Last, engagement in risk-taking behaviors may be an indicator of internal distress. It is well established that self-injury is commonly utilized by adolescents to reduce negative moods or relieve feelings of stress and anxiety. Although empirical research into the possible connection between SAB and self-injury has just begun, preliminary findings show an overlap of the behaviors and an increase in other risk-taking behaviors when both SAB and self-injury have been experimented with. If an adolescent is referred for participation in SAB, clinicians and school personnel should carefully assess for other risk-taking behaviors, including self-injury. Adolescents who are engaging in both types of behaviors may benefit from techniques that have been found to be effective for self-injury, such as cognitive-behavioral and problem-solving techniques.

CASE EXAMPLE WITH NO INTERVENTION

Kevin was a 14-year-old who lived in a somewhat rural area with his parents and younger sister. He was involved in school activities, including basketball and track, and had always been an average to above-average student. Kevin seemed to have a large peer group and spent lots of time with his teammates outside of school. One Saturday morning he came home from spending the night at a friend's home with several of his other friends from the track team. His mother noticed that he seemed quite tired, even for having been at his friend's home, and asked how the evening went. Kevin mumbled a response and continued to his room. Later his mother overhead him talking on the phone to one of his friends, laughing about posting something on YouTube. She also thought she heard him talk about playing "space monkey." When she asked him about the conversation later, Kevin shrugged it off and said it was nothing, "just a stupid game we played." She warned him about posting videos on YouTube and asked him not to post anything in the future.

In the next few weeks, Kevin spent a lot of time with his friends, but did not want to talk to his parents much. His parents figured he was "going through a phase" and left him alone. As the weeks went by, Kevin started spending a lot of time in his room when he was home, and started snapping more than usual at his sister and parents. One day he complained to his mother of a bad headache, and she recommended some Tylenol and rest. She followed him to his room and noticed some belts on the floor. Kevin usually only wore belts for special occasions, and she asked why they were out of the closet. Kevin snapped at his mother and rudely told her to leave him alone. She again assumed that he was "going through some kind of adolescent phase" and let him rest.

A few days later, Kevin's parents and sister came home from one of the sister's school functions and found the television on in the living room. Kevin was nowhere to be found, and his laptop was sitting on the coffee table, with several websites on the screen. His parents called for him and eventually went up to his room to check on him. They found him not breathing, with a belt around his neck and the other end tied to the bedpost. They called 911, but Kevin had been without oxygen for too long. His parents had no idea he had been playing "space monkey" with his friends at parties, and had then started to engage in the activity on his own as well. They found photos of him and his friends "passing out" on his cell phone, along with text messages about "playing the game." Similar posts were found on his Facebook page. His parents were shocked not only to learn about the "game," but also to learn that their son had been engaging in such a dangerous activity.

CASE EXAMPLE WITH EDUCATION AND INTERVENTION

Kristy is a 15-year-old high school freshman in a small Midwestern town. She has a few friends, but has always been a bit shy and reserved. She is not involved in extracurricular activities at school, even though her parents keep encouraging her to join clubs. Her parents have been worried about her for a few months because she seems to be growing more distant and withdrawn and spends a lot of time alone in her room. They know that she is introverted and want to give her privacy and space, but wonder if they should intervene a bit more. One day while doing laundry, her mother finds a piece of paper in the pocket of Kristy's jeans. At first it seems like another example of Kristy's many drawings and doodlings, but her mother realizes that the paper also includes some writing. She makes out the words "pain" and "gasp." She shows the paper to Kristy later that evening, and Kristy becomes very upset. She accuses her mother of invading her privacy and does not want to discuss the meaning of the drawings and writing. Her mother expresses concern and asks whether everything is okay at school. Kristy breaks down into tears and runs to her room.

The next day her mother looks around Kristy's room for any other clues about her daughter's apparent distress. She finds some razor blades in the desk drawer, and is immediately concerned that Kristy may be thinking about suicide. She talks with a good friend of hers, who also has a teenage daughter and works in a school as a counselor. Her friend educates her about self-injury and encourages her to talk with her daughter more. When Kristy's mother mentions the paper she found, her friend recognizes that Kristy may have been referring to the "choking game." Kristy's mother thinks she saw something about it on the news a few months ago, but is shocked that her daughter might both be self-injuring and engaging in this "game." That evening she talks with Kristy again, and this time Kristy opens up more. She is tearful again and admits to her mother that she has been feeling very stressed lately and having problems with some girls at school. A friend of hers told her about cutting to feel better, so she has tried that. She also remembers playing the "choking game" at a party in junior high with other girls and the "high" feeling it gave her, so she has tried that a few times lately too. They both agree that Kristy needs additional help with her stress and overwhelming emotions. Kristy's mom makes an appointment with a therapist, and they attend the first session together. As Kristy works with her therapist, she learns different, more effective ways to cope with her negative emotions.

CONCLUSION

- SAB, or the "choking game," is an activity that adolescents are experimenting with, usually in groups. SAB has harmful, and potentially fatal, consequences.
- Anecdotal information suggests that adolescents may encounter the behavior at a party or group function, and then engage in the behavior alone. Some have described the "high" or "rush" feeling they receive from SAB as addictive.
- Steps are being taken by activist groups such as GASP to provide education and prevention information to adolescents, parents, teachers, and other adults who work with adolescents professionally.
- Intervention techniques for SAB may depend on other concurrent risk behaviors and the functions of the behavior, making thorough assessment of all risk behaviors essential.

CHAPTER 23

Understanding, Managing, and Treating Foreign-Body Ingestion

with ARIANA PERRY

One of the more remarkable, even astonishing, self-harm behaviors is foreign-body ingestion (FBI). This activity consists of *intentionally* swallowing such items as pencils, toothbrushes, razor blades, nuts and bolts, coins, batteries, and many other objects. FBI is most commonly found in institutional settings involving some degree of confinement, such as psychiatric hospitals and correctional facilities. Over the last several years, I (Barent W. Walsh) have been asked to consult with various hospitals and prisons regarding individuals presenting with this very challenging behavior. In the process of providing these consultations, I have learned a great deal from the literature, the secure settings, and the patients or inmates themselves.

This chapter begins with a discussion of where FBI falls in relation to other forms of self-harm. Next, the literature on FBI is briefly reviewed. Nine cases of FBI are then discussed in terms of their adverse childhood experiences and current clinical profiles. The functions of the behavior are then examined, ranging from internal affect regulation to social and environmental influence and control. The chapter concludes with recommendations for preventing, managing, and treating the behavior.

314

CLASSIFYING FBI

In Chapter 3, I have discussed the distinction between direct and indirect self-harm and have reviewed myriad examples of behaviors within each category. FBI is somewhat puzzling to classify because it has unusual features. Many have asked this question: Is FBI an example of suicidal behavior, non-suicidal self-injury, or some other form of self-harm? I believe it to be *an atypical, severe form of nonsuicidal self-injury*, for these reasons:

- It is intentionally self-destructive, yet most individuals deny suicidal intent.
- Consistent with these reports, very few individuals die from FBI.
- Similar to other forms of self-injury, it does result in direct bodily harm. Most frequently, it causes gastritis, esophagitis, or gastroesophageal reflux disease (GERD); much more rarely, it can result in blockage, perforation, peritonitis, or other serious consequences (American Society for Gastrointestinal Endoscopy, 2002). In some cases, the amount of damage can be microscopic.

However, FBI is different from other forms of self-injury, in that the bodily harm is *not immediately visible to the perpetrator or others*. This is very different from all other forms of self-injury, for which wounds on extremities or other body areas are instantly evident. In fact, FBI can be invisible to self and others for hours, days, or even weeks. Nonetheless, most FBI does adhere to the definition of self-injury provided in Chapter 1: It is "intentional, self-effected, low-lethality bodily harm of a socially unacceptable nature, performed to reduce and/or communicate psychological distress."

THE LITERATURE ON FBI

Although many mental health professionals in community settings might work for an entire career without encountering a client with FBI, those employed in hospital or correctional settings report that the behavior is surprisingly common. There is an extensive literature on FBI, most of which consists of individual case reports. Some of the examples are so extreme as to test credulity, but there is ample confirmatory evidence via not only client self-report, but also independent medical data (via X-rays, magnetic resonance imaging, endoscopy reports, etc.).

Types of Objects Ingested

The range of foreign bodies ingested by individuals can be quite startling. Some of the more remarkable examples include the following:

- An individual who swallowed 204 live bullets (McNutt, Chambers, Dethlefsen, & Shah, 2001)
- An individual who ingested five iron rods 4–5 inches in length, plus two needles (Khan & Ali, 2006)
- A person who swallowed a wristwatch that, when retrieved by endoscopy, was still working 1 month after ingestion (Aggarwal & Sinha, 2006)
- An individual who ingested 71 metallic objects, including a wrench, wire springs, buttons, a lamp finial, and eyeglasses (Slovis, Tyler-Worman, & Solightly, 1982)
- A woman who ingested at least 21 sewing needles (Nicoll, 1908)
- An individual who swallowed 461 coins (Bennett et al., 1997)
- During the period of 1927–1929, a woman residing in a Missouri mental hospital ingested 453 nails, 9 bolts, 115 hairpins, 42 screws, assorted buttons, many pebbles, and 942 assorted pieces of metal (Capello, 2011); she died on an operating table, perhaps as much due to the primitive surgery she received as to the objects she ingested

Other objects reported in the FBI literature include open and closed safety pins, needles, tacks, push pins, razor blades, pens, batteries of diverse sizes, toothbrushes, paper clips, screws, bolts, nails, washers, rings, pendants, chains, hair pins, barrettes, game pieces, shards of glass, fragments from CDs or CD cases, pebbles, stones, spray can knobs, mattress vents, knives, and thermometers.

Demographic and Diagnostic Characteristics

Most persons who ingest objects are inpatients in psychiatric settings or inmates in correctional facilities, as noted earlier. Because of the lack of large-sample studies, gender differences are not clear. The age range appears to be primarily young adulthood to middle age, although some adolescents and a few elders have been reported. Prevalence estimates are not available. One study in Taiwan reported that 7 of 6,112 psychiatric inpatients (or 0.12% of the sample) presented with FBI (Tsai, 1997). However, others have reported high rates and social contagion episodes of FBI in inpatient (Hindley, Gordon, Newrith, & Mohan, 1999) or prison (Best, 1946) settings.

One hospital where I consulted indicated that 6 of 96 (or 6%) of inpatients presented with recurrent FBI. Many papers cite individuals with multiple incidents of FBI over time; for example, O'Sullivan et al. (1996) found that 14 of 36 clients (or 39%) presented with FBI recurrently.

The range of psychiatric diagnoses associated with FBI in the literature is broad. Individuals with FBI tend to fall into four main diagnostic groups in estimated order of prevalence: (1) personality disorders, especially, BPD and antisocial personality disorder; (2) major depression or bipolar disorders; (3) substance use disorders and/or eating disorders (with bulimia nervosa perhaps more common); and (4) schizophrenia or other psychoses. Another group, with a primary diagnosis of developmental disabilities, is not discussed here.

Medical Procedures and Course of Treatment

Not surprisingly, when individuals ingest things that are not digestible, medical procedures often ensue. The most common medical interventions described in the literature are (in reverse order of intrusiveness and risk) recurrent X-rays; use of laxatives; whole-bowel irrigation; endoscopy (via mouth/esophagus); laparotomy (surgery through the abdominal wall); and more extensive surgeries involving esophagus, stomach, and bowel.

Many reports state that 80–90% of foreign bodies pass through the digestive tract *without* medical intervention (e.g., Velitchkov, Grigorov, Losonoff, & Kjossev, 1996; Palta et al., 2009). More specifically, Palta et al. (2009) noted that 80–90% of foreign bodies pass spontaneously through the gastrointestinal (GI) tract; 10–20% require endoscopy; and only 1% require surgical exploration and extraction. Accordingly, most physicians recommend a *conservative approach* to medical management (Tsai, 1997; Palta et al., 2009). Frequent X-rays are recommended to monitor movement of objects versus obstruction. Sharp objects (e.g., pins, needles, razor blades, pens, and tacks) have the greatest potential for impaction, obstruction, and perforation.

Negative Caregiver Reactions

Negative caregiver reactions to FBI are commonly cited in the literature. Not surprisingly, professionals are likely to be shocked and dismayed to find that clients are so distressed as to intentionally swallow objects. FBI also frequently results in caregiver frustration, compassion fatigue, "negative countertransference," or "therapy-interfering behaviors" (Linehan, 1993a). Pejorative language is frequently found in the literature, including such terms as "malingerer," "manipulative," "attention-seeking," "controlling," and "responsibility-shirking." Physicians and other caregivers frequently complain that patients presenting with FBI are "taking time away from 'real' patients." They lament that they are forced to "do something" in order to appear decisive and proactive in response to FBI. As an example of how caregiver frustration can escalate, consider the following quotation:

> [FBI] carries a sense of insidiousness in the lack of outward evidence that harm has been done. . . . Furthermore, although a patient's environment can be controlled for objects used for cutting or burning, it is nearly impossible to prevent access to all potentially ingestible objects. . . . FBI . . . evokes more frustration from [these patients'] treaters who, if the object is not retrievable, are effectively "held hostage" . . . through the anxiety-provoking period until the object is safely passed. (Gitlin et al., 2007, pp. 162, 163)

In addition to the emotional reactions of caregivers, it is also important to note that coercive, intrusive interventions to prevent additional FBI are often the norm rather than the exception. In order to extinguish FBI, caregivers and correctional staffers have frequently resorted to such methods as restraint, seclusion, one-to-one or even two-to-one staff supervision, full-room and full-body searches, confiscation of all personal belongings, and a finger food diet (precluding the need for utensils). The inadvertent and perhaps iatrogenic consequences of these methods are discussed below in the section on management and treatment.

A SMALL-SAMPLE STUDY OF FBI

We recently completed an informal study of individuals who presented with FBI over the past several years. The findings obtained are obviously limited by the tiny sample size ($N = 9$); nonetheless, lessons learned from these individuals may have clinical utility. If nothing else, other clinicians and researchers may want to look at similar variables and expand the knowledge base about FBI over time.

Of the nine participants, all were interviewed for at least an hour. In some cases they were interviewed multiple times. I had also reviewed extensive case material for each of these individuals. All had been long-term residents in a state hospital, for periods ranging from 2 to more than 10 years. Their number of inpatient stays ranged from 7 to 30. Eight of the nine were female; all were European American. The eight females ranged in age from 20 to 29, with a mean age of 24 years; the lone male was 46 years old. The IQ for these individuals ranged from 72 to 108, but there were no IQ data for three of the nine patients.

Childhood Trauma

We wanted to look at what might have contributed to the emergence of FBI in these persons, so we examined their childhood histories. We discovered that all nine (or 100%) had been sexually abused as children. In addition, six of the nine (67%) had been physically abused. These individuals had clearly experienced extremely problematic childhoods.

Psychiatric and Medical Diagnoses

By the time these individuals reached adulthood, they had lengthy psychiatric histories. The number of psychiatric diagnoses ranged from 3 to 11 per individual. Seven of the nine (or 78%) had a diagnosis of PTSD. The same percentage was diagnosed with BPD. In addition, four of the nine (or 44%) were diagnosed with a mood disorder, including major depressive disorder or bipolar disorder. An identical percentage was diagnosed with schizoaffective disorder and/or schizophrenia. This rather inconsistent and confusing array of diagnoses may suggest that the professionals were grappling to understand and properly help these individuals.

The nine patients also carried multiple medical diagnoses, ranging from one to six per individual. These included GERD, reflux esophagitis, hypothyroid, pernicious anemia, angina, hypertension, aortic regurgitation, aortic aneurysm, asthma, chronic headaches, velocardiofacial syndrome, and fetal alcohol syndrome.

Self-Harm Behaviors (Other Than FBI)

In looking at these nine individuals, we were especially interested in learning more about their other self-harm behaviors besides FBI.

Suicidal and Aggressive Behavior

It was quite revealing that 100% of these individuals had made at least one prior suicide attempt. The range of attempts was one to four per subject. Their methods included overdose (seven of nine), self-strangulation (six of nine), hanging (four of nine), jumping from a height (two of nine), and one attempt at drowning. In addition to their suicidal behaviors, 100% had also been violent toward staff or other patients. This combination of behaviors helps explain why caregiver frustration often runs so high when individuals present with FBI. In addition to the ingesting behaviors, these individuals often presented with recurrent suicidality and violence toward others. Such behavior is very likely to result in caregiver fatigue and burnout.

Atypical and Common Nonsuicidal Self-Injury

Beyond suicide attempts and aggression, these individuals also presented with major or atypical self-injury as defined in Chapter 3. These forms of serious self-injury included cutting requiring more than 80 sutures; self-injury to the eyes, face, and breasts; multiple instances of breaking fingers intentionally; recurrent excoriation of an incision with suture removal; and recurrent insertion of objects into unhealed wounds. In addition, all nine of these individuals presented with more common forms of self-injury, such as cutting, head banging, scratching, excoriation, gouging, self-biting, and burning.

Indirect Self-Harm

The nine individuals also presented with multiple forms of indirect self-harm. More specifically, six of the nine (67%) had a history of substance abuse; four (44%) were diagnosed with an eating disorder; four (44%) had frequent problems with medication adherence or discontinuance; and two (22%) had taken physical and/or sexual risks.

In summary, these patients presented with what we have termed "poly-self-destructive behavior." Each had performed multiple forms of direct and indirect self-harm in combination. They were literally "walking invento-ries of self-harm behaviors." This is a topic that I have addressed at greater length in Chapter 17. When individuals present with such diverse and high rates of self-harm and aggression, it should be no surprise that caregivers will find them extremely challenging and fatiguing. This is why we have devoted Chapter 19 to managing the reactions of therapists and other care-givers. People who work with poly-self-destructive individuals need diverse forms of support and self-care in order to maintain a compassionate and skillful frame of mind.

FBI of the Study Participants

Of course, we were especially interested in the ingesting behaviors of the study participants. I found that two of the nine had ingested foreign objects only 1–2 times. The other seven ingested from 3 to 19 times. Altogether, the nine participants had ingested 69 objects (a mean of 7.7 per individual). Of these 69 ingestions, only 1 resulted in a perforation; 15 resulted in endo-scopic procedures; 1 in a gastrostomy and enterostomy; and 1 in bowel sur-gery with a portion of the bowel removed. The objects ingested included small (unopened) batteries ($n = 7$); game pieces ($n = 5$); razor blades ($n = 3$);

and CD fragments, unsharpened pencils, pins, screws, thumbtacks, stones/pebbles, and watch clasps ($n = 2$ for each of these).

Some of the patients engaged in FBI at very high rates. Three of the nine had done it 10 or more times, indicating a truly chronic problem. There was a wide range in the size of objects ingested (and associated risk), in that some patients swallowed objects that were sharp and/or large; these were more likely to result in medical complications. Others confined their ingestions to small, nonsharp objects exclusively. These patients seemed to have some awareness of medical risk and some motivation to avoid serious damage to the GI tract.

Staff Interventions

Consistent with the literature on FBI reviewed above, staff members at the various hospitals frequently employed intensive and coercive methods to try to prevent FBI. Six of the nine patients (67%) experienced frequent one-to-one staff observation and room restriction. Other interventions included stripped rooms, physical restraints, room searches with confiscation, two-to-one staff supervision, and eating restrictions with no access to utensils.

The Functions of FBI

In consulting with hospitals regarding these patients, we were especially interested in the functions of the FBI. What were the payoffs that would lead individuals to engage in this behavior? In assessing functions, we employed Nock and Prinstein's (2004) four-component model, as shown in Table 23.1. What was especially striking in looking at the functions of FBI in these individuals was that the social reinforcers were generally much more important than the internal reinforcers. This finding is very different from those in most other studies of self-injury (see, e.g., Klonsky, 2007, as well as earlier chapters of this book), where the primary motivation for FBI has been internal affect regulation. Only two of the nine patients cited internal affect regulation as a reason for their FBI, and this was of secondary importance.

The most common explanation voiced by patients was that they ingested foreign objects in order to be transferred from their psychiatric wards to medical facilities. In some cases, they sought this transfer because they found the medical staff to be more nurturing and compassionate than the ward staff. Other patients indicated that they "liked the scopes" or the sedatives associated with endoscopies. And many of the patients expressed a desire to escape their psychiatric wards because of ongoing interpersonal conflicts with staff members and other patients.

TABLE 23.1. Functions of FBI for Nine Individuals

Positive self-reinforcement	*Negative self-reinforcement*
"To have a sensation of food in my stomach."	"Sense of relief." "Thought battery would explode and kill me." "Same function as cutting."
Positive social reinforcement	*Negative social reinforcement*
"I was jealous of someone who got to go to the ER." "I like the scopes at the medical unit." "I get high off the sedatives they give me." "I want control of my treatment." "It's like playing Russian roulette and slapping God in the face."	"I don't want to be here: I want to go to the medical hospital." "When I swallow objects, I get transferred off the ward to a medical unit." "I get transferred from a psych ward to a medical hospital." "I want a sharp object lodged in my anus so that when someone rapes me, he will get his dick shredded."

RECOMMENDATIONS FOR MANAGEMENT AND TREATMENT

Reevaluating Coercive Interventions

For the individuals we studied, coercive interventions appeared to be common, yet ineffective in dealing with FBI. We frequently observed inpatient staff and patients engaged in bitter, escalating power struggles that culminated in FBI or other self-harm behaviors. It was notable that several patients were able to self-harm even when they received the most restrictive interventions. For example, one young female patient was placed in four-point restraint to prevent her from ingesting objects. In defiance of this intervention, she bit a mouthful of flesh from her shoulder. Her message was clear: "I can harm myself no matter how much you try to control me," and she appeared to be correct.

One problem in trying to reduce coercive interventions in treatment settings is that hospital policies and protocols need to be changed. Such modifications often require the approval of high-level administrators who may be concerned about liability and adverse incident reporting. These administrators need to be trained about FBI and convinced that changes in protocol will result in better care and a reduction in incidents of FBI and other forms of self-harm.

In addition, staff persons need considerable support and validation to work with such challenging clients. Regular staff supervision and team meetings need to be in place to manage and prevent staff burnout. A useful activity can be to review patient records episodically, to remind the staff of these individuals' extensive trauma histories. Patients do not become poly-self-destructive randomly or due to modest life frustrations; rather, they are often subject to extreme mistreatment and "poly-abuse" over many years. Reviewing the psychosocial histories of these patients can serve to rekindle compassion. However, when coercive interactions between staff members (via restrictions) and patients (via FBI and other self-harm) reach a crescendo, transferring the patients to another ward may offer a fresh start for both parties.

Another innovative approach that some psychiatric hospitals have used successfully is to develop the capacity to provide X-rays and endoscopies on site. This may markedly reduce the need for transfers to medical units, thereby managing both negative and positive social reinforcers more strategically.

Proactive Skills Training

Rather than trying to prevent FBI, a more helpful approach is to teach patients new skills. This moves away from prohibitive, coercive strategies and instead emphasizes collaborative skills practice and problem solving. For example, rather than having a staff person provide passive (often non-verbal) one-to-one supervision of a patient at risk of self-harm, a far more productive activity is to offer intensive skills training. Examples of these skills are discussed at length in Chapter 11. Some inpatient units have successfully implemented evidence-based practice models such as DBT (Linehan, 1993a) or IMR (Dartmouth Psychiatric Center, 2008). These treatments, both of which are discussed in Chapter 17, provide a wide array of skills to help patients manage urges to self-harm and interact more successfully with others.

Worth noting is that the patients in my small sample seemed to perform FBI in relation to social reinforcers much more often than to internal reinforcers. Given this finding, it may be especially important to target interpersonal effectiveness and conflict resolution skills, as opposed to the more common emphasis on emotion regulation skills.

CONCLUSION

In summary, FBI is an unusual form of self-harm behavior that falls within the category of atypical, severe nonsuicidal self-injury. Other key aspects of FBI covered in this chapter are as follows:

- FBI is a complex behavior often found to be associated with other forms of self-harm, such as suicide attempts, common forms of self-injury, and risk-taking behaviors.
- FBI is generally reported in psychiatric inpatient units or correctional facilities.
- Using a functional analysis to assess FBI is an important place to start.
- Unlike many other forms of nonsuicidal self-injury, FBI may be maintained primarily by social reinforcers.
- Coercive staff interventions (such as room restrictions and restraints) are very common, but are often ineffective, counterproductive, or even iatrogenic.
- Rather than forbidding behavior, it is more strategic to teach patients what to do (i.e., to provide very specific skills training).
- Skills training may need to prioritize interpersonal effectiveness and conflict resolution skills because FBI is strongly linked to social reinforcers.
- FBI should be responded to respectfully, with a low-key, dispassionate demeanor (see Chapter 7).
- Staff members need considerable training, support, and supervision to work effectively with patients who present with FBI.

CHAPTER 24

Self-Injury in Correctional Settings

KENNETH L. APPELBAUM

Self-injurious behavior in jails and prisons has many similarities to such behavior in community settings. Other chapters provide a detailed review of definitional, assessment, and treatment issues in the community that also have relevance to correctional settings. This chapter, however, examines some of the important contextual differences, including unique aspects of motives and management.

CONTEXT

Inmates who self-injure present one of the most challenging problems facing correctional systems. Their behaviors compromise health and safety, adversely affect operations and services, and drain fiscal resources. Each incident can cause significant institutional disruption. Custody and medical staff members may need to stop scheduled activities to respond to the event. Movement of other staff and inmates often comes to a standstill throughout the facility until the situation has resolved. In addition to the harm sustained by the inmate, staff responders and other inmates risk injury and potential exposure to body fluids. Transfer to the institutional infirmary adds to the drain on resources—and if the inmate has serious injuries, a transfer to an emergency room or an admission to a hospital create considerable security concerns, along with further diversion of staff and fiscal resources.

A recent survey of the mental health directors who oversee the nation's prison systems demonstrated the significance and challenges of self-injury in correctional settings (Appelbaum, Savageau, Trestman, Metzner, & Baillargeon, 2011). Over three-quarters of the 51 state and federal correctional systems responded to the survey, reflecting the importance of this issue. The survey found that although fewer than 2% of inmates per year engage in self-injurious behaviors, they do so with notable frequency. In 85% of responding state and federal prison systems, these behaviors occur at least weekly, with frequencies of several times per week, once per day, and more than once per day in 50%, 6%, and 15% of all systems, respectively. Self-injurious behaviors also cause substantial systemic difficulties. For example, 70% and 47% of respondents reported self-injury behaviors as moderately to extremely disruptive to mental health services and facility operations, respectively.

Despite the serious problems caused by inmate self-harm, the survey found that almost half of the nation's prison systems maintain no data on these events, and the remainder track data in a limited and inconsistent manner. Two aspects contribute to this deficiency. First, no consensus has emerged on which data to collect. The correctional field has yet to identify the individual, interpersonal, and environmental features that contribute most strongly to these behaviors. Similarly, no broad agreement exists on which outcome variables to track. As a result, we lack data on precipitating factors, severity of injuries to inmates and staff responders, medical interventions provided to inmates, disruptions to facility operations, or similar consequences. Second, correctional systems have not established a uniform method for data collection. Systems and researchers have yet to develop a practical and reliable approach for documenting something that currently occurs in a haphazard fashion, if at all.

The paucity of data regarding characteristics of self-injurious and suicidal inmates leaves correctional systems with little descriptive information on this population. Their attributes in broad clinical, demographic, and motivational areas have not been well established, and a useful classification system still needs development. With better data on potentially significant inmate characteristics, correctional systems might identify subgroups of inmates and match them to more carefully targeted interventions.

Despite the general lack of detailed quantitative data, findings from the national survey support two widely acknowledged observations. First, most self-injurious inmates have DSM-IV-TR psychiatric diagnoses: Cluster B personality disorders occur in over 50%, followed by mood disorders (15.5%), mixed personality disorders (12.2%), psychotic disorders (7.6%), and mental retardation/pervasive developmental disorders (3.2%). Second, segregation and other lock-down units have the highest rate of occurrence of self-injurious behaviors. These units typically confine inmates for disciplinary reasons to their cells for 23 hours a day, allowing them out only for showers and solitary exercise.

The higher prevalence of self-injury on lock-down units probably reflects not only the inherent characteristics of the inmates most likely to end up on them, but also the adverse effects of the environment itself. Conditions in correctional settings in general often exacerbate the symptoms of inmates with mental illness. As a class, they fare more poorly than their inmate peers, and they are more likely to decompensate and receive disciplinary reports for rule infractions, which may result in placement in punitive segregation (Morgan, Edwards, & Faulkner, 1993; Santamour & West, 1982; Toch & Adams, 1987). The prevalence of serious mental illness among inmates in these solitary confinement settings often greatly exceeds the prevalence found in prison general population units (Lovell, 2008; O'Keefe & Schnell, 2007). In some systems, over half of the inmates in segregation have serious mental disorders (Abramsky, Fellner, & Human Rights Watch, 2003). Conditions on the units themselves may lead to further deterioration. Prolonged isolation for any inmate can have detrimental psychological effects; these may include anxiety, mood disturbance, cognitive difficulties, perceptual distortions, or even psychosis (Grassian, 1983; Pizarro & Stenius, 2004; Rhodes, 2005; Smith, 2006). For inmates with underlying psychiatric disorders, isolation can cause further deterioration in behaviors, including self-injury (Abramsky et al., 2003).

Some inmates with repeated or severe disciplinary infractions may spend most, if not all, of their incarceration in segregation. Periods of isolation can last months or even years. In addition, some of these inmates continue to commit infractions while in segregation, resulting in added sanctions. For example, segregated inmates who misbehave may lose access to privileges and diversions, such as television, radio, or most reading materials. In more punitive correctional systems, loss of privilege time can accumulate into months or years. Sanctions this draconian quickly become meaningless and counterproductive. Another month of lost privileges provides little disincentive for misbehavior by inmates already deeply into cumulative loss, and the prospect of regaining privileges years down the road is too distant an incentive for good behavior.

MOTIVES

Self-injury by inmates can occur for many of the same reasons explored elsewhere in this book, but this chapter focuses primarily on motivations related to the correctional setting. Incarceration involves a substantial loss of autonomy. Inmates generally have limited ability to obtain what they want. Self-injury, however, returns some control to the inmate. These behaviors can serve as the means to desired ends. For example, serious incidents require transfer or admission to an infirmary or hospital, either of which may be more desirable than the setting from which the inmate came. Along with often nicer accommodations, the inmate will have contact with clinical staff. These encounters provide a typically welcomed contrast with prison routine. The trip alone to an outside medical facility may feel like a refreshing diversion. The transfer also can provide temporary respite from situational stressors, including, for example, threatened or actual sexual assault, contact with other predatory peers, or pressure to pay an outstanding debt. The desire to avoid these dangers produces an incentive to behave in a way that will remove the inmate from the risk.

Perhaps the greatest situational stressors, however, occur among inmates in long-term segregation. The detrimental psychological effects of isolation sometimes drive inmates to the brink of despair. When combined with harsh deprivations of privileges and diversions, prolonged periods of almost unremitting solitude take a toll. Inmates who initially tolerate the conditions may hit their limit after months or years. Having exhausted their coping abilities, they may resort to self-injury for several reasons. Physical pain and injury can provide a distraction and relief from their psychological distress. The ensuing staff response and commotion also break up the monotony and solitude of their existence. In extreme cases, the self-injury leads to a transfer to less draconian settings. As noted above, clinical settings typically offer services, privileges, and interpersonal contacts not found in segregation units. When an inmate is removed from the segregation environment, even severe dysphoric, anxious, or psychotic symptoms often rapidly resolve. Thus some inmates have powerful motivation to obtain the relief that self-injury and its consequences can offer.

Medication seeking may provide another motive for self-injury. Severe trauma or surgical interventions can lead to treatment with narcotic analgesics or other desirable substances. The psychological effects obtained from these medications serve as an inducement for some inmates to injure themselves. Others seek access to medications that they can divert for profit. Controlled substances and other medications are valuable commodities behind bars.

Anger can also fuel self-injurious behavior. In these instances, the inmate seeks to disrupt operations or cause distress to the staff. The behavior often serves as retaliation for a perceived insult or injustice, such as an undeserved sanction or loss of privileges. Incidents may be timed for maximum impact. For example, serious harm sustained late at night when the facility has little medical coverage is more likely to require a trip to an emergency room. This adds to the drain on staff and fiscal resources, as intended by some inmates. In addition, events like this frequently require notification of the prison superintendent or warden, to the delight of an inmate who hopes to disrupt the sleep of prison administrators. With little else to occupy time, payback may turn into an avocation.

MANAGEMENT

The management of seriously self-injurious inmates creates challenges for all correctional systems. Inmates may have powerful motivations to harm themselves, as described above. No easy solution exists in many cases. Even under the impoverished conditions found in many segregation settings, inmates still have access to their own bodies and the capacity to do damage to them. With enough time and ingenuity, they can fashion many readily available items into instruments of self-harm. Paint chips taken from a wall, for example, can provide cutting edges.

Unfortunately, self-injuring inmates sometimes become the focus of discord between the clinical and custodial staffs. Some of the reactions that these behaviors can engender in caregivers have been described in Chapter 19 of this volume. Correctional settings have the added potential for conflict among staff members over management responsibilities. Disputes may arise over whether the behaviors constitute a mental health or a security problem. Almost all cases, however, require a coordinated response, in which ongoing mental health service involvement is combined with responsive participation by custody staff.

Most cases of self-injurious behavior by inmates do not arise solely in response to underlying psychiatric disorders, and many occur in the context of the ulterior motives previously described. However, this does not negate the need for a shared response by medical, mental health, and custody staff. When divisiveness and splitting occur, interventions have little chance of success.

The most obvious initial role for mental health professionals involves an assessment of the underlying precipitants for the inmate's actions, including a diagnostic evaluation. This will help clarify the inmate's motives and any environmental factors contributing to or reinforcing the behavior. After elucidating these issues, staff members from all disciplines can work together in shaping a response.

Regardless of the reasons for self-injury, taking a punitive approach has contraindications. These behaviors have at times resulted in disciplinary sanctions for destruction of state property, under the theory that inmates belong to the state. This has occurred primarily in cases in which the behaviors have obvious underlying goals or occur as part of power struggles between inmates and staff. Such inmates are often labeled as "manipulative." This label, and the sanctions that sometimes accompany it, serve little purpose other than exacerbating the situation. Describing inmate behavior as "manipulative" tends to set up an adversarial relationship that portrays the inmate as demanding and personally challenging. This leads staff members to resist making sought-after concessions. Because the staffers are unwilling to lose what has now become a battle of wills, intransigence can set in, precluding a more dispassionate response. When accommodation feels like capitulation, professional perspective has been lost.

A more productive perspective accepts that inmates sometimes resort to self-injury when they see few if any alternatives. These behaviors get them attention and afford them leverage where otherwise they have none. Although they may have identifiable motives, real distress also often fuels their decision to self-injure. They may even be desperate enough to risk permanent injury or death to achieve their ends. An effective response begins by identifying the source of their distress, along with what they seek. Understanding their goals provides the basis for crafting management and treatment interventions.

Individualized behavior management plans can help diminish the frequency and severity of much self-injurious behavior. This approach, however, requires coordination and cooperation across disciplines. The custody staff typically controls access to the types of behavioral incentives and concessions likely to motivate inmates. Without flexibility in the use of such rewards, behavior becomes difficult if not impossible to reshape. This flexibility needs to include reasonable limits on the duration of punitive sanctions, so that rewards always appear attainable. This may require forgoing the addition of more lost privilege time for misbehavior by inmates who have already reached the maximum penalty.

An increasing number of states have been creating behavioral management units, especially as alternative settings for self-injurious inmates with aggressive behaviors who would otherwise be housed in lock-down segregation units. This trend has been driven by a series of influential federal court decisions mandating removal of some classes of inmates with mental disorders from prolonged segregation. The first of these cases, *Madrid v. Gomez* (1995), occurred in California in 1995 and led to the development of maximum-security, but less isolative, residential psychiatric treatment units within the prison. In addition to removing or diverting inmates with mental disorders from conditions of almost constant lock-down status, these units address the underlying behaviors and disorders that have led to the need for secure and segregated housing. Therapeutic programming attempts to provide inmates with alternative coping skills, with the overall goal of allowing them to function successfully in prison general population units and in the community after release from incarceration. Since 1995, many states in addition to California have undergone similar developments as the result of either court decisions or settlement agreements. Strong support for alternative settings to segregation that can address the needs of behaviorally disordered inmates with mental illness has come from government bodies (Collins & National Institute of Corrections, 2004), nongovernmental research and human rights organizations (Abramsky et al., 2003; Gibbons & Katzenbach, 2006), professional organizations (National Commission on Correctional Health Care, 2004), and individual commentators (Metzner & Fellner, 2010).

As with treatment plans in general, cooperation and flexibility are of great importance in the success of behavioral management units. Mental health professionals, in addition to custody staff, need to play active roles in the design and running of these units. This often requires relaxation of usual custody rules to allow use of positive reinforcement to change behaviors. Such reinforcements can include reduction or suspension of remaining disciplinary time; increased recreational and other out-of-cell time; provision of televisions or other sources of diversion; and access to programming and group therapeutic activities. Successful treatment may require a year or longer.

In the absence of specially designed behavioral intervention units, correctional systems typically face an unsolvable dilemma. Conditions on segregation units can fuel self-injurious behaviors. At the very least, these units are not well equipped to deal with inmates who have serious mental health needs. As a result, some inmates have a high risk of self-harm while in prolonged segregation. On the other hand, many of these same inmates also have predatory or aggressive tendencies that create significant safety concerns in less secure clinical and hospital settings. Too sick for secure segregation units and too dangerous for clinical settings, these inmates may bounce back and forth between two risky and unsuitable environments. In many systems, what they need does not exist: a secure and therapeutic housing option.

Correctional professionals (both clinical and custodial) sometimes object to modifications of sanctions or use of incentives for inmates who self-injure, due to fears that this may encourage imitative behaviors. They believe that other inmates may copy behaviors that have resulted in positive changes for their peers. Such concerns about contagion are understandable, but usually unwarranted. Most inmates simply do not have the stamina or desperation to resort to serious self-injury. They may share goals with their peers, but are unwilling or unable to adopt similar methods of achieving those goals. Even a risk of widespread mimicry, no matter how unlikely, would not contraindicate a more temperate use of behavioral interventions. It makes little sense to shun thoughtful and effective interventions if they ultimately achieve the desired results. The principles that work for more extreme cases have the same merit as the default approach.

Questions sometimes arise over the role of medications or mental health restraints during episodes of serious inmate self-injury. Using either of these interventions, however, as punitive or adverse stimuli has no place in clinical practice. Physicians who act otherwise breach basic ethical principles and jeopardize their licensure. Appropriate indications for psychotropic medications include treatment of underlying psychiatric disorders and, in rare instances, emergency chemical restraint necessary to prevent imminent harm. The latter justification also applies to the use of mechanical mental health restraints.

Unfortunately, correctional systems have at times had questionable standards regarding mental health restraints. In response, the American Psychiatric Association has produced a resource document that provides some guidance (Metzner et al., 2007). This document contends that correctional systems should be held to a similar standard of care as community health facilities. With a few exceptions, this requires following restraint practices in noncorrectional settings, in matters including indications, contraindications, location, techniques, time frames, observation, care, decision making, and staff training.

Even when the use of mental health restraints is limited to emergency situations and standards similar to those in the community, controversy persists over its role in correctional settings. The Metzner et al. (2007) resource document acknowledges some of the clinical challenges associated with this intervention in jails and prisons. Other commentators have elaborated upon the contraindications to clinical restraints in inherently nontherapeutic correctional environments. Because of these considerations, I have argued for limiting the use of mental health restraints primarily to the stabilization of unsafe situations during the time it takes to transfer an inmate to a psychiatric hospital (Appelbaum, 2007). For similar reasons, prisons in the United Kingdom do not typically use mental health restraints in their facilities (O'Grady, 2007).

CASE EXAMPLE

Mr. A is a 34-year-old man serving a life sentence for a murder he committed 10 years earlier. He has had a difficult adjustment to incarceration, with many disciplinary infractions ranging from disobeying orders of correctional officers to destruction of state property to assaults on staff and other inmates. After he seriously injured a correctional officer 7 years ago, prison authorities placed him in a long-term, maximum-security segregation unit. He spends 23 hours a day isolated in his cell, coming out for only an hour a day of solitary exercise, occasional showers, and other special reasons such as medical appointments.

Mr. A has continued to have disruptive behaviors, including conflicts with correctional officers, while in segregation. He claims that some officers have harassed him because he injured the other officer 7 years ago. He believes that much of his disruptive behavior in segregation has been a justified response to this alleged harassment. As a result of his ongoing misbehavior, however, he has accumulated additional sanctions that include loss of access to a television, radio, magazines, and most books. He has been without these items continuously for almost 5 years, and he currently has over 4 years of further sanction time remaining. Each episode of unacceptable behavior typically results in the addition of at least another 30 days to these accumulated sanctions. The prospect of receiving additional sanction time for misbehaviors does not deter him, because the 4 years remaining already feel like an eternity to him. He views the sanctions against him as unfair and as another example of his mistreatment.

About 6 months ago, Mr. A began to self-injure—primarily cutting, but also swallowing sharp objects, inserting foreign bodies into his urethra, and overdosing on secretly hoarded medications. The frequency of these acts has increased to at least daily. His injuries have often been severe, requiring transfer to a hospital or emergency room. For several weeks, he has regularly engaged in serious self-harm late at night or in the early hours of the morning.

Prison mental health services have assessed Mr. A and determined that he has antisocial personality disorder. Although he presents as anxious, dysphoric, and angry, he has no suicidal intent. Instead, he states that self-injuring is his only way to protest the sanctions against him. He enjoys causing distress to officers and disruption to the facility's operations. He knows that prison policy requires immediate notification of the facility superintendent whenever a serious incident occurs, which includes inmates' being sent out for emergency medical treatment. He feels delighted that he can disrupt the sleep of the superintendent every night as revenge for his own suffering. He also acknowledges that the prolonged isolation and loss of privileges have taken a toll on him, and he can no longer tolerate the boredom and distress. He looks forward to his trips to local emergency rooms or even to the prison infirmary. The commotion and movement out of his cell provide some relief for his boredom and dysphoria.

Although the prison administrators are loath to give Mr. A what he seeks, they agree to some changes in response to recommendations from the mental health staff. Except for 30 days, authorities waive the sanctions depriving Mr. A of forms of diversion. They also agree to try a cap of no more than 30 days on accumulation of such sanctions, to provide a more timely incentive for good behavior. In addition, the administrators take some steps to lessen the potential for mistreatment of Mr. A by the correctional staff. After these changes are instituted, the frequency and severity of Mr. A's self-injurious and other disruptive behaviors noticeably decrease.

CONCLUSION

Although only a few inmates engage in self-injurious behavior, they create serious health, safety, operational, and fiscal problems for correctional systems. Despite many similarities to such events in the community, the correctional setting has some unique contextual, motivational, and management aspects. Nevertheless, the characteristics of these inmates, and their behaviors and management, have received relatively little research attention.

Some reasons why inmates, who generally have few means of getting what they need or want, may self-injure include the following:

- Respite from stressful situations through transfer to an infirmary or hospital
- Coping with psychological distress from prolonged isolation in segregation units
- Obtaining narcotics or other desired medications
- Causing facility disruptions as an expression of anger at authorities

Effective management of self-injurious inmates requires the following:

- Shared responsibility and a coordinated approach by mental health, medical, and custody staffs
- Avoidance of punitive or adversarial responses
- Understanding and accepting the inmate's motives
- Individualized behavior management plans
- Creation of secure behavioral management units
- Flexible use of behavioral rewards and incentives
- Use of medications only for appropriate clinical indications
- Limits on the use of mental health restraints, and only with standards similar to those in community health facilities

CHAPTER 25

Treating Major Self-Injury

This chapter is one of the most disturbing to read in the book, because it focuses on *major* self-injury. This is *not* a relevant chapter for those working in school or university settings or in other locations where the clientele is high-functioning. It can be useful for those employed in correctional facilities, psychiatric hospitals, group homes, supported housing programs, Program of Assertive Community Treatment teams, clubhouses, and other programs that serve persons with serious mental illness or severe personality disorders.

DEFINITION

Favazza (1996, p. 233) stated that "major self-injury refers to infrequent acts—such as eye enucleation, castration, and limb amputation—that result in the destruction of significant body tissue." This type of self-injury can properly be referred to as "self-mutilation" because it meets a dictionary definition for the word "mutilate," meaning "to cut up or alter radically so as to make imperfect" and "to maim, cripple" (Merriam-Webster Dictionary, 1995, p. 342). In this chapter, the terms "major self-injury" and "self-mutilation" are used interchangeably.

INTENT

Although major self-injury, by definition, involves significant tissue damage, such behavior usually does not involve suicidal intent. Persons who perform major self-injury are generally in very acute distress and/or states of intoxication. The extreme behavior often indicates that they are trying to solve a major life problem, to transform themselves, or to follow perceived instructions from a powerful external force (e.g., God or the devil). Noticeably absent in the intent of such persons is a desire to die (Menninger, 1938/1966; Walsh & Rosen, 1988; Favazza, 1996; Grossman, 2001). The case examples provided below describe the type of idiosyncratic intent that often accompanies major self-injury.

PREVALENCE

The overall prevalence of major self-injury is unknown. Fortunately, the behavior appears to be quite rare. For example, Grossman (2001, p. 53) noted that only "115 cases of male genital self-mutilation have been reported in English, German, and Japanese literature since the end of the nineteenth century." He also identified 90 cases of ocular self-mutilation in the modern literature during the same time period. Because it is a rare behavior, the literature on major self-injury consists almost entirely of individual case reports. I am not aware of any empirical studies of major self-injury. Some authors (e.g., Greilsheimer & Groves, 1979; Kennedy & Feldman, 1994; Grossman, 2001; Large et al., 2008) have provided summative discussions of case reports for such categories as genital or ocular self-mutilation. These articles are the best available for trying to generalize across the population of individuals who commit major self-injury.

FORMS OF THE BEHAVIOR

Grossman (2001) noted that four main types of major self-injury have been reported in the literature:

- Genital (e.g., transection of the penis, castration, removal of the penis; female laceration of the urethra and vagina)
- Ocular (e.g., enucleation, puncture, laceration, self-blinding through self-hitting)
- Digit and limb amputation (e.g., finger and limb removal)
- Other especially rare forms (e.g., major self-injury to the nose, tongue, mouth, face, autocannibalism)

DIAGNOSTIC DIVERSITY

When people hear of such horrific acts, they understandably jump to the conclusion that the behaviors must be associated almost exclusively with psychosis. In actuality, the literature describes many examples of major self-injury by individuals with a startlingly wide range of psychiatric diagnoses. Favazza (1996) has stated that the major forms of self-injury are "most commonly associated with psychosis (acute psychotic episodes, schizophrenia, mania and depression)" (p. 234). However, he has also noted that major self-injury has been reported in states of "acute intoxication" and "carefully planned transsexual castration" (p. 234) in which psychosis played no part.

Based on his review of the literature, Grossman (2001) noted that approximately 80% of persons committing genital self-mutilation have been in a psychotic state at the time of the act. He summarized the diversity of diagnoses and circumstances for such persons, indicating that they fall into five generalized groups (Grossman, 2001, p. 53):

1. Young males with acute psychoses
2. Violence-prone males during acute intoxication
3. Transgender males seeking a sex change
4. Older males with psychotic depression and somatic illness
5. Individuals with severe personality disorders acting out rageful feelings

The findings of Large et al. (2008) also point to the strong association between major self-injury and psychosis. They found in reviewing 189 cases of major self-mutilation (including removal of an eye or testicle, severing of the penis, or amputation of a limb) that 143 (or 75.6%) of these individuals were diagnosed with a psychotic illness. Of the 143, 119 (or 83.2%) carried a diagnosis of "schizophrenia spectrum psychosis" (Large et al., 2098, p. 1012). Also important in the Large et al. report is their finding that 53.5% of the cases reviewed were experiencing "first-episode psychosis." Thus they recommend that "earlier treatment of psychotic illness may reduce the incidence of major self-mutilation" (p. 1012).

Grossman (2001) indicated that 75% of those who commit ocular self-mutilation have been described as psychotic at the time of the act. The remaining 25% have had such diagnoses as depressive disorder, Munchausen syndrome, substance abuse, and OCD (Grossman, 2001; Kennedy & Feldman, 1994). Thus individuals who perform major self-injury exhibit a broad range of psychiatric diagnoses, including the psychoses, personality disorders, substance use disorders, PTSD, OCD, and even comorbid Tourette's disorder with OCD (Hood, Baptista-Neto, Beasley, Lobis, & Pravdova,

2004). For thorough reviews of this diagnostic information, see Greilsheimer and Groves (1979), Kennedy and Feldman (1994), and Grossman (2001).

To these findings I would add, from my own experience, that clients who have been repeatedly sexually abused and are suffering from PTSD (and related states of dissociation) also may present with major self-injury. In some cases their symptoms of dissociation may at first look like psychosis, but they are not. Rather, these clients genuinely have PTSD and should be treated as such (see Chapter 16). A case example of this type is provided below.

PREVENTION AND RISK ASSESSMENT

The primary goal in working with persons capable of major self-injury is to prevent the behavior from happening in the first place. Warning signs for major self-mutilation have not been precisely defined, in part because the literature is based on case reports rather than empirical studies. Moreover, the majority of work in performing risk assessments has focused on those with psychotic disorders rather than other diagnoses. As noted by Grossman (2001),

> It should be clearly acknowledged that accurate prediction of major SIB [self-injurious behavior] is not possible but that certain factors should heighten the clinician's level of concern with regard to the probability of such behavior occurring. In general, as positive symptoms of psychosis increase, so does the risk of SIB. (p. 58)

Rosen and I presented a protocol (Walsh & Rosen, 1988) for assessing self-injury associated with psychosis. This protocol is similar to the list of risk factors presented by Grossman (2001), but is more extensive and inclusive. I have updated this protocol and present it below. The protocol is not empirically validated, but is informed by clinical experience and knowledge of the literature on major self-injury/self-mutilation.

PROTOCOL FOR ASSESSING RISK OF MAJOR SELF-INJURY

1. Key points of historical information
   - History of previous self-injury and major self-injury
   - History of impulsive violence directed at self and/or others
   - History of childhood deprivation, physical abuse, or sexual abuse
   - Recent interpersonal loss or major change in life circumstances
   - Recent self-imposed change in physical appearance (e.g., shaving one's head, donning military garb)

2. Assessment of mental status
   - Presence of auditory hallucinations with self-injurious content (e.g., hearing a voice stating, "You must hurt yourself because you deserve it; you are no good")
   - Belief in the credibility of the source of the hallucinations (e.g., "The voice comes from God and must be obeyed"; it could be the voice of a deceased parent, an angel, or some other figure perceived as powerful/omniscient)
   - Presence of delusions with self-injurious content (e.g., "My self-injury is part of the plan for the universe")
   - Presence of religious delusions, especially any regarding sinfulness, expiation of sins, unworthiness, etc. (e.g., "I must assault or remove this body part to atone for my sins")
   - Presence of persecutory delusions (e.g., "People are after me and will stop only if I remove my eye")
   - Presence of somatic delusions (e.g., "My penis is rotting and must be removed," "My vagina is dirty and disgusting; it must be cleansed and punished")
   - Presence of delusions of grandiosity (e.g., "If I remove my eye, I will experience no pain and will sit at the right hand of God")
   - Belief in the credibility of any of these delusions (e.g., "The nature of reality has been revealed to me and only me," "God must be obeyed," "My father told me I was no good for so long, it must be true")
   - Magical thinking (e.g., "If I hurt myself, all my problems will be solved")
   - Substance use or intoxication that exacerbates any of the above-described mental status conditions
   - Unauthorized discontinuance of psychotropic medication that triggers decompensation and exacerbation of any of the above-described symptoms
3. Details related to major self-injury
   - Presence of rituals associated with self-injury
   - Preoccupation with any body areas or body parts
   - Preoccupation with any tools or methods of self-injury
   - Preoccupation with or quoting of biblical passages with self-injury content, such as "And if thy right eye offend thee, pluck it out . . . And if thy right hand offend thee, cut it off" (Matthew 5: 29–30)
   - Preoccupation with any historical or mythological self-injurers (e.g., van Gogh, Bodhidharma, Oedipus)
   - Preoccupation with transgender issues (especially desire for a sex change)

- Preoccupation and discomfort with unwanted sexual fantasies, impulses, behaviors
- An absence of physical pain related to any previous self-injury

CASE EXAMPLE RELEVANT TO ASSESSMENT

I have previously described in detail a case of self-enucleation (Walsh & Rosen, 1988). I initially became aware of this individual when I was asked to conduct a critical-incident investigation immediately after the act. Subsequently, this individual came into care at my agency, residing in a group home for adults with serious and persistent mental illness. His residency in this program provided an unusual opportunity to follow a person for many years after a major self-injury. I discuss this case in two parts: (1) as an illustrative case example related to the protocol presented above, and (2) by providing an update regarding the life (and death) of this individual after his self-enucleation.

At the time of his self-enucleation (circa 1986), Mr. M was a single 31-year-old European American male well known to the local mental health system. He had an extended history of mental illness and many admissions to the local state hospital. Mr. M's first psychiatric hospitalization had occurred at age 18. Since that time, he had lived at home with his mother when he was not hospitalized. Mr. M's primary diagnosis was paranoid schizophrenia, although he had acquired others over the years. During the previous 13 years, his pattern was to experience recurrent psychotic decompensations, chronic unemployment, poor compliance with treatment programs and medication regimens, limited social relationships, and episodic poor self-care in such areas as money management and personal hygiene. His strengths included good intelligence, a sense of humor, an interest in art, and a generally pleasant demeanor.

During his most recent state hospital stay, plans had been made to place Mr. M, upon discharge, in a community residential program with another agency. The reason for the change was that he was becoming increasingly difficult for his mother to manage because of his dangerous smoking behavior, inconsistent sleeping habits, refusal to do chores, poor personal hygiene, and isolation. Thus, at the time of Mr. M's self-enucleation, he was living in a supervised community residence. Despite his participation in the program, his mental status had deteriorated over the previous several months. As we learned subsequently, he had periodically stopped taking his psychotropic medication.

Two days before the act, his outreach worker perceived him to be "more paranoid than usual." However, he did not present with any self-destructive ideation or behavior. In fact, Mr. M had no history of self-destructive behavior whatsoever.

Staff members were alerted to be attentive to his medication ingestion, because it seemed likely that his deterioration was due in part to his "cheeking" his medications (i.e., tucking pills into his cheeks and subsequently spitting them out). Record material indicated that Mr. M seemed depressed and required reassurance that he was safe and that no one wanted to harm him in the residence.

On the morning of his self-enucleation, an overnight counselor found notes written by Mr. M that were puzzling and vague, but ominous in content. The notes read: (1) "Julie forgive me"; (2) "Perhaps it was a good home . . . it was the best"; (3) "Good bye Julie"; (4) "Always try to live in a good home . . . I'm a coward." (Julie was an acquaintance from high school whom he had not seen for over 10 years.)

Mr. M left the residence unaccompanied that morning and went to a local psychiatric emergency room. When he arrived, he asked that he be given "a lethal dose of poison." At this point Mr. M was readmitted to the state hospital.

He arrived on the ward during the 3–11 P.M. shift and was given a low dose of Prolixin for agitation. In a nursing assessment note, Mr. M was described as saying, "I want something lethal—a lethal injection," and "I'm a dirty bastard." Due to his restlessness and preoccupation with death-oriented thoughts, he was given an additional low dose of Prolixin, again without noticeable positive effect. Subsequent low doses of Prolixin produced no improvement.

Throughout the night, Mr. M talked in a rambling, deluded fashion. At one point he ran down the hall of the ward screaming, turned over a table, and had to be physically restrained. He spoke repeatedly about crucifying a girlfriend, said that he was a murderer and rapist of young girls, and stated that he had fathered multiple illegitimate children. He also stated that he was soon to die and to be reincarnated as a "Jewish black prince." However, when he was asked whether he planned to hurt himself, he emphatically said, "No."

Mr. M remained psychotic and bizarre over the next 12 hours and was being watched closely by the staff. However, at one point he slipped into a bathroom unaccompanied. The staff then heard Mr. M scream. Upon opening the door to the bathroom, the staff found Mr. M standing with one hand covering his right eye, which was bleeding profusely. Asked what he had done, Mr. M stated he had flushed the eye down the toilet. Mr. M was then transferred to an intensive care medical unit.

ASSESSING THE RISK OF MAJOR SELF-INJURY

The case of Mr. M provides a good example regarding the assessment of risk for major self-injury. Mr. M presented with many warning signs from the protocol, although there were also many other items that did not apply. For example, if we look at section 1 of the protocol (historical information), we see that Mr. M met only two of the five criteria. He had no history of prior self-injury. He also had no history of abuse or deprivation; nor had he made any recent changes to physical appearance. He did present with some relatively modest physical violence on the ward prior to his self-injury, and he certainly had experienced a recent loss in being placed away from his mother for the first time. Mr. M clearly seemed to be grieving for this loss in his statements about the importance of "living in a good home" and perhaps referring to his mother's home as "the best."

In regard to assessing Mr. M's mental status, as delineated in section 2 of the protocol, he presented with multiple problems indicative of serious risk. His rambling verbal content included religiosity ("Jewish black prince," crucifying girls, condemnation of his immorality), sexual preoccupations (committing rape and fathering illegitimate children), and persecutory ideas (requiring reassurance at the group home as to his safety). He also presented with a variety of highly unusual self-destructive thoughts, in that he requested a lethal dose of poison or medication on multiple occasions. Another warning sign was that he had discontinued his psychotropic medication surreptitiously. He had not used or abused any substances. Thus, in the second category of the protocol, there were many "hits" that should have alarmed someone conducting a professional assessment. This portion of the protocol is the one that pointed most directly to the risk of major self-injury posed by Mr. M's mental status.

The third and final section of the protocol concerns details regarding the self-injury. This section would not have been especially helpful with Mr. M, because he had no prior history of self-harm. Also, he did not present with any preoccupations with body parts, tools, or transgender issues. At one point Mr. M did quote the passage from the Bible regarding plucking out one's eye, but this was several days *after the fact*. He certainly did present with preoccupation about sexuality and seemed to be experiencing guilt about imagined sexual offenses.

Mr. M provided additional information about his motivations to remove his eye in the days following the act. For example, he described some homosexual fears and wishes related to having a roommate at his group home. He remained preoccupied with harming and impregnating young girls. In the end, he seemed to have struck some sort of "psychic bargain" by removing his eye to expiate his sins and being allowed to survive (Menninger, 1938/1966). He also disclosed some persecutory ideation, saying that he "needed to remove his eye, or the bomber pilot would have gotten it." Much of his ideation was so floridly psychotic that others could not decipher its meaning. It is important to note that most of this content emerged only several days *after* the self-enucleation. Unless this ideation had been elicited prior to the act, it would not have helped in prevention.

In summary, the case of Mr. M demonstrates that the protocol for assessing major self-injury can be a useful tool in alerting clinicians to danger. However, it is far from being as precise as a thermometer measuring temperature. The protocol provides some useful guidelines, but only a very astute team of professionals might have been able to prevent Mr. M's self-enucleation. Identifying precise predictors of major self-injury is regrettably still a long way off.

UPDATE ON THE CASE OF MR. M

Shortly after his self-enucleation, Mr. M entered a residential program operated by my agency. His life thereafter was generally stable. He continued to suffer from schizophrenia, but he became more compliant regarding his medication and treatment program participation. His compliance seemed to improve as his mother became less involved in his day-to-day care. Mr. M gradually came to accept living away from his mother and eventually took pride in his greater level of independence. He became active in a local clubhouse program for people with mental illness.

Occasionally Mr. M presented with increased levels of agitation, anger, and restlessness. At these times, Mr. M sometimes stated that his "good eye hurt." He also made what seemed to be veiled self-threats, such as, "I hope nothing happens to my good eye." At these times, staff members in the residential program became appropriately alarmed and hypervigilant. They encouraged him to talk about whatever frustrations he might be experiencing. They also used the protocol presented above. In addition, without exception, a consultation regarding medication was immediately arranged. Increases were usually prescribed for relatively short periods. During the 10 years he lived in the program, Mr. M never presented with another self-harm behavior. He passed away from natural causes (a heart attack) in the mid-1990s.

TREATMENT OF CLIENTS WITH PSYCHOSES

Psychopharmacology

For individuals suffering from psychoses, the treatment of choice to prevent major self-injury is psychopharmacological. As noted in Chapter 14 by Gordon Harper, trials of antipsychotic agents are indicated for clients with delusional self-injury. He describes the possible benefits of using antipsychotic agents, such as risperidone (Risperdal), clozapine (Clozaril) and others. Grossman (2001) has discussed the pharmacotherapy of major self-injury at length. He has suggested that the basic principles of medication treatment in preventing self-injury are (1) rapid treatment of the psychosis, (2) establishment of a regimen that optimizes medication compliance, and (3) sedation during acute periods of agitation. (Note that these are exactly the principles we followed in treating Mr. M in our residential program.) Grossman (2001) has also discussed the use of benzodiazepines, mood stabilizers, and antidepressants in the treatment of major self-injury.

Psychological Therapies

Psychological therapies are designed both to prevent major self-injury and to manage it in those for whom it is ongoing. Some clients have extended histories of performing major self-injury. The psychological treatments provided to those at risk of novel or recurrent major self-injury depend in part on the diagnosis. As noted by Grossman (2001), in the majority of cases the diagnosis is one of the psychoses. For these individuals, the treatment of choice (in addition to medication) is often a symptom management skills training approach (Liberman, 1999; Mueser et al., 2006). For example, Liberman (1999) employs an empirically validated manualized treatment that teaches symptom management and relapse prevention skills to individuals with psychoses. He employs four skills modules: (1) medication management, (2) recreation for leisure, (3) symptom management, and (4) conversational skills. If clients learn to manage their medication properly, to identify warning signs of decompensation, to cope with persistent symptoms, and to avoid alcohol and drugs (Liberman, 1999), they are far more likely to avoid relapse into psychosis. When psychotic decompensation is avoided, related risk of major self-injury is thereby reduced. A more elaborate model than Liberman's, IMR (Mueser et al., 2006), is described in Chapter 17.

Cognitive-Behavioral Therapy

The symptom management approach is sometimes combined with cognitive-behavioral therapy. The basics of cognitive treatment have been described in Chapter 12. As noted there, cognitive therapy (1) targets the automatic thoughts, intermediate beliefs, and core beliefs that support self-injury; (2) collects information about these types of cognitions; and (3) elicits from the client evidence in support of and counter to the dysfunctional cognitions that support the behavior. When the evidence falls counter to the dysfunctional thoughts, the client is assisted in creating a new, more accurate, and more helpful thought. Prognosis in working with psychotic delusions may be linked to how firmly the individual believes in the delusions, how flexible the delusions are in accommodating new information, and how pervasive the delusions are in the person's daily experience (Kingdon & Turkington, 2005). Some basic modifications to the cognitive therapy approach often need to be made in working with people with psychoses (Kingdon & Turkington, 2005; Merlo, Perris, & Brenner, 2004). For example, Kingdon and Turkington (2005) have identified four steps in working with delusional material in clients who have schizophrenia:

1. Target the less strongly held beliefs first.
2. Avoid direct confrontation of the delusional material.
3. Focus on the evidence for the delusion, not the content of the delusion itself.
4. Encourage the client to voice his or her own doubts about, or arguments against, the beliefs.

An example of such therapy with a man whose schizophrenia led to major self-injury is provided below.

Also worth noting is that psychological treatments are now targeting "first-episode psychosis" (Penn et al., 2011). These treatments focus on social and role functioning and quality of life. Early intervention is thought to have potential in reducing cognitive distortions, forestalling social isolation, and delimiting severity of psychotic symptoms. If psychosis does not progress, major self-injury may be prevented as well.

Cognitive Therapy with Mr. Z

I first met Mr. Z, a 45-year-old European American, as part of a consultation I provided to a residential treatment program. Mr. Z's self-harm behaviors included hitting his legs, arms, and chest—and, more alarmingly, punching his eyes. The eye-punching behavior had resulted in significant loss of sight for Mr. Z over the years, to the extent that he was now legally blind. Mr. Z could still read, but only when he held text within inches of his face.

When I interviewed Mr. Z as part of the consultation, I uncovered some important information. A standard part of my interview with persons who engage in recurrent or chronic self-mutilation is to ask them about the six dimensions of body image, as discussed in Chapter 15. I therefore asked him about the dimensions of (1) attractiveness, (2) effectiveness (athleticism), (3) health, (4) sexual characteristics, (5) sexual behavior, and (6) body integrity.

When I asked Mr. Z about sexual behavior, he shared information that his caregivers at the residential program had not heard before. Mr. Z stated that he had "consorted with prostitutes" a number of times when he was a college student, and had also looked at pornographic magazines. He considered these to be grievous sins for which he was still being punished. When asked who was punishing him, Mr. Z replied, "The devils." The program staff was very familiar with this delusional material.

At the conclusion of this consultation, I made two recommendations. The first was that the staff should differentiate between two categories of self-harm for Mr. Z: the hitting that caused little tissue damage, versus the eye punching that was blinding him. The new plan was to call for evaluation for a respite placement outside his residential program whenever the eye punching occurred, whereas the other, less damaging self-harm behaviors would continue to be handled internally. This simple contingency management technique was designed to provide aversive consequences for Mr. Z for the major self-injury. We hoped that this would shape his responses in the direction of less severe self-injury.

I also recommended that the staff collect data for the two categories of self-injury on a daily basis at the program, and that his therapist pursue the sexual material and related guilt in therapy. The goal in therapy was to try to lessen his irrational thoughts and guilt about past "sins," and thereby reduce his motivation to self-injure.

About a year later I was asked to provide individual therapy with Mr. Z, because his long-time therapist had left the program. Thereafter I met with Mr. Z twice a month for several years. Sessions with Mr. Z generally lasted about 30 minutes, which was as much time as he could tolerate. During the sessions, Mr. Z was cooperative; he sincerely tried to answer all my questions, and gave direct, honest, and thoughtful replies. The only time he became uncooperative was when I pursued information regarding his relationship with the devils too extensively. Then Mr. Z would say that he was "not supposed to talk about the devils so much," whereupon he would change the subject and refuse to return to it.

Of interest is that in my first therapy meeting with Mr. Z, he brought up the topic of the prostitutes to me, even though he had not seen me in about 14 months. A bit taken aback, I pursued the topic and learned that he continued to believe he was being punished for his sexual indiscretions from some 20 years earlier. Since this behavior was causing Mr. Z considerable discomfort, and it appeared to have a direct link with his self-harm behaviors, I decided to pursue it at each session if possible.

Over time, Mr. Z continued to discuss the punishment he was receiving via the devils. More specifically, he indicated that the devils "took over [his] body and punished [him] for having had sex with prostitutes." At these times, Mr. Z said, the devils had complete control of his body, and he was powerless to resist them or the self-harming acts inflicted by them.

Intrigued by this content regarding devils, I explored his religious background with him and learned that Mr. Z had been raised a Roman Catholic. He indicated that he had practiced his religion quite faithfully throughout his childhood, but that his practice had lapsed since he had been in residential treatment.

The conversation regarding Mr. Z's religious background led to a treatment strategy, which I proposed to the residential program staff. I suggested that Mr. Z meet with a priest in order to confess his "sins." The speculation on my part was that if Mr. Z were willing to confess his sins and then to receive absolution, he might gain some much-needed relief and reduce his motivation for self-injury.

When I shared this proposal with the treatment team, I emphasized that it was a speculative one at best, and that I had no idea whether it would work. My goal was to alter Mr. Z's core beliefs about his basic sinfulness and need for punishment. The team agreed to the plan, but it took months to locate a priest who was comfortable hearing the confession of a man with psychotic delusions. Finally, Mr. Z and I located a local priest who was willing. At this meeting, all three of us were present for the first part of the discussion. I explained to the priest (with previously obtained permission from Mr. Z) about his experiences with prostitutes and pornography. I also stated that Mr. Z believed that he was still being punished for these sins. With this introduction concluded, the priest spoke with Mr. Z directly. When Mr. Z referred to his behavior as adultery, "one of the worst sins," the priest corrected him, saying that it was not adultery since it seemed unlikely that any of the involved parties was married. The priest also clarified for Mr. Z that if he decided to confess his sins and did so in a sincere manner, his sins would be forgiven in the eyes of God forever. After some additional discussion, I left the room, and the priest heard Mr. Z's confession and administered absolution.

When I met with Mr. Z a week later, he indicated that he was pleased with both the meeting and the confession, and that he felt they had done him some good. He also stated that he believed he was harming himself less since the confession. However, over the next several months, data collected at the program indicated (1) no decrease in his rate of self-harm, and (2) no decrease in his assaults to the head. It became clear that modifying Mr. Z's fixed delusions would be no easy task. His delusions were especially hard to change in that, as noted by Kingdon and Turkington (2005), they were characterized by great conviction, flexibility, and pervasiveness.

He also became agitated if he was pushed too much regarding his conviction in his "relationship with the devils." In fact, the only two times I saw him assault himself was when I had pushed too long or too hard about his delusional material. In addition, he sometimes spoke positively about the devils, saying that they "granted [him] mercy and taught [him] positive things." The fact that the devils were sometimes "helpful" to him made challenging his belief system all the more difficult.

Another strategy I pursued with Mr. Z was exploring the "evidence for his beliefs," as recommended by Kingdon and Turkington (2005) and Mueser et al. (2009). Mr. Z had received training in the sciences as an undergraduate. He had a good understanding of biology and chemistry. I pursued a strategy in which we discussed the scientific explanations for schizophrenia and the symptom of delusions. Mr. Z participated actively in these discussions, as long as they were general and not applied to himself. When the conversation got more personal, he simply changed the subject or asserted emphatically, "The devils cause my self-injury," and "Brain chemistry has nothing to do with it." Thus my efforts at CR using this approach failed as well.

The most productive strategy in working with Mr. Z focused on skills training. I decided to try some replacement skills training, since the cognitive strategies had not been productive. First I attempted to teach him a couple of breathing techniques, as presented in Chapter 11. He was initially cooperative in learning these, but he failed to practice and eventually refused to do them any longer, saying that the devils disapproved of them.

Next, I decided to pursue a visualization strategy; frankly, I was grasping at straws by now. In each session, I would create for him a visualization that was relevant to his daily experience. For example, I would describe a day in which he was sitting in the living room of the residence, feeling peaceful, relaxed, and self-injury-free. Mr. Z reported that he liked hearing these visualizations and found them relaxing. However, he was not able or willing to practice them on his own. He relied on me for each "new chapter."

To my surprise, after several months of therapy that invariably involved a visualization, Mr. Z started to repeat back to me the language used in the exercises. For example, he reported feeling "more peaceful" in the residence, "more relaxed," and relatively "self-injury-free." It appeared as if *indirectly* suggesting a different way of experiencing himself and the world was more productive than *directly* challenging his core delusional beliefs.

I am not clear whether Mr. Z's improvement was temporary or sustained, as he moved to a new location shortly thereafter, and our therapy ceased. What this case example is designed to demonstrate is that altering the delusions that support major self-injury can be very difficult. Many different techniques may need to be tried until one is identified that is congruent with, and not too challenging of, the individual's highly idiosyncratic world view.

THERAPY WITH CLIENTS WHO ARE NOT PSYCHOTIC

For self-mutilating clients who are not psychotic, the treatment strategies described in Part II of this book are generally appropriate without substantial modification. Clients with diagnoses such as BPD, PTSD, antisocial personality disorder, OCD, other anxiety disorders, or depression will usually benefit from some combination of contingency management, replacement skills training, cognitive therapy, and psychopharmacology. For those who have endured trauma, body image work and exposure treatment may also be important. This chapter concludes with one such case example of a self-mutilating individual who was not psychotic:

Rosa was a woman in her 30s who had had a very difficult life. Sexually abused for years as a child, she had learning problems and did not complete high school. She began using substances as a teen, including alcohol, marijuana, and cocaine. She became addicted to crack and began engaging in prostitution to support her habit. During her late teens and 20s, she had three children by three different men. All of the children were removed by state protective services.

Eventually, Rosa ended up in prison for cocaine possession, dealing, and prostitution. She did not adjust well to prison, frequently assaulting other inmates and harming herself. Her self-injury generally took the form of cutting her arms and thighs with sharp objects. However, when she was especially distressed, she would violently bite her forearms. These wounds required many sutures and skin grafts and left deep, half-dollar-sized scars.

Rosa was eventually transferred to a state hospital forensic unit because of her increasingly bizarre behavior. She continued to assault others and to bite and scratch herself. The heart of Rosa's problem was the horrific abuse she had suffered at the hands of her aunt's boyfriend and others. She frequently experienced flashbacks and nightmares that tended to be followed by assaults and major self-injury. Before she could deal with her trauma, Rosa desperately needed some skills to manage her intense rage, shame, guilt, and self-loathing. In group and individual treatment on the forensic unit, Rosa learned a number of breathing skills. She particularly liked a visualization from her childhood when she went to the beach with her aunt. She also used art as a release and found that stroking her arms with a cosmetic brush was a soothing activity. These skills allowed Rosa to reduce her assaults on herself and others over time. Her major self-injury (self-biting) stopped, but her cutting episodically continued.

Eventually Rosa made productive use of cognitive therapy. She began to look at her incredibly negative core beliefs, which supported much of her self-loathing, rage, and violence. She also started working on her body image and developed some strategies whereby she "pampered" her body rather than destroying it. The goal is for Rosa eventually to be ready for CR for PTSD (Mueser et al., 2009) or PET (Foa et al., 2000), as described in Chapter 16. If she can resolve some major aspects of her trauma history, there is still hope for Rosa to have a productive life in the community after her sentence is completed.

CONCLUSION

- Major self-injury, such as self-enucleation or autocastration, is among the most challenging behaviors faced by clinicians.

- The greatest ally in preventing the behavior is often antipsychotic or other psychotropic medication.
- Ancillary treatments that can be helpful are cognitive therapy, replacement skills training, and, in cases involving trauma, CR for PTSD or PET (see Chapter 16).
- Fortunately, cases of major self-injury are rare. When acts of such extreme self-mutilation are encountered, they are often unforgettable.
- At least in the large majority of cases, the clients survive their extreme acts of self-harm—which provides some small solace to the individuals, families, and treaters involved.

Afterword

Two of the most well-known stories in Zen Buddhism involve extreme self-injury. They both feature Bodhidharma, a monk who is said to have brought Zen from India to China about 526 C.E. This Zen master was so committed to attaining enlightenment that he retreated in solitude to a cave for 9 years to practice meditation. Frustrated by his tendency to doze off and thereby "neglect" his practice, he cut off his eyelids. With such fierce dedication, he eventually obtained his goal of a clear, complete *satori*.

Some years later, a monk named Hui K'o came to Bodhidharma's cave, seeking to learn from the master. Bodhidharma turned him away. Again and again this monk appealed for admission as a disciple, and Bodhidharma's answer was always the same: refusal. One day, standing in a blizzard outside Bodhidharma's cave, the monk cut off his arm and presented it to the master as a token of his resolve and conviction. He was then accepted as a disciple and eventually became heir to Bodhidharma's teaching lineage.

Certainly eyelid removal or arm amputation should be imitated by no one. However, there may be a symbolic significance in these mythical actions. Individuals who self-injure can be viewed as pursuing a quest that has a fervor beyond most mortal pursuits. Whether the goal is release from pain, the resolution of trauma, or an altered state of consciousness, self-injuring persons are willing to pursue actions that most others eschew. They bring their seeking to a level of conviction that takes on physical proportions. Bodily transformation may have as its goal psychological or even spiritual renewal. We should respect their intensity as indicative of great resolve and promise.

My work with persons who self-injure has taught me, again and again, that great things are possible from those who are able to transform pain into affirmation. The life stories of these persons often move from anguish, isolation, and bodily harm to accomplishment, affiliation, and self-protection. We professionals are fortunate to play some role in assisting these seekers to find a higher ground.

Appendices

Breathing Manual

This manual presents a number of breathing techniques that can be used to manage distress and eliminate self-injury. The examples come from different traditions, including psychology, psychotherapy, social work, and Buddhist meditation. The first five techniques are simpler; after that, the different types of breathing are listed in no particular order. The suggestion is to find a few that are comfortable and useful, and to practice those frequently. None will work without practice; all can be helpful tools in reducing and eliminating self-harm behaviors. For all the techniques, it is best to practice for at least 20 minutes three times a week to achieve a beneficial effect.

Thich Nhat Hanh (1991) has said:

> While we practice conscious breathing, our thinking will slow down, and we can give ourselves a real rest. Most of the time, we think too much, and mindful breathing helps us to be calm, relaxed and peaceful. It helps us stop thinking so much and stop being possessed by sorrows of the past and worries about the future. It enables us to be in touch with life, which is wonderful in the present moment. (p. 11)

Nhat Hanh (1991) has also stated:

> Our breathing is the link between our body and our mind. Sometimes our mind is thinking of one thing and our body is doing another, and mind and body are not unified. By concentrating on our breathing, "In" and "Out," we bring body and mind back together, and become whole again. Conscious breathing is an important bridge. (p. 9)

BREATHING TECHNIQUES

"In . . . Out" Breathing

As you breathe in, say "in" inside your mind; as you breathe out, say "out" inside your mind. Continue for several minutes.

    Comment: This simplest of breathing exercises appeals to many as an introduction to mindful breathing. Its simplicity can also be its weakness, because attention may wander. This technique is especially useful for cognitively limited individuals who have trouble remembering more complex techniques. However, people of all abilities have used this technique effectively.

"I Am Here . . . I Am Calm"

This breathing exercise requires some explanation. "I am here" is shorthand for the longer sentence "I am here in the present moment without judgment." This sentence means "As I am breathing, I am not thinking about the past, and I am also not anticipating the future; I'm residing in the present moment." "Without judgment" means "I am suspending judgment right now about myself and others. I am taking a complete break, a vacation, from criticizing myself and other people." With this exercise, as you breathe in, you say to yourself, "I am here." As you breathe out, you say, "I am calm."

    Comment: For whatever reason, this breathing exercise is the all-time favorite of clients at my agency, The Bridge. I believe people like it because it conveys the essence of mindfulness in a brief, concise way. It is complex enough to hold a client's attention and meaningful enough to foster conviction.

1 through 10 Exhale Breathing

As you breathe in, focus on the physical sensation of breathing; as you breathe out, say "1." Next, as you breathe in, focus on your breath again, and as you breathe out, say "2." Continue in this manner up to 10, counting only on the exhalations. When you reach 10, return to 1. If you lose count or go beyond 10, return to 1 and start over.

    Comment: This is a good alternative introductory exercise to "in . . . out" breathing. It is more complex and requires more attention; however, it is still quite simple and easily remembered. This technique is 2,500 years old and is often the first one taught in various traditions of meditation.

1 through 10 Inhalation and Exhalation Breathing

Start with 1 on the inhalation and continue with 2 on the exhalation, alternating up to 10. Then continue the breathing in reverse: 9 on the inhalation, 8 on the exhalation, back down to 1 and then up again, and so on.

Comment: Many people like this exercise because of its soothing up-and-down rhythm. It is complicated enough to hold a client's attention, but simple enough to support relaxation.

Deeper Breathing

Most of us breathe throughout the day in a fairly shallow way, using only a modest percentage of lung capacity. This exercise involves intentionally deepening the breath. Taking deeper breaths in a calm manner increases relaxation. Alertness is also enhanced as more oxygen reaches the brain. Begin by focusing on your breath. Deliberately slow down the breath and make your in-breath fuller. Next, as you breathe out, do so more fully; deliberately expel more of the air from your lungs than you typically do. As you practice this exercise, find a comfortable new rhythm for breathing deeply.

Comment: Some people can end up light-headed with this type of breathing. Return to typical "shallow" breathing if you start to feel any shortness of breath or other discomfort. With practice, a good rhythm can be found.

Bamboo Breathing

To learn bamboo breathing, see Figure A.1. This breathing technique comes from Sekida (1985). It is called "bamboo breathing" because bamboo grows in

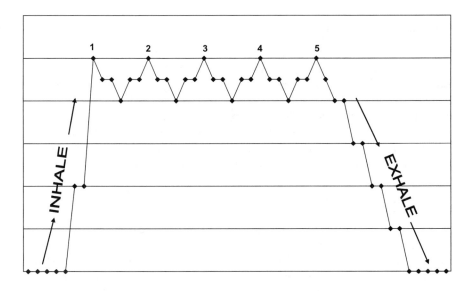

FIGURE A.1. Bamboo breathing.

clearly delineated sections, as shown in the figure. The horizontal lines on the chart represent brief pauses in breathing. The long diagonal lines represent long, deep breaths; the short diagonal lines represent short, shallow breaths. More specifically, the breathing begins with two long in-breaths and is followed by two brief out-breaths, then two brief in-breaths. This occurs for five cycles, concluding with four long out-breaths.

Comment: This exercise is complex and requires a good memory and concentration to complete and repeat successfully. People who have persistent trouble with becoming distracted find this exercise quite helpful. When you are first learning bamboo breathing, it may be necessary to look at the diagram.

This exercise can be too difficult for some. Others initially may find themselves gasping for breath if they are unable to establish a good rhythm. Return to typical, comfortable breathing if you experience shortness of breath or other discomfort. In general, people who smoke heavily or who have asthma may have trouble with more complex breathing techniques.

"Breathing In, I Calm My Body; Breathing Out, I Smile"

This is another breathing exercise from Nhat Hanh (1991). Say, "Breathing in, I calm my body; breathing out, I smile" recurrently.

Comment: Nhat Hanh states that smiling relaxes all the muscles in the face, and he recommends it for this reason.

"Letting Go of . . . " Breathing

As you breathe in, say, "Mindfully breathing." As you breathe out, say, "Letting go of X . . . " (insert for X whatever you'd like to have less of, such as anxiety, tension, anger, judgments, memories, perfectionism, etc.). You can select one thing to let go of and say that recurrently, or you can let go of different emotions with each successive out-breath. The idea is not to "drive out" or forbid any thoughts or feelings, but rather to notice them and then let them go on their way.

Comment: Many individuals identify this exercise as a favorite way to release unwanted, persistent negative thoughts or feelings.

"Cultivating X . . . " Breathing

This exercise is similar to "letting go of X . . . " breathing, but instead of letting go, you "cultivate" something positive (patience, calmness, relaxation, mindfulness, compassion, etc.). In this case, breathe out as you say, "Cultivating," and breathe in as you say, "Patience" (or whatever you are cultivating). The metaphor is that as you breathe in, the desired state is entering your body and increasing.

Comment: It's usually better to teach this technique after the preceding one, "letting go of X . . ." breathing.

"Letting Be, Letting Go" Breathing

This form of breathing comes from Kabat-Zinn (1990). It is designed to assist in dealing with emotions as they emerge. As you become aware of feelings, you say internally:

> On the in-breath: "Seeing [insert the relevant feeling—e.g., anger, anxiety]."
> On the out-breath: "Letting be."
> On the in-breath: "Seeing [insert the same feeling name]."
> On the out-breath: "Letting go."

Comment: This exercise conveys a fundamentally important message about psychotherapy and mental health. Over the course of therapy (and in life in general), feelings must be encountered and experienced (letting them be). They cannot just be negated, ignored, or repressed. Such a strategy never works; the feelings just return to haunt us. However, at some point, after fully experiencing the feelings, we also need to let them go.

Wave Breathing

This form of breathing was also inspired by Kabat-Zinn (1990). In his "Guided Mindfulness Meditation" recording, he uses the phrase "riding the wave of the breath." I found this phrase suggestive and used it to create a visualization. As you breathe in, imagine the ocean gently lapping on the beach; as you breathe out, the ocean gently recedes. In imagining the ocean's movement, you can include sight, sound, smell, and touch.

Pleasant-Word Breathing

Select a word that appeals to you, and repeat it each time you exhale. A colleague of mine, perhaps uniquely, likes the word "onomatopoeia." Others have selected such words as "calm," "ocean," "peaceful," "soothing," "relax," and the like.

Breathing with Tapping

Some prefer to make breathing a more active, tactile experience. One way to do this is to tap your left finger gently on your left leg as you breathe in, and tap your right finger on your right leg as you breathe out. Decide on a rhythm of tapping that is comfortable for you.

Raised-Arm Breathing

A variation of breathing with movement involves sitting with an arm comfortably resting on each leg, with the fingertips near the knees. As you inhale, slowly raise both arms up to a comfortable position close to the shoulders; as you exhale, return the arms and hands to your legs. Repeat.

Body Scan Breathing

This is a type of breathing that involves progressive body awareness. I learned it from Issho Fujita, a Soto Zen priest. Begin by bringing your attention gently to the areas of your body that are supported by the chair, floor, or cushion. After noticing these sensations, turn your attention to where your feet and legs are supported. After several minutes, shift your attention to focusing on the rise and fall of the abdomen with each in-breath and out-breath. After several more minutes, turn your attention to the rise and fall of the upper chest with each in- and out-breath. After several minutes, bring your attention to the nostrils, and become aware of the air going in and out with each breath. You may notice that the air is cooler going in and warmer going out. After several minutes, turn your attention to the full body. Imagine that a single membrane surrounds your body. Imagine that your body is a single cell, a one-celled amoeba. Become aware of the full body. After several minutes of this focusing, the exercise concludes.

   Comment: This technique is good for physical grounding. It is especially helpful for those who are easily distracted, because it provides multiple steps on which to focus.

Pause Breathing

In this exercise, you begin by finding a comfortable rhythm of deeper breathing (see above). Once you have this rhythm, concentrate on the gap or pause between the end of the inhalation and the beginning of the exhalation. It is often helpful to deliberately extend the pause beyond its usual length.

   Some suggest that this brief moment between breaths symbolizes a break in the constant striving for survival (e.g., taking in oxygen, food, information, expelling carbon dioxide, producing work, speaking to others). It represents an interlude from the effort of balancing inner and outer worlds.

   Comment: This type of breathing can produce some unusual thoughts, feelings, or insights. However, some find it initially difficult to locate or hold the pause.

Walking Meditation

Nhat Hanh (1975) strongly recommends walking meditation as a complement to meditative breathing in a seated position. Walking meditation involves walking at a slower-than-usual pace. It also entails focusing on the breath as your body moves through its paces. One way to do walking meditation is to place your right hand on your sternum in a fist with your thumb tucked inside. Then place your left hand over the right, covering it (Issho Fujita, personal communication). As you begin walking, extend your left leg very slowly, touching down first on the heel. Focus quite deliberately on the physical sensations in your leg and foot. Continue focusing as you gradually shift your weight first to the instep, then to the ball of the foot, and finally to the toes of the left foot. Continue for the right leg, foot, and toes. After several moments, a rhythm is established.

As you are walking, it is useful to synchronize your breath with your steps. One way to do this is to take one step for each in-breath and out-breath. However, you should discover your own natural synchrony.

Stoplight or Telephone Breathing

Nhat Hanh (1975) suggests using stoplights or ringing phones as meditation bells that signal brief moments of mindful breathing. This is an excellent way to build some self-soothing and mindful concentration into daily activities.

Return-to-Health Breathing

The late psychologist Cindy Sanderson once taught this type of breathing at an intensive DBT training. She reported learning it when she was being treated for cancer. She has since died from a recurrence of the disease, making the second half of the mantra all the more meaningful.

In-breath: "Let me be one with the heart."
Out-breath: "Let me be healed."
In-breath: "Let me be free from suffering."
Out-breath: "Let me be at peace."

Comment: Repetitive phrases, sometimes referred to as "mantras," are part of many mindful breathing and meditative exercises. They are both relaxing and focusing.

Empty-Mind Breathing

This technique is generally for those with more experience in mindful breathing. As you focus on your breathing, try to think of absolutely nothing. Release all thoughts, feelings, memories, images, anticipations, sensations. Do and think of nothing.

Comment: To get to the point of an empty mind, you may have to breathe mindfully for extended periods of time.

Distress Tolerance Breathing

Derived from Nhat Hanh (1991), this exercise seems very consistent with the concept of "distress tolerance" from DBT (Linehan, 1993b). The instructions are to say the following to oneself:

"Breathing in, I'm aware of my anger [or whatever feeling]."
"Breathing out, I'm aware of my anger."
"Breathing in, I sit with my anger."
"Breathing out, I sit with my anger."
"Breathing in, I know my anger will pass."
"Breathing out, I know my anger will pass."
"Breathing in, I will transform my anger into something positive."
"Breathing out, I will transform my anger into something positive."

Comment: As with other exercises, this one can be modified to meet the needs of each individual (simplified, shortened, extended, etc.).

Breathing Retraining

This technique is used by Foa and colleagues (Foa & Rothbaum, 1998; Meadows & Foa, 1998) in their treatment of trauma survivors.

As you inhale slowly, you count (silently) to 4. As you exhale slowly, you say the word "calm" or "relax" in a long, drawn-out fashion—for example, "caaalllmmmm." When the breath is fully exhaled, you pause and count to 4 before inhaling again. Then repeat for at least 10 minutes. This technique is designed to help manage anxiety, calm the body physiologically, and teach mastery over unpleasant emotions.

"White Light, Black Smoke" Breathing

I learned this technique from the Venerable Lobsang Phuntsok, a Tibetan monk. As you breathe in, imagine a column of white light entering your body and purifying and cleansing your thoughts, feelings, habits, and behaviors. Then as you breathe out, envision black smoke leaving your body. This black smoke carries with it all the toxins, negative thoughts, judgments, feelings, behaviors, and habits. This exercise can be simplified by saying to yourself, as you breathe in, "White light, compassion," and as you breathe out, "Black smoke, anger" or "judgments" or "frustration." Phuntsok emphasizes that it is important to visualize the light entering the body and the black smoke exiting the lungs as vividly as possible.

Comment: The metaphoric images of "white light" and "black smoke" are especially evocative and therefore appeal to many.

"This Too Shall Pass" Breathing

As you breathe in, say, "This too," and as you breathe out, say, "shall pass."

Just Breathing

With practice, you may find that you get to the point where you just breathe. There is no need for counting, words, phrases, sentences, images, or other techniques. You focus on the breath and just breathe.

Body Attitudes Scale (BAS)

This questionnaire concerns body image and satisfaction. Please write the appropriate number on the line next to each question.

1	2	3	4	5
Strongly disagree	Disagree	Neither agree nor disagree	Agree	Strongly agree

____ 1. Most people find me attractive.

____ 2. I try never to do anything that threatens my health.

____ 3. Sometimes I feel disconnected from my body.

____ 4. Most days I feel physically sick.

____ 5. I am good at most sports activities.

____ 6. I often seem to damage my health without meaning to.

____ 7. Everyone deserves to have sexual pleasure.

____ 8. I am not a good-looking individual.

____ 9. I have never had the experience of feeling outside my body.

____ 10. Good health is one of the most important things in my life.

____ 11. Sometimes my body feels out of control.

____ 12. I do not have good physical endurance.

_____ 13. I take care of myself when I feel sick.

_____ 14. My body is sexually appealing.

_____ 15. Sometimes my body feels like an enemy.

_____ 16. I hate being touched by others.

_____ 17. I am currently at an attractive weight.

_____ 18. I like my looks just the way they are.

_____ 19. I can imagine having a satisfying sex life in the future.

_____ 20. Most of the time when I look in the mirror, I feel ugly.

_____ 21. I would prefer to live without a body.

_____ 22. I like the idea of having a physically mature body.

_____ 23. I enjoy being sexually aroused.

_____ 24. I liked my body much better before it matured.

_____ 25. I am not a physically coordinated individual.

_____ 26. I am presently at a healthy weight.

_____ 27. I have to work hard to make myself attractive to others.

_____ 28. Sexual experiences give me pleasure.

_____ 29. My looks often disgust me.

_____ 30. People consider me a very good athlete.

_____ 31. I frequently wish I were more sexually attractive.

_____ 32. I often feel at war with my body.

_____ 33. I am physically ill more often than I am well.

_____ 34. I prefer to avoid sexual experiences.

_____ 35. I feel that my body is strong.

_____ 36. I think of myself as sexually appealing.

Clinical Scales to Assess Self-Injury

FUNCTIONAL ASSESSMENT OF SELF-MUTILATION (FASM)

A. In the *past year*, have you engaged in the following behaviors to *deliberately harm yourself* (check all that apply)

	No	Yes	How many times?	Have you gotten medical treatment?
1. cut or carved on your skin				
2. hit yourself on purpose				
3. pulled your hair out				
4. gave yourself a tattoo				
5. picked at a wound				
6. burned your skin (i.e., with a cigarette, match or other hot object)				
7. inserted objects under your nails or skin				

	No	Yes	How many times?	Have you gotten medical treatment?
8. bit yourself (e.g., your mouth or lip)				
9. picked areas of your body to the point of drawing blood				
10. scraped your skin				
11. "erased" your skin				
12. other: _____				

B. If not in the past year, have you EVER done any of the above acts?

_____ Yes

_____ No

If yes to any of the above behaviors in the past year, please complete the questions (C–H) below:

C. While doing any of the above acts, were you trying to kill yourself?

_____ Yes

_____ No

D. How long did you think about doing the above act(s) before actually doing it?

_____ none

_____ "a few minutes"

_____ <60 minutes

_____ >1 hour but <24 hours

_____ more than 1 day but less than a week

_____ greater than a week

E. Did you perform any of the above behaviors while you were taking drugs or alcohol?

_____ Yes

_____ No

F. Did you experience pain during this self-harm?

          ____ severe pain

          ____ moderate pain

          ____ little pain

          ____ no pain

G. How old were you when you first harmed yourself in this way? _____

H. Did you harm yourself for any of the reasons listed below? (check all reasons that apply):

0	1	2	3
Never	**Rarely**	**Some**	**Often**

Reasons:	Rating
1. to avoid school, work, or other activities	
2. to relieve feeling "numb" or empty	
3. to get attention	
4. to feel something, even if it was pain	
5. to avoid having to do something unpleasant you don't want to do	
6. to get control of a situation	
7. to try to get a reaction from someone, even if it's a negative reaction	
8. to receive more attention from your parents or friends	
9. to avoid being with people	
10. to punish yourself	
11. to get other people to act differently or change	
12. to be like someone you respect	
13. to avoid punishment or paying the consequences	
14. to stop bad feelings	
15. to let others know how desperate you were	

Reasons:	Rating
16. to feel more a part of a group	
17. to get your parents to understand or notice you	
18. to give yourself something to do when alone	
19. to give yourself something to do when with others	
20. to get help	
21. to make others angry	
22. to feel relaxed	
23. other:	

Thank you for your responses!

ALEXIAN BROTHERS URGE TO SELF-INJURE SCALE (ABUSI)

The questions below apply to *the last week*. Place *an "X" in the box* next to the most appropriate statement.

1. **How often have you thought about injuring yourself or about how you want to injure yourself?**

   ☐ **Never,** 0 times in the last week

   ☐ **Rarely,** 1–2 times in the last week

   ☐ **Occasionally,** 3–4 times in the last week

   ☐ **Sometimes,** 5–10 times in the last week, or 1–2 times a day

   ☐ **Often,** 11–20 times in the last week, or 2–3 times a day

   ☐ **Most of the time,** 20–40 times in the last week, or 3–6 times a day

   ☐ **Nearly all of the time,** more than 40 times in the last week, or more than 6 times a day.

From Washburn, Juzwin, Styer, and Aldridge (2010). Reprinted with permission from the authors in Walsh (Guilford Press, 2012). This scale is in the public domain and may be photocopied freely. Purchasers may download a larger version of this scale from the book's page on The Guilford Press website.

2. **At the most severe point, how strong was your urge to self-injure in the last week?**

   ☐ **None** at all.

   ☐ **Slight**, that is, a very mild urge.

   ☐ **Mild** urge.

   ☐ **Moderate** urge.

   ☐ **Strong** urge, but **easily** controlled.

   ☐ **Strong** urge, but **difficult** to control.

   ☐ **Strong** urge **and would have self-injured if able to.**

3. **How much time have you spent thinking about injuring yourself or about how you want to injure yourself?**

☐	☐	☐	☐	☐	☐	☐
None.	Less than 20 min.	21–45 min.	46–90 min.	90 min to 3 hrs.	3–6 hrs.	More than 6 hrs.

4. **How difficult was it to *resist* injuring yourself in the last week?**

☐	☐	☐	☐	☐	☐	☐
Not difficult at all	Very mildly difficult	Mildly difficult	Moderately difficult	Very difficult	Extremely difficult	Was not able to resist

5. **Keeping in mind your responses to the previous questions, please rate your *overall average* urge or desire to injure yourself in the last week.**

   ☐ **Never** thought about it and **never** had the urge to self-injure.

   ☐ **Rarely** thought about it and **rarely** had the urge to self-injure.

   ☐ **Occasionally** thought about it and **occasionally** had the urge to self-injure.

   ☐ **Sometimes** thought about it and **sometimes** had the urge to self-injure.

   ☐ **Often** thought about it and **often** had the urge to self-injure.

   ☐ Thought about self-injury **most** of the time and had the urge to do it **most** of the time.

   ☐ Thought about self-injury **nearly all** the time and had the urge to do it **nearly all** the time.

Helpful Websites Related to Self-Injury

www.crpsib.com

The website for the Cornell Research Program on Self-Injurious Behavior. It offers current research-informed information on self-injury; it is not a website for those looking for immediate help or support. The program is directed by Janis Whitlock, PhD, MPH.

www.selfinjury.com

A website run by Wendy Lader, PhD, MEd, Karen Conterio, and Michelle Seliner, MSW, LCSW. The site promotes their treatment programs, webinars, and book; their treatment model is known as S.A.F.E. The website also offers referral links to therapists nationwide and a call-in number (1-800-DONT-CUT).

www.insync-group.ca

The website for the Interdisciplinary National Self-Injury in Youth Network Canada. A multifaceted website with research information as well as support for youth, families, and professionals. Major contributors include Nancy Heath, PhD, Mary K. Nixon, MD, FRCPC, and several others.

www.wjh.harvard.edu/~nock/nocklab

The website of the Laboratory for Clinical and Developmental Research at Harvard University, directed by Matthew Nock, PhD. Dr. Nock is a leading researcher on suicide and self-injury, and almost all of his publications are available under the "Publications" tab on this website.

www.mentalhealthscreening.org

The website for Screening for Mental Health, Inc., of Wellesley, Massachusetts. It offers a variety of prevention programs related to suicide and one for self-injury.

www.isssweb.org

The website for the International Society for the Study of Self-Injury. This website is still its infancy, but given the society's international professional membership, the site should develop into an important resource.

www.helpguide.org/mental/self_injury.htm

A concise, reasonably helpful webpage that recounts some basic information about self-injury, its warning signs, and how to respond to it, plus some self-help tips.

Bill of Rights for People Who Self-Harm

PREAMBLE

An estimated one percent of Americans use physical self-harm as a way of coping with stress; the rate of self-injury in other industrial nations is probably similar. Still, self-injury remains a taboo subject, a behavior that is considered freakish or outlandish and is highly stigmatized by medical professionals and the lay public alike. Self-harm, also called self-injury, self-inflicted violence, or self-mutilation, can be defined as self-inflicted physical harm severe enough to cause tissue damage or leave visible marks that do not fade within a few hours. Acts done for purposes of suicide or for ritual, sexual, or ornamentation purposes are not considered self-injury. This document refers to what is commonly known as moderate or superficial self-injury, particularly repetitive SI; these guidelines do not hold for cases of major self-mutilation (i.e., castration, eye enucleation, or amputation).

Because of the stigma and lack of readily available information about self-harm, people who resort to this method of coping often receive treatment from physicians (particularly in emergency rooms) and mental-health professionals that can actually make their lives worse instead of better. Based on hundreds of negative experiences reported by people who self-harm, the following Bill of Rights is an attempt to provide information to medical and mental-health personnel. The goal of this project is to enable them to more clearly understand the emotions that underlie self-injury and to respond to self-injurious behavior in a way that protects the patient as well as the practitioner.

THE BILL OF RIGHTS FOR THOSE WHO SELF-HARM

1. **The right to caring, humane medical treatment.** Self-injurers should receive the same level and quality of care that a person presenting with an identical but accidental injury would receive. Procedures should be done as gently as they would be for others. If stitches are required, local anesthesia should be used. Treatment of accidental injury and self-inflicted injury should be identical.

2. **The right to participate fully in decisions about emergency psychiatric treatment (so long as no one's life is in immediate danger).** When a person presents at the emergency room with a self-inflicted injury, his or her opinion about the need for a psychological assessment should be considered. If the person is not in obvious distress and is not suicidal, he or she should not be subjected to an arduous psych evaluation. Doctors should be trained to assess suicidality/homicidality and should realize that although referral for outpatient follow-up may be advisable, hospitalization for self-injurious behavior alone is rarely warranted.

3. **The right to body privacy.** Visual examinations to determine the extent and frequency of self-inflicted injury should be performed only when absolutely necessary and done in a way that maintains the patient's dignity. Many who SI have been abused; the humiliation of a strip-search is likely to increase the amount and intensity of future self-injury while making the person subject to the searches look for better ways to hide the marks.

4. **The right to have the feelings behind the SI validated.** Self-injury doesn't occur in a vacuum. The person who self-injures usually does so in response to distressing feelings, and those feelings should be recognized and validated. Although the care provider might not understand why a particular situation is extremely upsetting, she or he can at least understand that it *is* distressing and respect the self-injurer's right to be upset about it.

5. **The right to disclose to whom they choose only what they choose.** No care provider should disclose to others that injuries are self-inflicted without obtaining the permission of the person involved. Exceptions can be made in the case of team-based hospital treatment or other medical care providers when the information that the injuries were self-inflicted is essential knowledge for proper medical care. Patients should be notified when others are told about their SI and as always, gossiping about any patient is unprofessional.

6. **The right to choose what coping mechanisms they will use.** No person should be forced to choose between self-injury and treatment. Outpatient therapists should never demand that clients sign a no-harm contract; instead, client and provider should develop a plan for dealing with self-injurious impulses and acts during the treatment. No client should feel [that he or she] must lie about SI or be kicked out of outpatient therapy. Exceptions to this may be made in

hospital or ER treatment, when a contract may be required by hospital legal policies.

7. **The right to have care providers who do not allow their feelings about SI to distort the therapy.** Those who work with clients who self-injure should keep their own fear, revulsion, anger, and anxiety out of the therapeutic setting. This is crucial for basic medical care of self-inflicted wounds but holds for therapists as well. A person who is struggling with self-injury has enough baggage without taking on the prejudices and biases of [his or her] care providers.

8. **The right to have the role SI has played as a coping mechanism validated.** No one should be shamed, admonished, or chastised for having self-injured. Self-injury works as a coping mechanism, sometimes for people who have no other way to cope. They may use SI as a last-ditch effort to avoid suicide. The self-injurer should be taught to honor the positive things that self-injury has done for him [or] her as well as to recognize that the negatives of SI far outweigh those positives and that it is possible to learn methods of coping that aren't as destructive and life-interfering.

9. **The right not to be automatically considered a dangerous person simply because of self-inflicted injury.** No one should be put in restraints or locked in a treatment room in an emergency room solely because his or her injuries are self-inflicted. No one should ever be involuntarily committed simply because of SI; physicians should make the decision to commit based on the presence of psychosis, suicidality, or homicidality.

10. **The right to have self-injury regarded as an attempt to communicate, not manipulate.** Most people who hurt themselves are trying to express things they can say in no other way. Although sometimes these attempts to communicate seem manipulative, treating them as manipulation only makes the situation worse. Providers should respect the communicative function of SI and assume it is not manipulative behavior until there is clear evidence to the contrary.

References

Abramsky, S., Fellner, J., & Human Rights Watch. (2003). *Ill-equipped: U.S. prisons and offenders with mental illness*. New York: Human Rights Watch.

Aggarwal, N., & Sinha, D. (2006). An amazing case of working wrist watch in the esophagus. *Indian Journal of Otolaryngology and Head and Neck Surgery, 58*, 105–106.

Alderman, T. (1997). *The scarred soul: Understanding and ending self-inflicted violence*. Oakland, CA: New Harbinger.

American Association of Suicidology (AAS). (2008). Suicide in the USA. Retrieved from *http://suicidology.org/c/document_library/get_file?folderId=232&name=DLFE-244.pdf*

American Association of Suicidology (AAS). (2011). Survivors of suicide fact sheet. Retrieved from *http://suicidology.org/c/document_library/get_file?folderId=229&name=DLFE-82.pdf*

American Psychiatric Association. (2010). *DSM-5 development: Non-suicidal self-injury*. Retrieved from *www.dsm5.org/ProposedRevisions/Pages/proposed-revision.aspx?rid=443*

American Society for Gastrointestinal Endoscopy. (2002). Guideline for the management of ingested foreign bodies. *Gastrointestinal Endoscopy, 55*, 802–806.

Appelbaum, K. L. (2007). Commentary: The use of restraint and seclusion in correctional mental health. *Journal of the American Academy of Psychiatry and the Law, 35*(4), 431–435.

Appelbaum, K. L., Savageau, J., Trestman, R. L., Metzner, J., & Baillargeon, J. (2011). A national survey of self-injurious behavior in American prisons. *Psychiatric Services, 62*(3), 285–290.

Arnold, E. L., Vitiello, B., McDougle, C., Scahill, L. M., Shah, B., Gonzalez, N. M., et al. (2003). Parent-defined target symptoms respond to risperidone in RUPP autism study: Customer approach to clinical trials. *Journal of the American Academy of Child and Adolescent Psychiatry, 42,* 1443–1450.

Ashford, J. B., LeCroy, C. W., & Lortie, K. L. (2001). *Human behavior in the social environment* (2nd ed.). Belmont, CA: Brooks/Cole.

Baetens, I., Claes, L., Muehlenkamp, J. J., Grietens, H., & Onghena, P. (2011). Non-suicidal and suicidal self-injurious behavior among Flemish adolescents: A web-survey. *Archives of Suicide Research, 15,* 56–67.

Bandura, A. (1977). *Social learning theory.* Englewood Cliffs, NJ: Prentice-Hall.

Barley, W. D., Buie, S. E., Peterson, E. W., Hollingsworth, A. S., Griva, M., & Hickerson, S. C. (1993). Development of an inpatient cognitive-behavioral treatment program for borderline personality disorders. *Journal of Personality Disorder, 7,* 232–240.

Bateman, A., & Fonagy, P. (2006). *Mentalization-based treatment for borderline personality disorder: A practical guide.* New York: Oxford University Press.

Bayda, E. (2002). *Being Zen: Bringing meditation to life.* Boston: Shambhala.

Beck, A. T., Freeman, A., Davis, D. D., & Associates. (2003). *Cognitive therapy of personality disorders* (2nd ed.). New York: Guilford Press.

Beck, A. T., Rush, A. J., Shaw, B. F., & Emery, G. (1979). *Cognitive therapy of depression.* New York: Guilford Press.

Beck, J. S. (2005). *Cognitive therapy for challenging problems: What to do when the basics don't work.* New York: Guilford Press.

Beck, J. S. (2011). *Cognitive therapy behavior: Basics and beyond* (2nd ed.). New York: Guilford Press.

Beherec, L., Lambrey, S., Quilici, G., Rosier, A., Falissard, B., & Guillin, O. (2011). Retrospective review of clozapine in the treatment of patients with autism spectrum disorder and severe disruptive behaviors. *Journal of Clinical Psychopharmacology, 31*(3), 341–344.

Bennett, D. R., Baird, C. J., Chan, K., Crookes, P. F., Bremner, C. G., Gottlieb, M. M., et al. (1997). Zinc toxicity following massive coin ingestion. *American Journal of Forensic Pathology, 18,* 148–153.

Berman, A. L., Jobes, D. A., & Silverman, M. M. (2006). *Adolescent suicide: Assessment and intervention* (2nd ed.). Washington, DC: American Psychological Association.

Berman, M. E., & Walley, J. C. (2003). Imitation of self-aggressive behavior: An experimental test of the contagion hypothesis. *Journal of Applied Social Psychology, 33,* 1036–1057.

Best, R. R. (1946). Management of sharp pointed foreign bodies in the gastrointestinal tract. *American Journal of Surgery, 72,* 545–549.

Blake, B. L., Muehlmann, A. M., Egami, K., Breese, G. R., Devine, D. P., & Jinnah, H. A. (2007). Nifedipine suppresses self-injurious behaviors in animals. *Developmental Neuroscience, 29*(3), 241–250.

Bohus, M., Haaf, B., Simms, T., Limberger, M., Schmahl, C., & Unckel, C. (2004). Effectiveness of inpatient dialectical behavior therapy for borderline personality disorder: A controlled trial. *Behaviour Research and Therapy, 42,* 487–499.

Bohus, M., Haaf, B., Stiglmayr, C., Pohl, U., Bohme, R., & Linehan, M. (2000). Evaluation of inpatient dialectical-behavior therapy for borderline personality disorder: A prospective study. *Behaviour Research and Therapy, 38,* 875–879.

Bohus, M., Limberger, M., Ebner, U., Glocker, F. X., Schwarz, B., Wernz, M., et al. (2000). Pain perception during self-reported distress and calmness in patients with borderline personality disorder and self-mutilating behavior. *Psychiatry Research, 95,* 251–260.

Boiko, I., & Lester, D. (2000). Deliberate self-injury in female Russian inmates. *Psychological Reports, 87*(3), 789–790.

Bower, P., & Gilbody, S. (2005). Stepped care in psychological therapies: Access, effectiveness and efficiency. *British Journal of Psychiatry, 186,* 11–17.

Brausch, A. M. (2011). *Exploring prevalence and functions of asphyxial risk taking behavior in adolescents.* Unpublished manuscript.

Brausch, A. M., Decker, K. M., & Hadley, A. G. (2011). Risk of suicidal ideation in adolescents with both self-asphyxial risk taking behavior and non-suicidal self-injury. *Suicide and Life-Threatening Behavior, 41*(4), 424–434.

Brenner, H. D., Roder, V., Hodel, B., Kienzle, N., Reed, D., & Liberman, R. P. (1994). *Integrated psychological therapy for schizophrenic patients.* Cambridge, MA: Hogrefe & Huber.

Briere, J., & Gil, E. (1998). Self-mutilation in clinical and general population samples: Prevalence, correlates, and functions. *American Journal of Orthopsychiatry, 68*(4), 609–620.

Brown, M. (1998). The behavioral treatment of self-mutilation. In *Self-mutilation: Treatment and research.* Symposium conducted at the XVI Congress of the World Association for Social Psychiatry, Vancouver, British Columbia, Canada.

Brown, M. (2002). *The impact of negative emotions on the efficacy of treatment for parasuicide in borderline personality disorder.* Unpublished doctoral dissertation, University of Washington, Seattle.

Brown, M., Comtois, K. A., & Linehan, M. M. (2002). Reasons for suicide attempts and nonsuicidal self-injury in women with borderline personality disorder. *Journal of Abnormal Psychology, 111*(1), 198–202.

Capello, M. (2011). *Swallow: Foreign bodies, their ingestion, inspiration, and the curious doctor who extracted them.* New York: New Press.

Cash, T. F. (2004). Body image: Past, present, and future. *Body Image: An International Journal of Research, 1,* 1–5.

Cash, T. F., & Pruzinsky, T. (Eds.). (1990). *Body images: Development, deviance, and change.* New York: Guilford Press.

Cash, T. F., & Pruzinsky, T. (Eds.). (2002). *Body image: A handbook of theory, research, and clinical practice.* New York: Guilford Press.

Cassano, P., Lattanzi, L., Pini, S., Dell'Osso, L., Battistini, G., & Cassano, G. B. (2001). Topiramate for self-mutilation in a patient with borderline personality disorder. *Bipolar Disorders, 3,* 161.

Centers for Disease Control and Prevention (CDC). (2008). Unintentional strangulation deaths from the "choking game" among youths aged 6–19 years—United States, 1995–2007. *Morbidity and Mortality Weekly Report, 57,* 141–144.

Centers for Disease Control and Prevention (CDC). (2010). *Web-based Injury Statistics Query and Reporting System (WISQARS).* Available from *www.cdc.gov/injury/wisqars/index.html*

Chengappa, K. N., Ebeling, T., Kang, J. S., Levine, J., & Parepally, H. (1999). Clozapine reduces severe self-mutilation and aggression in psychotic patients with borderline personality disorder. *Journal of Clinical Psychiatry, 60,* 477–484.

Chowanec, G. D., Josephson, A. M., Coleman, B., & Davis, H. (1991). Self-harming behavior in incarcerated male delinquent adolescents. *Journal of the American Academy of Child and Adolescent Psychiatry, 30,* 202–207.

Clark, D. M. (1986). A cognitive approach to panic. *Behaviour Research and Therapy, 24,* 461–470.

Clendenin, W. W., & Murphy, G. E. (1971). Wrist cutting. *Archives of General Psychiatry, 25,* 465–469.

Cloutier, P. F., & Nixon, M. K. (2003). The Ottawa Self-Injury Inventory: A preliminary evaluation. Abstracts to the 12th International Congress European Society for Child and Adolescent Psychiatry. *European Child and Adolescent Psychiatry, 12*(Suppl. 1), I/94.

Collins, W. C., & National Institute of Corrections. (2004). *Supermax prisons and the Constitution: Liability concerns in the extended control unit.* Washington, DC: U.S. Department of Justice, National Institute of Corrections.

Comtois, K. A. (2002). A review of interventions to reduce the prevalence of parasuicide. *Psychiatric Services, 53*(9), 1138–1144.

Connor, D. F., Doerfler, L. A., Toscano, P. F., Volungis, A. M., & Steingard, R. J. (2004). Characteristics of children and adolescents admitted to a residential treatment center. *Journal of Child and Family Studies, 13*(4), 497–510.

Connors, R. E. (2000). *Self-injury.* Northvale, NJ: Aronson.

Conterio, K., & Lader, W. (1998). *Bodily harm.* New York: Hyperion.

Cookson, M. R. (2003). Pathways to parkinsonism. *Neuron, 37,* 7–10.

Crabtree, L. H., & Grossman, W. K. (1974). Administrative clarity and redefinition for an open adolescent unit. *Psychiatry, 37,* 350–359.

Darche, M. A. (1990). Psychological factors differentiating self-mutilating and non-self-mutilating adolescent inpatient females. *Psychiatric Hospital, 21,* 31–35.

Dartmouth Psychiatric Research Center. (2008, December). Integrated illness management and recovery for older adults with SMI. Retrieved from *http://dms.dartmouth.edu/prc/aging/projects/older_smi/iimr*

Davis, M., Eshelman, E. R., & McKay, M. (1982). *The relaxation and stress reduction workbook* (2nd ed.). Oakland, CA: New Harbinger.

Deiter, P. J., Nicholls, S. S., & Pearlman, L. A. (2000). Self-injury and self-capacities: Assisting an individual in crisis. *Journal of Clinical Psychology, 56*(9), 1173–1191.

Denys, D., van Megan, H. J., & Westenberg, H. G. (2003). Emerging skin-picking behavior after serotonin reuptake inhibitor-treatment in patients with obsessive–compulsive disorder: Possible mechanisms and implications for clinical care. *Journal of Psychopharmacology, 17,* 127–129.

Dimeff, L. A., Koerner, K., & Linehan, M. M. (2007). *Dialectical behavior therapy in clinical practice: Applications across disorders and settings.* New York: Guilford Press.

Drews, D. R., Allison, C. K., & Probst, J. R. (2000). Behavioral and self-concept differences in tattooed and nontattooed college students. *Psychological Reports, 86*(2), 475–481.

Dulit, R. A., Fyer, M. R., Leon, A. C., Brodsky, B. S., & Frances, A. J. (1994). Clinical correlates of self-mutilation in borderline personality disorder. *American Journal of Psychiatry, 151,* 1305–1311.

Dworkin, A. (1974). *Woman hating.* New York: Dutton.

D'Zurilla, T. J., & Goldfried, M. R. (1971). Problem solving and behavior modification. *Journal of Abnormal Psychology, 78,* 107–126.

D'Zurilla, T. J., & Nezu, A. M. (2001). Problem solving therapies. In K. Dobson (Ed.), *Handbook of cognitive-behavioral therapies* (2nd ed.). New York: Guilford Press.

Earl, T. (2010, September). Talking therapies and the stepped care model. *Journal of the New Zealand College of Clinical Psychologists.* Retrieved from *www. tepou.co.nz/knowledge-exchange/research/view/publication/571*

Ellis, A. (1962). *Reason and emotion in psychotherapy.* New York: Lyle Stuart.

Farber, S. K. (2000). *When the body is the target: Self-harm, pain, and traumatic attachments.* Northvale, NJ: Aronson.

Farberow, N. L. (Ed.). (1980). *The many faces of suicide: Indirect self-destructive behavior.* New York: McGraw-Hill.

Favaro, A., & Santonastaso, P. (1998). Impulsive and compulsive self-injurious behavior in bulimia nervosa: Prevalence and psychological correlates. *Journal of Nervous and Mental Disease, 186,* 157–165.

Favaro, A., & Santonastaso, P. (2000). Self-injurious behavior in anorexia nervosa. *Journal of Nervous and Mental Disease, 188,* 537–542.

Favazza, A. (1987). *Bodies under siege.* Baltimore: Johns Hopkins University Press.

Favazza, A. (1989). Why patients mutilate themselves. *Hospital and Community Psychiatry, 40,* 137–145.

Favazza, A. (1996). *Bodies under siege* (2nd ed.). Baltimore: Johns Hopkins University Press.

Favazza, A. (1998). The coming of age of self-mutilation. *Journal of Nervous and Mental Disease, 186,* 259–268.

Favazza, A., & Conterio, K. (1988). The plight of chronic self-mutilators. *Community Mental Health Journal, 24*(1), 22–30.

Favazza, A., DeRosear, L., & Conterio, K. (1989). Self-mutilation and eating disorders. *Suicide and Life-Threatening Behaviors, 19*(4), 352–361.

Favazza, A., & Rosenthal, R. J. (1990). Varieties of pathological self-mutilation. *Behavioural Neurology, 3*, 77–85.

Fisher, S. (1970). *Body experience in fantasy and behavior.* New York: Appleton-Century-Crofts.

Foa, E., Hembree, E., & Rothbaum, B. O. (2007). *Prolonged exposure therapy for PTSD: Emotional processing of traumatic experiences: Therapist guide.* New York: Oxford University Press.

Foa, E. B., Keane, T. M., & Friedman, M. J. (Eds.). (2000). *Effective treatments for PTSD.* New York: Guilford Press.

Foa, E. B., & Rothbaum, B. O. (1998). *Treating the trauma of rape: Cognitive-behavioral therapy for PTSD.* New York: Guilford Press.

Fontana, D. (2001). *Discover Zen: A practical guide to personal serenity.* San Francisco: Chronicle Books.

Freeman, A., & Reinecke, M. A. (1993). *Cognitive therapy of suicidal behavior.* New York: Springer.

Gardner, A. R., & Gardner, A. J. (1975). Self-mutilation: Obsessionality and narcissism. *British Journal of Psychiatry, 127*, 127–132.

Gardner, D. L., & Cowdry, R. W. (1985). Suicidal and parasuicidal behavior in borderline personality disorder. *Psychiatric Clinics of North America, 8*, 389–403.

Garnefski, N., & Diekstra, R. F. W. (1996). Perceived social support from family, school, and peers: Relationship with emotional and behavioral problems among adolescents. *Journal of the American Academy of Child and Adolescent Psychiatry, 35*, 1657–1664.

Garner, D. M., & Garfinkel, P. E. (Eds.). (1997). *Handbook of treatment for eating disorders* (2nd ed.). New York: Guilford Press.

Garner, D. M., Vitousek, K. M., & Pike, K. M. (1997). Cogntive-behavioral therapy for anorexia nervosa. In D. M. Garner & P. E. Garfinkel (Eds.), *Handbook of treatment for eating disorders* (2nd ed.). New York: Guilford Press.

Geist, R. (1979). Onset of chronic illness in children and adolescents. *American Journal of Orthopsychiatry, 52*, 704–711.

Gibbons, J. J., & Katzenbach, N. D. (2006). *Confronting confinement: A report of the Commission on Safety and Abuse in America's Prisons.* New York: Vera Institute of Justice.

Gitlin, D. F., Caplan, J. P., Rogers, M. P., Avni-Barron, O., Braun, I., & Barsky, A. J. (2007). Foreign-body ingestion in patients with personality disorders. *Psychosomatics, 48*, 162–166.

Glassman, L. H., Weierich, M. R., Hooley, J. M., Deliberto, T. L., & Nock, M. K.

(2007). Child maltreatment, non-suicidal self-injury, and the mediating role of self-criticism. *Behaviour Research and Therapy, 45,* 2483–2490.

Gough, K., & Hawkins, A. (2000). Staff attitudes to self-harm and its management in a forensic psychiatric service. *British Journal of Forensic Practice, 2*(4), 22–28.

Grant, B. F., Harford, T. C., Dawson, D. A., Chou, P., Dufour, M., & Pickering, R. (1994). Epidemiologic Bulletin No. 35: Prevalence of DSM-IV alcohol abuse and dependence, United States, 1992. *Alcohol Health and Research World, 18,* 243–248.

Grassian, S. (1983). Psychopathological effects of solitary confinement. *American Journal of Psychiatry, 140*(11), 1450–1454.

Gratz, K. L. (2001). Measurement of deliberate self-harm: Preliminary data on the Deliberate Self-Harm Inventory. *Journal of Psychopathology and Behavioral Assessment, 23,* 253–263.

Gratz, K. L., Conrad, S. D., & Roemer, L. (2002). Risk factors for deliberate self-harm among college students. *American Journal of Orthopsychiatry, 72*(1), 128–140.

Gratz, K. L., Lacroce, D. M., & Gunderson, J. G. (2006). Measuring changes in symptoms relevant to borderline personality disorder following short-term treatment across partial hospital and intensive outpatient levels of care. *Journal of Psychiatric Practice, 12,* 153–159.

Green, A. H. (1968). Self-destructive behavior in physically abused schizophrenic children. *Archives of General Psychiatry, 18,* 171–179.

Greilsheimer, H., & Groves, J. E. (1979). Male genital self-mutilation. *Canadian Psychiatric Association Journal, 36,* 441–446.

Grossman, R. (2001). Psychotic self-injurious behaviors: Phenomenology, neurobiology, and treatment. In D. Simeon & E. Hollander (Eds.), *Self-injurious behaviors: Assessment and treatment.* Washington, DC: American Psychiatric Association.

Grossman, R., & Siever, L. (2001). Impulsive self-injurious behaviors, neurobiology and psychopharmacology. In D. Simeon & E. Hollander (Eds.), *Self-injurious behaviors: Assessment and treatment.* Washington, DC: American Psychiatric Association.

Gutierrez, P. M., & Osman, A. (2008). *Adolescent suicide: An integrated approach to the assessment of risk and protective factors.* DeKalb: Northern Illinois University Press.

Gutierrez, P. M., Osman, A., Barrios, F. X., & Kopper, B. A. (2001). Development and initial validation of the Self-Harm Behavior Questionnaire. *Journal of Personality Assessment, 77,* 475–490.

Haines, J., & Williams, C. (1997). Coping and problem solving of self-mutilators. *Journal of Clinical Psychology, 53*(2), 177–186.

Haw, C., Houston, K., Townsend, E., & Hawton, K. (2002). Deliberate self harm patients with depressive disorders: Treatment and outcome. *Journal of Affective Disorders, 70,* 57–65.

Hawton, K., Arensman, E., Townsend, E., Bremner, S., Feldman, E. Goldney, R. et al., (1998). Deliberate self-harm: Systematic review of efficacy of psychosocial and pharmacological treatments in preventing repetition. *British Medical Journal, 317,* 441–447.

Hawton, K., Townsend, E., Arensman, E., Gunnell, D., Hazell, P., House, A., et al. (2009, January). Psychosocial and pharmacological treatments for deliberate self harm. *Cochrane Summaries.* Retrieved from *summaries.cochrane.org/ CD001764/psychosocial-and-pharmacological-treatments-for-deliberate-self-harm.*

Hayes, S. C. (2004). Acceptance and commitment therapy and the new behavior therapies. In S. C. Hayes, V. M. Follette, & M. M. Linehan (Eds.), *Mindfulness and acceptance: Expanding the cognitive-behavioral tradition.* New York: Guilford Press.

Heath, N. L., Baxter, A. L., Toste, J. R., & McLouth, R. (2010). Adolescents' willingness to access school-based support for nonsuicidal self-injury. *Canadian Journal of School Psychology, 25,* 260–276.

Heath, N. L., Schaub, K., Holly, S., & Nixon, M. K. (2009). Self-injury today: Review of population and clinical studies. In M. K. Nixon & N. L. Heath (Eds.), *Self-injury in youth: The essential guide to assessment and intervention.* New York: Routledge.

Heath, N. L., Toste, J. R., Nedecheva, T., & Charlebois, A. (2008). An examination of nonsuicidal self-injury among college students. *Journal of Mental Health Counseling, 30,* 137–156.

Heinsz, S. V. (2000). Self-mutilation in child and adolescent group home populations. *Dissertation Abstracts International, 61*(4), 2201B.

Himber, J. (1994). Blood rituals: Self-cutting in female psychiatric inpatients. *Psychotherapy, 31,* 620–631.

Hindley, N., Gordon, H., Newrith, C., & Mohan, D. (1999). The management of cylindrical battery ingestion in psychiatric settings. *Psychiatric Bulletin, 23,* 224–226.

Holdin-Davis, D. (1914). An epidemic of hair-pulling in an orphanage. *British Journal of Dermatology, 26,* 207–210.

Hollander, M. (2008). *Helping teens who cut.* New York: Guilford Press.

Hood, K. K., Baptista-Neto, L., Beasley, P. J., Lobis, R., & Pravdova, I. (2004). Case study: Severe self-injurious behavior in comorbid Tourette's disorder and OCD. *Journal of the American Academy of Child and Adolescent Psychiatry, 43*(10), 1298–1303.

Howard League for Penal Reform. (1999). *Scratching the surface: The hidden problem of self-harm in prison.* London: Author.

Hughes, M. (1982). Chronically ill children in groups: Recurrent issues and adaptations. *American Journal of Orthopsychiatry, 52,* 704–711.

Hyman, J. (1999). *Women living with self-injury*. Philadelphia: Temple University Press.

Ireland, J. L. (2000). A descriptive analysis of self-harm reports among a sample of incarcerated adolescent males. *Journal of Adolescence, 23*, 605–613.

Jacobs, D. G., Brewer, M., & Klein-Benheim, M. (1999). Suicide assessment. In D. G. Jacobs (Ed.), *The Harvard Medical School guide to suicide assessment and intervention*. San Francisco: Jossey-Bass.

Jacobs, D. G., Walsh, B. W., & Pigeon, S. (2009). Signs of Self-Injury Prevention Program. Wellesley, MA: Screening for Mental Health and The Bridge. Retrieved from *www.mentalhealthscreening.org/programs/youth-prevention-programs/sosi*.

Jacobson, C. M., & Gould, M. (2007). The epidemiology and phenomenology of non-suicidal self-injury among adolescents: A critical review of the literature. *Archives of Suicide Research, 11*, 129–147.

Joiner, T. (2005). *Why people die by suicide*. Cambridge, MA: Harvard University Press.

Kabat-Zinn, J. (1990). *Full catastrophe living: Using the wisdom of your body and mind to face stress, pain and illness*. New York: Dell.

Katz, L. Y., Cox, B. J., Gunasekara, S., & Miller, A. L. (2004). Feasibility of dialectical behavior therapy for suicidal adolescent inpatients. *Journal of the American Academy of Child and Adolescent Psychiatry, 43*(3), 276–282.

Kazdin, A. E. (1994). *Behavior modification in applied settings*. Pacific Grove, CA: Brooks/Cole.

Kennedy, B. L., & Feldman, T. B. (1994). Self-inflicted eye injuries: Case presentations and a literature review. *Hospital and Community Psychiatry, 45*, 470–474.

Kettlewell, C. (1999). *Skin game: A memoir*. New York: St. Martin's Press.

Keuthen, N. J., Stein, D. J., & Christenson, G. A. (2001). *Help for hair pullers: Understanding and coping with trichotillomania*. Oakland, CA: New Harbinger.

Khan, A. S., & Ali, U. (2006). Case report: Ingestion of metallic rods and needles. *Journal of the College of Physicians and Surgeons—Pakistan, 16*, 305–306.

Kingdon, D. G., & Turkington, D. (2005). *Cognitive therapy of schizophrenia*. New York: Guilford Press.

Klonsky, E. D. (2007). The functions of deliberate self-injury: A review of the evidence. *Clinical Psychology Review, 27*, 226–239.

Klonsky, E. D. (2009). The functions of self-injury in young adults who cut themselves: Clarifying the evidence for affect-regulation. *Psychiatry Research, 166*, 260–268.

Klonsky, E. D., & Glenn, C. R. (2009a). Assessing the functions of non-suicidal self-injury: Psychometric properties of the Inventory of Statements about Self-Injury (ISAS). *Journal of Psychopathology and Behavioral Assessment, 31*, 215–219.

Klonsky, E. D., & Glenn, C. R. (2009b). Non-suicidal self-injury: What independent practitioners should know. *The Independent Practitioner.* Retrieved from *www.42online.org/node/163*

Klonsky, E. D., & May, A. (2010, April). *The relationship between non-suicidal self-injury and attempted suicide in three samples.* Paper presented at the annual meeting of the Ameican Association of Suicidology, Orlando, FL.

Klonsky, E. D., Oltmanns, T. F., & Turkheimer, E. (2003). Deliberate self-harm in a nonclinical population: Prevalence and psychological correlates. *American Journal of Psychiatry, 160,* 1501–1508.

Kreitman, N. (1976). The coal gas story. United Kingdom suicide rates, 1960–71. *British Journal of Preventive and Social Medicine, 30*(2), 86–93.

Kreitman, N. (Ed.). (1977). *Parasuicide.* Chichester, UK: Wiley.

Kroll, J. C. (1978). Self-destructive behavior on an inpatient ward. *Journal of Nervous Mental Disease, 166,* 429–434.

Langbehn, D. R., & Pfohl, B. (1993). Clinical correlates of self-mutilation among psychiatric inpatients. *Annals of Clinical Psychiatry, 5,* 45–51.

Large, M., Babidge, N., Andrews, D., Storey, P., & Nielssen, O. (2008). Major self-mutilation in the first episode of psychosis. *Schizophrenia Bulletin, 35*(5), 1012–1021.

Laye-Gindhu, A., & Schonert-Reichl, K. A. (2005). Nonsuicidal self-harm among community adolescents: Understanding the 'whats' and 'whys' of self-harm. *Journal of Youth and Adolescence, 34,* 447–457.

Lester, D. (1972). Self-mutilating behavior. *Psychological Bulletin, 2,* 119–128.

Levenkron, S. (1998). *Cutting: Understanding and overcoming self-mutilation.* New York: Norton.

Levey, J., & Levey, M. (1991). *The fine arts of relaxation, concentration and meditation.* Boston: Wisdom.

Levey, J., & Levey, M. (1999). *Simple meditation and relaxation.* Berkeley, CA: Conari Press.

Lewis, S. P., Heath, N. L., St. Denis, J. M., & Noble, R. (2011 February). The scope of nonsuicidal self-injury on YouTube. *Pediatrics, 127*(3), e552–e557.

Liberman, R. (1999). *Social and independent living skills* (UCLA skills training video series). Cambridge, MA: Hogrefe & Huber.

Lightfoot, C. (1997). *The culture of adolescent risk-taking.* New York: Guilford Press.

Linehan, M. M. (1993a). *Cognitive-behavioral treatment of borderline personality disorder.* New York: Guilford Press.

Linehan, M. M. (1993b). *Skills training manual for treating borderline personality disorder.* New York: Guilford Press.

Linehan, M. M., Armstrong, H. E., Suarez, A., Allmon, D., & Heard, H. L. (1991). Cognitive-behavioral treatment of chronically parasuicidal borderline patients. *Archives of General Psychiatry, 48,* 1060–1064.

Linehan, M. M., Comtois, K. A., Brown, M. Z., Heard, H. L., & Wagner, A. (2006).

Suicide Attempt Self-Injury Interview (SASII): Development, reliability, and validity of a scale to assess suicidal attempts and intentional self-injury. *Psychological Assessment, 18,* 303–312.

Linkletter, M., Gordon, K., & Dooley, J. (2010). The choking game and YouTube: A dangerous combination. *Clinical Pediatrics, 49*(3), 274–279.

Lloyd, E. E., Kelley, M. L., & Hope, T. (1997, March). *Self-mutilation in a community sample of adolescents: Descriptive characteristics and provisional prevalence rates.* Poster presented at the annual meeting of the Society for Behavioral Medicine, New Orleans, LA.

Lloyd-Richardson, E. E., Perrine, N., Dierker, L., & Kelley, M. L. (2007). Characteristics and functions of non-suicidal self-injury in a community sample of adolescents. *Psychological Medicine, 37,* 1183–1192.

Lovell, D. (2008). Patterns of disturbed behavior in a supermax population. *Criminal Justice and Behavior, 35*(8), 985–1004.

Low, G., Jones, D., MacLeod, A., Power, M., & Duggan, C. (2000). Childhood trauma, dissociation and self-harming behaviour: A pilot study. *British Journal of Medical Psychology, 73,* 269–278.

Mace, F. C., Blum, N. J., Sierp, B. J., Delaney, B. A., & Mauk, J. E. (2001). Differential response of operant self-injury to pharmacologic versus behavioral treatment. *Journal of Developmental and Behavioral Pediatrics, 22,* 85–91.

Macnab, A., Deevska, M., Gagnon, F., Cannon, W., & Andrew, T. (2009). Asphyxial games or 'the choking game': A potentially fatal risk behaviour. *Injury Prevention, 15*(1), 45–49.

Macy, J. D., Beattie, T. A., Morgenstern, S. E., & Arnsten, A. F. (2000) Use of guanfacine to control self-injurious behavior in two rhesus macaques (*Macaca mulatta*) and one baboon (*Papio anubis*). *Comparative Medicine, 50,* 419–425.

Madrid v. Gomez, 889 F. Supp. 1146 (N. D. California 1995).

Maltsberger, J. T. (1986). *Suicide risk.* New York: New York University Press.

Marlatt, G. A. (2012). *Harm reduction: Pragmatic strategies for managing high-risk behaviors* (2nd ed.). New York: Guilford Press.

Marlatt, G. A., & Vandenbos, G. R. (1997). *Addictive behaviors: Readings on etiology, prevention and treatment.* Washington, DC: American Psychological Association.

Massachusetts Department of Elementary and Secondary Education. (2008). *Health and risk behaviors of Massachusetts youth: The report.* Retrieved from *www.doe.mass.edu/cnp/hprograms/yrbs*

Matthews, P. C. (1968). Epidemic self-injury in an adolescent unit. *International Journal of Social Psychiatry, 14,* 125–133.

McCracken, J. T., McGough, J., Shah, B., Cronin, P., Hong, D., Aman, M. G., et al. (2002). Risperidone in children with autism and serious behavioral problems. *New England Journal of Medicine, 347,* 314–321.

McKay, D., Kulchycky, S., & Dankyo, S. (2000). Borderline personality disorder and obsessive–compulsive symptoms. *Journal of Personality Disorders, 14*(1), 57–63.

McKerracher, D. W., Loughnane, T., & Watson, R. A. (1968). Self-mutilation in female psychopaths. *British Journal of Psychiatry, 114*, 829–832.

McNutt, T. K., Chambers, J., Dethlefsen, M., & Shah, R. (2001). Bite the bullet: Lead poisoning after ingestion of 206 lead bullets. *Veterinary and Human Toxicology, 43*, 288–289.

Meadows, E. A., & Foa, E. B. (1998). Intrusion, arousal, avoidance: Sexual abuse survivors. In V. M. Follette, J. I. Ruzek, & F. R. Abueg (Eds.), *Cognitive-behavioral therapies for trauma.* New York: Guilford Press.

Medinfo.co.uk. (2012). SSRIs. Retrieved from *www.medinfo.co.uk/drugs/ssris. html.*

Menninger, K. (1966). *Man against himself.* New York: Harcourt Brace Jovanovich. (Original work published 1938)

Merlo, M., Perris, C., & Brenner, H. (2004). *Cognitive therapy with schizophrenic patients.* Cambridge, MA: Hogrefe & Huber.

Merriam-Webster dictionary: Home and office edition. (1995). Springfield, MA: Merriam-Webster.

Metzner, J. L., & Fellner, J. (2010). Solitary confinement and mental illness in U. S. prisons: A challenge for medical ethics. *Journal of the American Academy of Psychiatry and the Law, 38*(1), 104–108.

Metzner, J. L., Tardiff, K., Lion, J., Reid, W. H., Recupero, P. R., Schetky, D. H., et al. (2007). Resource document on the use of restraint and seclusion in correctional mental health care. *Journal of the American Academy of Psychiatry and the Law, 35*(4), 417–425.

Miller, A. L., Rathus, J. H., & Linehan, M. M. (2007). *Dialectical behavior therapy with suicidal adolescents.* New York: Guilford Press.

Miller, A. L., Rathus, J. H., Linehan, M. M., Wetzler, S., & Leigh, E. (1997). Dialectical behavior therapy for suicidal adolescents. *Journal of Practical Psychiatry and Behavioral Health, 3*(2), 78–86.

Miller, D. (1994). *Women who hurt themselves: A book of hope and understanding.* New York: Basic Books.

Milnes, D., Owens, D., & Blenkiron, P. (2002). Problems reported by self-harm patients: Perception, hopelessness and suicidal intent. *Journal of Psychosomatic Research, 53*(3), 819–822.

Morgan, D. W., Edwards, A. C., & Faulkner, L. R. (1993). The adaptation to prison by individuals with schizophrenia. *Bulletin of the American Academy of Psychiatry and the Law, 21*(4), 427–433.

Motz, A. (2001). *The psychology of female violence: Crimes against the body.* Hove, UK: Brunner-Routledge.

Muehlenkamp, J. J. (2006). Empirically supported treatments and general therapy guidelines or non-suicidal self-injury. *Journal of Mental Health Counseling, 28*, 166–185.

Muehlenkamp, J. J., Claes, L., Smits, D., Peat, C. M., & Vandereycken, W. (2011). Non-suicidal self-injury in eating disordered patients: A test of a conceptual model. *Psychiatry Research, 188*(1), 102–108.

Muehlenkamp, J. J., Cowles, M., & Gutierrez, P. M. (2010). Validation of the Self-Harm Behavior Questionnaire for use with adolescents of different ethnicities. *Journal of Psychopathology and Behavioral Assessment, 32,* 236–245.

Muehlenkamp, J. J., Engel, S. G., Crosby, R. D., Wonderlich, S. A., Simonich, H., & Mitchell, J. E. (2009). Emotional states preceding and following acts of non-suicidal self-injury in bulimia nervosa patients. *Behaviour Research and Therapy, 47,* 83–87.

Muehlenkamp, J. J., & Gutierrez, P. M. (2007). Risk for suicide attempts among adolescents who engage in non-suicidal self-injury. *Archives of Suicide Research, 11,* 69–82.

Muehlenkamp, J. J., Walsh, B. W., & McDade, M. (2009). Preventing non-suicidal self-injury in adolescents: The Signs of Self-Injury Program. *Journal of Youth and Adolescence, 39,* 306–314.

Mueser, K. T., Meyer, P. S., Penn, D. L., Clancy, R., Clancy, D. M., & Salyers, M. P. (2006). The illness management and recovery program: Rationale, development, and preliminary findings. *Schizophrenia Bulletin, 32,* 32–43.

Mueser, K. T., Rosenberg, S. D., & Rosenberg, H. J. (2009). *Treatment of post-traumatic stress disorder in special populations.* Washington, DC: American Psychological Association Press.

Murphy, M. (2002). *One bird one stone: 108 American Zen stories.* New York: Renaissance Books.

Nada-Raja, S., Skegg, K., Langley, J., Morrison, D., & Sowerby, P. (2004). Self-harmful behaviors in a population-based sample of young adults. *Suicide and Life-Threatening Behavior, 34,* 177–186.

National Commission on Correctional Health Care. (2004). *Clinical guidelines for correctional facilities: Treatment of schizophrenia in correctional institutions.* Chicago: Author.

Newman, F. L., Rugh, D., & Ciarlo, J. A. (2004). Guidelines for selecting psychological instruments for treatment planning and outcomes assessment. In M. E. Marush (Ed.), *The use of psychological testing for treatment planning and outcomes assessment: Vol. 1. General considerations* (3rd ed., pp. 197–214). Mahwah, NJ: Lawrence Erlbaum Associates.

New Zealand Ministry of Health. (2009). *Towards optimal primary mental health care in the primary care environment: A draft guidance paper.* Wellington: Author.

Nhat Hanh, T. (1975). *The miracle of mindfulness.* Boston: Beacon Press.

Nhat Hanh, T. (1991). *Peace is every step: The path of mindfulness in every day life.* New York: Bantam Books.

Nicoll, A. (1908). A remarkable case of persistent ingestion of needles. *Lancet, 171*(4411), 772–778.

Nixon, M. K., & Heath, N. L. (Eds.). (2009). *Self-injury in youth: The essential guide to assessment and intervention.* New York: Routledge.

Nock, M. K. (2008). Actions speak louder than words: An elaborated theoretical model of the social functions of self-injury and other harmful behaviors. *Applied and Preventive Psychology, 12,* 159–168.

Nock, M. K. (Ed.). (2009a). *Understanding nonsuicidal self-injury: Origins, assessment, and treatment.* Washington, DC: American Psychological Association.

Nock, M. K. (2009b). Why do people hurt themselves?: New insights into the nature and functions of self-injury. *Current Directions in Pschological Science, 18*(2), 78–83.

Nock, M. K. (2010). Self-injury. *Annual Review of Clinical Psychology, 6,* 339–363.

Nock, M. K., Holmberg, E. B., Photos, W. I., & Michel, B. D. (2007). The Self-Injurious Thoughts and Behaviors Interview: Development, reliability, and validity in an adolescent sample. *Psychological Assessment, 19,* 309–317.

Nock, M. K., Joiner, T. E., Gordon, K., Lloyd-Richardson, E., & Prinstein, M. J. (2006). Non-suicidal self-injury among adolescents: Diagnostic correlates and relation to suicide attempts. *Psychiatry Research, 144,* 65–72.

Nock, M. K., & Kessler, R. C. (2006). Prevalence of and risk factors for suicide attempts versus suicide gestures: Analysis of the National Comorbidity Survey. *Journal of Abnormal Psychology, 115,* 616–623.

Nock, M. K., & Prinstein, M. J. (2004). A functional approach to the assessment of self-mutilative behavior. *Journal of Consulting and Clinical Psychology, 72,* 885–890.

Offer, D. O., & Barglow, P. (1960). Adolescent and young adult self-mutilation incidents in a general psychiatric hospital. *Archives of General Psychiatry, 3,* 194–204.

O'Grady, J. C. (2007). Commentary: A British perspective on the use of restraint and seclusion in correctional mental health care. *Journal of the American Academy of Psychiatry and the Law, 35*(4), 439–443.

O'Keefe, M., & Schnell, M. (2007). Offenders with mental illness in the correctional system. *Journal of Offender Rehabilitation, 45*(1–2), 81–104.

O'Leary, K. D., & Wilson, G. T. (1987). *Behavior therapy: Application and outcome* (2nd ed.). Englewood Cliffs, NJ: Prentice-Hall.

Orbach, I., Lotem-Peleg, M., & Kedem, P. (1995). Attitudes toward the body in suicidal, depressed and normal adolescents. *Suicide and Life-Threatening Behavior, 25,* 211–221.

Orbach, I., Milstein, I., Har-Even, D., Apter, A., Tiano, S., & Elizur, A. (1991). A multi-attitude suicide tendency scale for adolescents. *Psychological Assessment, 3,* 398–404.

Osuch, E. A., Noll, J. G., & Putnam, F. W. (1999). The motivations for self-injury in psychiatric inpatients. *Psychiatry, 62,* 334–345.

Osuch, E. A., & Payne, G. W. (2009). Neurobiological perpectives on self-injury. In M. K. Nixon & N. L. Heath (Eds.), *Self-injury in youth: The essential guide to assessment and intervention*. New York: Routledge.

O'Sullivan, R. L., Phillips, K. A., Keuthen, N. J., & Wilhelm, S. (1999). Near-fatal skin picking from delusional body dysmorphic disorder responsive to fluvoxamine. *Psychosomatics, 40*, 79–81.

O'Sullivan, S. T., Reardon, C. M., McGreal, G. T., Hehir, D. J., Kirwan, W. O., & Brady, M. P. (1996). Deliberate ingestion of foreign bodies in institutionalized psychiatric hospital patients and prison inmates. *International Journal of Medical Sciences, 165*, 294–296.

Palta, R., Sahota, A., Bemarki, K., Salama, P., Simpson, N., & Layne, L. (2009). Foreign-body ingestion: Characteristics and outcomes in a lower socioeconomic population with predominantly intentional ingestion. *Gastrointestinal Endoscopy, 69*, 426–433.

Pao, P. E. (1969). The syndrome of delicate self-cutting. *British Journal of Medical Psychology, 42*, 195–206.

Patterson, G. (1975). *Professional guide for families and living with children*. Portland, OR: Research Press.

Pattison, E. M., & Kahan, J. (1983). The deliberate self-harm syndrome. *American Journal of Psychiatry, 140*, 867–872.

Paul, T., Schroeter, K., Dahme, B., & Nutzinger, D. O. (2002). Self-injurious behavior in women with eating disorders. *American Journal of Psychiatry, 159*, 408–411.

Penn, D. L., Uzenoff, S. R., Perkins, D., Mueser, K. T., Hamer, R. M., Waldheter, E. J., et al. (2011). A pilot investigation of the Graduated Recovery Intervention Program (GRIP) for first episode psychosis. *Schizophrenia Research, 125*, 247–256.

Penn, D. L., Waldheter, E. J., Perkins, D. O., Mueser, K. T., & Lieberman, J. A. (2005). Psychosocial treatment for first episode psychosis: A research update. *American Journal of Psychiatry, 162*, 2220–2232.

Phillips, R. H., & Alkan, M. (1961). Some aspects of self-mutilation in the general population of a large psychiatric hospital. *Psychiatric Quarterly, 35*, 421–423.

Pizarro, J., & Stenius, V. M. K. (2004). Supermax prisons: Their rise, current practices, and effect on inmates. *Prison Journal, 84*(2), 248–264.

Plener, P. L., Libal, G., & Nixon, M. K. (2009). In M. K. Nixon & N. L. Heath (Eds.), *Self-injury in youth: The essential guide to assessment and intervention*. New York: Routledge.

Podvoll, E. M. (1969). Self-mutilation within a hospital setting: A study of identity and social compliance. *British Journal of Medical Psychology, 42*, 213–221.

Ponton, L. E. (1997). *The romance of risk: Why teenagers do the things they do*. New York: Basic Books.

Ramowski, S., Nystrom, R., Chaumeton, N., Rosenberg, K., & Gilchrist, J. (2010). "Choking game" awareness and participation among 8th graders—Oregon, 2008. *Morbidity and Mortality Weekly Report, 59*(1), 1–5.

Rapaport, J. L., Ryland, D. H., & Kriete, M. (1992). Drug treatment of canine acral lick: An animal model of obsessive–compulsive behavior. *Archives of General Psychiatry, 49,* 517–521.

Rhodes, L. A. (2005). Pathological effects of the supermaximum prison. *American Journal of Public Health, 95*(10), 1692–1695.

Rodham, K., & Hawton, K. (2009). Epidemiology and phenomenology of nonsuicidal self-injury. In M. K. Nock (Ed.), *Understanding nonsuicidal self-injury: Origins, assessment, and treatment.* Washington, DC: American Psychological Association.

Rodham, K., Hawton, K., & Evans, E. (2004). Reasons for deliberate self-harm: Comparison of self-poisoners and self-cutters in a community sample of adolescents. *Journal of the American Academy of Child and Adolescent Psychiatry, 43,* 80–87.

Rodriguez-Srednicki, O. (2001). Childhood sexual abuse, dissociation and adult self-destructive behavior. *Journal of Child Sexual Abuse, 10*(3), 75–90.

Rosen, D. M., & Hoffman, A. (1972). Focal suicide: Self-mutilation in two young psychotic individuals. *American Journal of Psychiatry, 128,* 1367–1368.

Rosen, P., & Walsh, B. (1989). Relationship patterns in episodes of self-mutilative contagion. *American Journal of Psychiatry, 146,* 656–658.

Rosenberg, L. (1998). *Breath by breath: The liberating practice of insight meditation.* Boston: Shambhala.

Ross, R. R., & McKay, H. R. (1979). *Self-mutilation.* Lexington, MA: Lexington Books.

Ross, S., & Heath, N. (2002). A study of the frequency of self-mutilation in a community sample of adolescents. *Journal of Youth and Adolescence, 1,* 67–77.

Rothbaum, B. O., Meadows, E. A., Resick, P., & Foy, D. W. (2000). Cognitive-behavioral therapy. In E. B. Foa, T. M. Keane, & M. J. Friedman (Eds.), *Effective treatments for PTSD.* New York: Guilford Press.

Rothbaum, B. O., & Ninan, P. T. (1999). Manual for the cognitive-behavioral treatment of trichotillomania. In D. J. Stein, G. A. Christenson, & E. Hollander (Eds.), *Trichotillomania.* Washington, DC: American Psychiatric Press.

Rush, A. J., & Nowels, A. (1994). Adaptation of cognitive therapy for depressed adolescents. In T. C. R. Wilkes, G. Belsher, A. J. Rush, E. Frank, & Associates (Eds.), *Cognitive therapy for depressed adolescents.* New York: Guilford Press.

Russ, M. J., Roth, S. D., Kakuma, T., Harrison, K., & Hull, J. W. (1994). Pain perception in self-injurious borderline patients: Naloxone effects. *Biological Psychiatry, 35,* 207–209.

Russ, M. J., Roth, S. D., Lerman, A., Kakuma, T., Harrison, K., Shindledecker, R.

D., et al. (1992). Pain perception in self-injurious patients with borderline personality disorder. *Biological Psychiatry, 32*(6), 501–511.

Ryckman, R. M., Robbins, M., Thornton, B., & Cantrell, P. (1982). Development and validation of a physical self-efficacy scale. *Journal of Personality and Social Psychology, 42*, 891–900.

Sandman, C. A. (2009). Psychopharmacologic treatment of nonsuicidal self-injury. In M. K. Nock (Ed.), *Understanding non-suicidal self-injury: Origins, assessment, and treatment*. Washington, DC: American Psychological Association.

Sandman, C. A., Hetrick, W., Taylor, D. V., Marion, S. D., Touchette, P., Barron, J. L., et al. (2000). Long-term effects of naltrexone on self-injurious behavior. *American Journal on Mental Retardation, 105*, 103–117.

Santamour, M. B., & West, B. (1982). The mentally retarded offender: Presentation of the facts and a discussion of the issues. In M. B. Santamour & P. S. Watson (Eds.), *The retarded offender*. New York: Praeger.

Schilder, P. (1935). *The image and appearance of the human body*. New York: International Universities Press.

Schwartz, A. E. (1995). *Guided imagery for groups*. Duluth, MN: Whole Person Associates.

Secord, P. F., & Jourard, S. M. (1953). The appraisal of body cathexis: Body cathexis and the self. *Journal of Consulting Psychology, 17*(5), 343–347.

Segal, Z. V., Williams, J. M. G., & Teasdale, J. D. (2002). *Mindfulness-based cognitive therapy for depressions*. New York: Guilford Press.

Sekida, K. (1985). *Zen training: Methods and philosophy*. New York: Weatherill.

Seligman, M. E. P. (1992). *Helplessness: On depression, development, and death* (with a new introduction by the author). New York: Freeman.

Shapira, N. A., Lessig, M. C., Murphy, T. K., Driscoll, D. J., & Goodman, W. K. (2002). Topiramate attenuates self-injurious behaviour in Prader–Willi syndrome. *International Journal of Neuropsychopharmacology, 5*, 141–145.

Shapiro, S., & Dominiak, G. M. (1992). *Sexual trauma and psychopathology*. New York: Lexington Books.

Shaw, S. N. (2002). *The complexity and paradox of female self-injury: Historical portrayals, journeys toward stopping, and contemporary interventions*. Unpublished doctoral dissertation, Harvard University Graduate School of Education, Cambridge, Masschusetts.

Shea, C. S. (1999). *The practical art of suicide assessment*. New York: Wiley.

Sher, L., & Stanley, B. H. (2008). The role of endogenous opioids in the pathophysiology of self-injurious and suicidal behavior. *Archives of Suicide Research, 12*(4), 299–308.

Sher, L., & Stanley, B. H. (2009). Biological models of nonsuicidal self-injury. In M. K. Nock (Ed.), *Understanding nonsuicidal self-injury: Origins, assessment, and treatment*. Washington, DC: American Psychological Association.

Shneidman, E. S. (1985). *Definition of suicide*. New York: Wiley.

Shneidman, E. S. (1993). *Suicide as psychache.* New York: Wiley.

Simeon, D., & Favazza, A. (2001). Self-injurious behaviors, phenomenology and assessment. In D. Simeon & E. Hollander (Eds.), *Self-injurious behaviors: Assessment and treatment.* Washington, DC: American Psychiatric Association.

Simeon, D., & Hollander, E. (Eds.). (2001). *Self-injurious behaviors: Assessment and treatment.* Washington, DC: American Psychiatric Association.

Slovis, C. M., Tyler-Worman, R., & Solightly, D. P. (1982). Massive foreign object ingestion. *Annals of Emergency Medicine, 11,* 433–435.

Smith, P. S. (2006). The effects of solitary confinement on prison inmates: A brief history and review of the literature. *Crime and Justice, 34,* 441–528.

Symons, F. J., Sutton, K. A., & Bodfish, J. W. (2001). Preliminary study of altered skin temperature at body sites associated with self-injurious behavior in adults who have developmental disabilities. *American Journal on Mental Retardation, 106,* 336–343.

Taiminen, T. J., Kallio-Soukainen, K., Nokso-Koivisto, H., Kaljonen, A., & Helenius, H. (1998). Contagion of deliberate self-harm among adolescent inpatients. *Journal of the American Academy of Child and Adolescent Psychiatry, 37*(2), 211–217.

Thompson, J. K., Berland, N. W., Linton, P. J., & Weinsier, R. L. (1987). Utilization of self-adjusting light beam in the objective assessment of body distortion in seven eating disorder groups. *International Journal of Eating Disorders, 5*(11), 113–120.

Tiefenbacher, S., Novak, M. A., Lutz, C. K., & Meyer, J. S. (2005). The physiology and neurochemistry of self-injurious behavior: A nonhuman primate model. *Frontiers in Bioscience, 10,* 1–11.

Toch, H., & Adams, K. (1987). The prison as dumping ground: Mainlining disturbed offenders. *Journal of Psychiatry and Law, 15,* 539–553.

Tsai, S.-J. (1997). Foreign body ingestion in psychiatric inpatients. *International Medical Journal, 4,* 309–311.

Tsiouris, J. A., Cohen, I. L., Patti, P. J., & Korosh, W. M. (2003). Treatment of previous undiagnosed psychiatric disorders in persons with developmental disabilities decreased or eliminated self-injurious behavior. *Journal of Clinical Psychiatry, 64,* 1081–1090.

Tucker, L. A. (1981). Internal structure, factor satisfaction, and reliability of the body cathexis scale. *Perceptual and Motor Skills, 53,* 891–896.

Tucker, L. A. (1983). The structure and dimensional satisfaction of the body cathexis construct of males: A factor analytic investigation. *Journal of Human Movement Studies, 9,* 189–194.

Tucker, L. A. (1985). Dimensionality and factor satisfaction of the body image construct: A gender comparison. *Sex Roles, 12*(9), 931–937.

Turell, S. C., & Armsworth, M. W. (2000). Differentiating incest survivors who self-mutilate. *Child Abuse and Neglect, 24,* 237–249.

U.S. Census Bureau. (2010). Resident population by sex and age: 1980 to 2008. Retrieved from *www.census.gov/compendia/statab/2010/tables/10s0007.pdf*

Vale, V., & Juno, A. (1989). *Modern primitives*. San Francisco: Re/Search Publications.

van der Kolk, B. A., McFarlane, A. C., & Weisaeth, L. (Eds.). (1996). *Traumatic stress*. New York: Guilford Press.

van der Kolk, B. A., Perry, C., & Herman, J. L. (1991). Childhood origins of self-destructive behavior. *American Journal of Psychiatry, 148*, 1665–1671.

Velazquez, L., Ward-Chene, L., & Loosigian, S. R. (2000). Fluoxetine in the treatment of self-mutilating behavior [Letter]. *Journal of the American Academy of Child and Adolescent Psychiatry, 39*, 812–814.

Velitchkov, N. G., Grigorov, G. I., Losonoff, J. E., & Kjossev, K. T. (1996). Ingested foreign bodies of the gastrointestinal tract: Retrospective analysis of 542 cases. *World Journal of Surgery, 20*, 1001–1005.

Villalba, R., & Harrington, C. J. (2000). Repetitive self-injurious behavior: A neuropsychiatric perspective and review of pharmacologic treatments. *Seminars in Clinical Neuropsychiatry, 5*, 215–226.

Virkkunen, M. (1976). Self-mutilation in antisocial personality disorder. *Acta Psychiatrica Scandinavica, 54*, 347–352.

Walser, R. D., & Hayes, S. C. (1998). Acceptance and trauma survivors: Applied issues and problems. In V. M. Follette, J. I. Ruzek, & F. R. Abueg (Eds.), *Cognitive-behavioral therapies for trauma*. New York: Guilford Press.

Walsh, B. W. (1987). *Adolescent self-mutilation: An empirical study*. Unpublished doctoral dissertation, Boston College Graduate School of Social Work.

Walsh, B. W. (2001). Self-mutilation. In C. D. Bryant (Ed.), *Encyclopedia of criminology and deviant behavior* (Vol. 4). London: Taylor & Francis.

Walsh, B. W. (2006). *Treating self-injury: A practical guide*. New York: Guilford Press.

Walsh, B. W., & Doerfler, L. A. (2009). Residential treatment of self-injury. In M. K. Nock (Ed.), *Understanding nonsuicidal self-injury: Origins, assessment, and treatment*. Washington, DC: American Psychological Association.

Walsh, B. W., & Frost, A. K. (2005). *Attitudes regarding life, death, and body image in poly-self-destructive adolescents*. Unpublished manuscript.

Walsh, B. W., & Rosen, P. (1985). Self-mutilation and contagion: An empirical test. *American Journal of Psychiatry, 142*, 119–120.

Walsh, B. W., & Rosen, P. (1988). *Self-mutilation: Theory, research, and treatment*. New York: Guilford Press.

Warren, F., Dolan, B., & Norton, K. (1998). Bloodletting, bulimia nervosa and borderline personality disorder. *European Eating Disorders Review, 6*, 277–285.

Washburn, J. J., Juzwin, K. R., Styer, D. M., & Aldridge, D. (2010). Measuring the urge to self-injure: Preliminary data from a clinical sample. *Psychiatry Research, 178*, 540–544.

Weintrob, A. (2001). Paxil and self-scratching [Letter]. *Journal of the American Academy of Child and Adolescent Psychiatry, 40,* 5.

Weissman, M. (1975). Wrist cutting. *Archives of General Psychiatry, 32,* 1166–1171.

Whitlock, J. L., Eckenrode, J. E., & Silverman, D. (2006). Self-injurious behavior in a college population. *Pediatrics, 117*(6), 1939–1948.

Whitlock, J., Eells, G., Cummings, N., & Purington, A. (2009). Nonsuicidal self-injury in college populations: Mental health provider assessment of prevalence and need. *Journal of College Student Psychotherapy, 23*(3), 172–183.

Whitlock, J. L., Muehlenkamp, J., & Eckenrode, J. (2008). Variation in non-suicidal self-injury: Identification of latent classes in a community population of young adults. *Journal of Clinical Child and Adolescent Psychology, 37*(4), 725–735.

Whitlock, J. L., Purington, A., & Gershkovich, M. (2009). Influence of the media on self-injurious behavior. In M. Nock (Ed.), *Understanding non-suicidal self-injury: Current science and practice.* Washington, DC: American Psychological Association Press.

Williams, M., Teasdale, J., Segal, Z., & Kabat-Zinn, J. (2007). *The mindful way through depression: Freeing yourself from chronic unhappiness.* New York: Guilford Press.

Wilson, G. T., Fairburn, C. G., & Agras, W. S. (1997). Cognitive-behavioral therapy for bulimia nervosa. In D. M. Garner & P. E. Garfinkel (Eds.), *Handbook of treatment for eating disorders* (2nd ed.). New York: Guilford Press.

Wolpe, J. (1969). *The practice of behavior therapy.* New York: Pergamon Press.

Zweig-Frank, H., Paris, J., & Guzder, J. (1994). Psychological risk factors for dissociation and self-mutilation in female patients with borderline personality disorder. *Canadian Journal of Psychiatry, 39,* 259–264.

Index

Page numbers followed by *f* or *t* indicate figures and tables.